AF439913

Progress in Respiratory Research

Vol. 43

Series Editor

Felix J.F. Herth Heidelberg

Tuberculosis and War

Lessons Learned from World War II

Volume Editors

John F. Murray San Francisco, CA

Robert Loddenkemper Berlin

95 figures, 19 in color, 20 tables, 2018

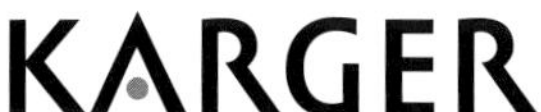

Basel · Freiburg · Paris · London · New York · Chennai · New Delhi ·
Bangkok · Beijing · Shanghai · Tokyo · Kuala Lumpur · Singapore · Sydney

Prof. Emeritus John F. Murray
University of California San Francisco
P.O. Box 0841
San Francisco, CA 94143-0841 (USA)

Prof. Dr. Robert Loddenkemper
German Central Committee against Tuberculosis
Hertastrasse 3
14169 Berlin (Germany)

Library of Congress Cataloging-in-Publication Data

Names: Murray, John F. (John Frederic), 1927- editor. | Loddenkemper, Robert,
   editor.
Title: Tuberculosis and war : lessons learned from World War II / volume
   editors, John F. Murray, Robert Loddenkemper.
Other titles: Progress in respiratory research ; v. 43. 1422-2140
Description: Basel ; New York : Karger, 2018. | Series: Progress in
   respiratory research, ISSN 1422-2140 ; vol. 43 | Includes bibliographical
   references and indexes.
Identifiers: LCCN 2017051894| ISBN 9783318060942 (hard cover : alk. paper) |
   ISBN 9783318060959 (e-ISBN)
Subjects: | MESH: Tuberculosis, Pulmonary--history | Tuberculosis,
   Pulmonary--epidemiology | World War II
Classification: LCC RA644.T7 | NLM WF 11.1 | DDC 614.5/4209044--dc23 LC record
available at https://lccn.loc.gov/2017051894

© Copyright 2018 by S. Karger AG, P.O. Box, CH–4009 Basel (Switzerland)
www.karger.com
Printed on acid-free and non-aging paper (ISO 9706)
ISSN 1422–2140
e-ISSN 1662–3932
ISBN 978–3–318–06094–2
e-ISBN 978–3–318–06095–9

Contents

Conclusion

Preface

Tuberculosis and War – Lessons Learned from World War II

For centuries, tuberculosis (TB) has remained the largest cause of adult deaths from any single infectious disease, and still ranks among the top 10 causes of death worldwide. When TB and war overlap, their partnership spreads disease, heightens misery, worsens suffering, and intensifies mortality. Accordingly, TB is one of the most frequent and deadly diseases to complicate the special circumstances of warfare.

In *Tuberculosis and War – Lessons Learned from World War II*, the impact of war on TB is investigated using the example of World War II (WWII), the worst man-made disaster in history with its 60 million military and civilian casualties. In his post-war summary in 1949, Daniels concludes that TB was the major health disaster of the war years, but notes that not all belligerent countries sustained the same pattern of TB mortality during the war years, 1939 to 1945. Three variations were observed: (1) countries in which there was virtually no wartime increase (e.g., Denmark and Norway); (2) countries in which TB mortality increased during the first few years of the war but then decreased (e.g., England and Wales, Belgium, and France); and (3) countries/cities in which death rates increased from the beginning to after the end of the war (e.g., especially in capital cities like Berlin, Warsaw, Budapest, Vienna, Rome, and Amsterdam). Furthermore, it became unquestioned that the increase of TB during WWII was closely related to the severity of war conditions.

Written by internationally acclaimed experts, this book provides for the first time a comprehensive analysis of the status of TB before, during, and after WWII in the 25 belligerent countries that were chiefly involved (chapters 5–19). In the first of the 4 introductory chapters, chapter 1 summarizes the 70,000-year-old history of TB up to the present. In even earlier times, our hunter-gatherer kindred survived for 2–3 million years of peaceful life before wars began during the Neolithic Revolution. The downside to the amenities of civilization – wars with their human butchery and property destruction – were already taking place before written languages were available to document their existence. The escalation of weapons and means of killing people in the race to annihilation seems to have currently reached a threshold of success with the availability of abundant hydrogen bombs and the steady creation of more and more of them.

Further important background information is conveyed about the history of TB and war in general, including the difficulties of collecting exact epidemiological data (chapter 2), and the risk factors that hasten the spread of TB and its mortality during wartime (chapter 3). A special feature (chapter 4) on "Nazi medicine, TB and genocide" examines the horrendous, inhuman Nazi ideology, which during WWII used TB as a justification for murder, and targeted the disease by eradicating millions who had it.

The main risk factors for TB in wartime include malnutrition/starvation, which weaken host immune defenses. Overcrowding at the front, in concentration camps, prisoner of war quarters, and slave labor facilities worsens the transmission of tubercle bacilli. And disruption of medical and public health services limit treatment and control. All played a major role during WWII in most of the belligerent countries, both in the civilian population and in the military service.

The final chapter, number 20, summarizes the lessons learned from WWII and more recent wars and describes potential anti-TB measures for future conflicts. Today, HIV/TB-coinfection has created a significant additional risk factor. A major step forward after WWII has been the foundation of several international governmental organizations (WHO, UNICEF, UNRRA) as well as non-governmental affiliations, which initiated or supported measures to improve post-war TB diagnosis and treatment.

Thanks to the pure coincidence of timing, in the midst of all the chaos and destruction during the last several months that terminated WWII in 1945, the first 2 effective drugs for the treatment of TB: para-aminosalicylic acid (PAS) and streptomycin were discovered almost simultaneously. When the war was over, the world's reception to this monumental, long-awaited revelation – to some extent – quieted memories of and attention to the WWII-related outburst of TB. Heightened interest of patients, commitment by TB specialists, and researchers all sought to find the optimum way of using these promising new drugs. In 1952, the miraculous solution to the search for the missing element in the treatment of TB was discovered, isoniazid – highly effective, low toxicity, cheap, could not be patented – was soon combined with PAS and streptomycin to create "triple therapy," the regimen that reliably cured TB for the first time ever and saved millions of lives. New antibiotics have subsequently been developed, but resistance against anti-TB drugs has become a serious problem.

The original observation established once and for all that the presence of World War I caused an explosion of TB during the 4-year period of warfare, plus another 2 or three years because of the overlapping end of the Spanish Flu epidemic. Roughly 20 years later, an identical recrudescence of TB occurred during WWII. And now of course, everyone recognizes that the ongoing war in Syria has kindled another obvious worsening of TB. These unmistakable messages keep reminding us: war exacerbates TB. Is not there something we could or should do about it?

We hope that our book provides useful and practical information, not only to TB specialists and pulmonologists but also to readers interested in public health, infectious diseases, and epidemiology. The partnership between war, military-related issues, and TB should be noted in the history of medicine. We believe it should also be of interest to non-medical readers like journalists, historians, and politicians.

Finally, we want to thank all our authors who represent so many countries and organizations for their dedicated participation. We are grateful for the contributions of Prof. Annette Finley-Croswhite for ensuring accuracy of historical facts and of Prof. Hans Rieder for his guidance about epidemiological issues. Special thanks go to Clare Pierard who read and revised numerous chapters and dealt with queries concerning much of the book. We thank Karger Publishers, notably Thomas Nold for his constant support and the Editorial staff, in particular Freddy Brian and Magdalena Mühlemann, for the superior production of this volume. Thanks also go to the two foundations that provided financial support for our work: the Oskar-Helene-Heim Foundation and the Günther Labes Foundation, both in Berlin.

John F. Murray, San Francisco, CA
Robert Loddenkemper, Berlin

Background Information about Essential Material

Murray JF, Loddenkemper R (eds): Tuberculosis and War. Lessons Learned from World War II.
Prog Respir Res. Basel, Karger, 2018, vol 43, pp 2–19 (DOI: 10.1159/000481471)

History of Tuberculosis and of Warfare

John F. Murray

University of California San Francisco, San Francisco, CA, USA

Abstract

It all started back in the Pliocene epoch, 5.3 million years ago, when Lucy and her primate accomplices first stood erect. That marvel launched a random, several million-years-long evolutionary upgrading that featured bigger brains, upright bodies, primitive weapons, and the management of fire. Our ancestor *Homo sapiens* started life about 200,000 years ago, but needed time to expand in sufficient numbers to leave Africa and start migrating to Eurasia. Accompanying this Great Expansion, around 70,000 years ago, *Mycobacterium tuberculosis* began to infect humans and cause tuberculosis (TB). Early human history was dominated by small groups of hunter-gatherers, who survived chiefly by foraging. Then 10,000 years ago, everything changed when *H. sapiens* switched from their nomadic pursuits to permanent lifestyles of farming and taming animals. Continued population growth, including a doubling of birth rates, brought new administrative and professional roles, royalty, and private property. With these furnishings of "civilization" came its opposite: war, the organized, deliberate killing of humans, with armies and weapons. Later, *M. tuberculosis* matured from a low-density to an epidemic disease and for several 100 years was the world's most common cause of mortality. Together, the TB and war partnership has become a major cause of death and destruction.   © 2018 S. Karger AG, Basel

Two independent calamities – tuberculosis (TB) and war – usually rage on different paths without any connection to each other: TB causes disease and death; war causes destruction and death. But when the 2 disasters overlap, their partnership spreads disease, heightens misery, worsens suffering, and produces exceptional mortality. This introductory chapter tells the story about TB and war, which occur most often as separate tragedies, but at times combine with unprecedented catastrophe.

Robert Koch, discoverer of the bacterium that causes TB, *Mycobacterium tuberculosis*, declared in his famous lecture in 1882 that

If the importance of a disease for mankind is measured by the number of fatalities it causes, then TB must be considered much more important than those feared infectious diseases, plague, cholera, and the like. One in 7 of all human beings dies from TB.

That was famously true in 1882, but mortality from TB was actually much higher roughly 80 years earlier in Germany when death rates had already peaked and were steadily dropping. Around 1800, 1 in 4 deaths in the city of London was caused by the disease; and TB still causes more adult deaths than any other single infectious disease in the world, and has been doing so for a very long time. In Western Europe, during the 17th, 18th, and 19th centuries, TB was by far the most important cause of all human deaths, and during its 300-year swath of colossal mortality, is believed to have killed more than 1 billion people of all ages.

TB did not begin during the Neolithic Demographic Revolution (10,000–7,000 years ago), as previously believed. Moreover, it probably comes as a total surprise for many to learn that TB started roughly 70,000 years ago. This large gap of time has been partially filled in by advances in new techniques of genomic sequencing and genetic analyses that have greatly advanced knowledge about the transmissibility and pathogenicity of current and historical lineages of TB.

In marked contrast to the 70,000 years that TB has been causing disease and death, warfare is practically brand new. No one knows exactly when wars originated, but it was certainly long before recorded history could keep track of them. A reasonable estimate is sometime during the already mentioned Neolithic Revolution, when hunter-gatherers had almost finished switching to growing plants, domesticating animals, and commenced having political issues or territorial disputes to fight about. During their relatively short historical lifetime, wars have been virtually endless and increasingly deadly and destructive, and now, of course, they are crowned by nuclear weapons that threaten the end of civilization.

Evolution of Humans

Prehistory

From time to time, curious people, both young and old, ask the question "when did humans show up in the history of the world?" That's a great question, but the answer is complicated and experts still are not certain about exactly how human evolution unfolded. A good place to start is the recently refined definition of *hominids* and their family tree, which includes modern human beings and several extinct ancient species plus their direct ancestors. Hominids originated during the Pliocene epoch, which began 5.3 million years ago, and is celebrated by the presence of the first primates who stood erect. This important discovery was made in 1974 by paleoanthropologist Johanson et al. [1] in Ethiopia, and included the spectacular finding of the nearly intact skeleton of a 3-foot-plus tall young adult female, who was promptly named Lucy and became widely famous. Four years later, Mary Leakey [2] discovered similar bony remains and numerous prehumen footprints more than 1,000 km away in Tanzania. Today, nearly 400 specimens of *Australopithecus afarensis* have been studied and securely dated from 3.9 to 3.0 million years ago.

A major transition from prehuman to human hominids occurred a few million years after the onset of the Pleistocene epoch, or last Great Ice Age, 2.6 million years ago. The new descendants were the first humans who warranted the name *"Homo,"* which means *"man,"* and were designated *Homo habilis,* or "Handy Man" [3]. *H. habilis* had both ape-like physical features and manner of walking, but the species knew how to make and use primitive stone (mainly flint) tools. Within the next half a million years or so, *Homo erectus* appeared

showing off its human-like body and larger brain; moreover, it walked fully upright and probably could run [4]. *H. erectus* originated in Kenya and Tanzania in sub-Saharan Africa, but then migrated widely in Eurasia and as far away as Indonesia. A talented species, *H. erectus* invented specialized stone tools and weapons, hand axes, clubs, awls, harpoons, and cleavers. Though there was competition over who won the contest, *H. erectus* is often credited as discovering "the controlled use of fire." Other precursor human species are known but less well characterized. Archaic *Homo neanderthalensis,* evolved more than 350,000 years ago and achieved "full-blown" structure 130,000 years ago [5]. *H. neanderthalensis* had genetic similarities with *Homo sapiens,* but was shorter, stockier, and had similar or even larger cranial cavities and brains [6]. Until becoming extinct around 30,000 years ago, *H. neanderthalensis* overlapped in time with *H. sapiens*, and DNA evidence suggests they may have interbred with modern humans.

The sole surviving species of humans, *H. sapiens*, first appeared in Africa around 200,000 years ago, but remained geographically isolated for the first 100,000 or so years, possibly owing to the prevailing and always menacing climatic upheavals. New evidence suggests up to 300,000 years ago [7]. Their predecessors, probably *H. erectus*, had migrated out of Africa "during a warm interglacial period," between 130,000 and 80,000 years ago in the Near East, which was subsequently taken over by Neanderthals [8]. Paleo archaeologists are not certain exactly when, but once the opportunity opened up, probably because the climate mellowed a little, successive waves of migration took place, which was called the Great Expansion [8]. Not long before and then accompanying the earliest migrations – the newly established time table estimates that around 70,000 years ago, *M. tuberculosis* began to infect and cause TB in *H. sapiens* – initially in Africa, then in Eurasia [9].

Hunter-Gatherers

Most of human history, to the limits that are known, was inhabited by hunter-gatherers, foragers who survived by hunting and killing animals, both large and small, and eating whatever foods they could pick from trees, find in nests or ponds, dig up, or scavenge. Before becoming extinct, groups of *H. erectus* survived as hunter-gatherers for around 2 million years – far longer than *H. sapiens* relatively brief existence thus far [4]. Dwellings, mostly temporary, were built and caves were commonly used for shelter and refuge. *H. sapiens* started out as nomadic hunter-gatherers, but as described in the next section, Neolithic Demographic Revolution, began to settle down in a single location, growing plants and domesticating animals.

A global marker of both the wide distribution and creativity of early *H. sapiens* culture are examples of Stone Age cave art. First recognized in Spain and France, outstanding decorative paintings were later discovered in Indonesia, some as early as 25,000–40,000 years ago. Before *H. neanderthalensis* became extinct, they also contributed to cave art. Most early cave paintings depict everyday animals – but some infrequent ones, such as mammoths, lions, and rhinoceros – and stencils of cave men's (and women's?) fingers and hands. Far less frequent were simple representations of human beings, often stylized.

Life expectancy was undoubtedly short, one educated guess is 35 years or less, and human survival remained treacherous for millions of years. Violence was epidemic. Competition between and among groups of hunter-gatherers seeking food, mating rights, and places of refuge must have led to violence. Many, but by no means all, anthropologists seem to agree that at least *H. sapiens*, and possibly earlier hominids, possess innate, genetically programmed lethal violence. Experts debate whether chimpanzees, our closest living relatives, have a similar violent predisposition. Other authorities agree that killing by apes does occur but nearly always from ordinary attacks of aggression. In contrast, as living conditions improved during the end of the Pleistocene period, the prehistoric human population of hunter-gatherers enlarged during the Great Expansion as serial colonization may have caused hunting territory to become crowded; competition seems to have triggered a few episodes of organized killing of humans by humans, which have been documented as shown below.

Human warfare is rarely illustrated in cave art, but one painting in Caugnac, France, dated roughly 25,000 years ago shows a "wounded man" with 3 spears protruding from his back and upper thigh, perhaps depicting some sort of interpersonal violence [10]. More scenes of war and battles show up in the rock art of Arnhem Land, N.T., Australia, dated "as early as 10,000 years ago" [11]. Another "unique evidence of a warfare event among hunter-gatherers" was reported recently (2016) by Mirazon et al. [12] in the late Pleistocene-early Holocene period in Kenya, Africa, at an "estimated age of –9,500 to 10,500 years (ago)." These authors describe the remains of a "minimum of 27 individuals," 10 of whose 12 skeletons were found to have serious traumatic, presumably lethal injuries; in addition, there was evidence of arrow wounds, and other signs of "deliberate violent trauma." These examples of warfare among nomadic hunter-gatherers overlap the early origins of newly settled human groupings. (See also later section on Prehistory of warfare.)

Neolithic Demographic Revolution

Hunting and gathering kept ancient *H. habilis* and descendant humans alive and surviving for nearly all the 2 million-plus years of human's total existence. But it all changed, rather rapidly during the Neolithic Demographic Revolution (or Transition): a major turning point in human history [13]. It all started roughly 10,000 years ago, when *H. sapiens* began to slowly change from their nomadic lifestyles and settle down permanently and start farming and taming animals. According to Diamond [14], "Plant and animal domestication is the most important development in the past 13,000 years of human history"; it started not long before the beginning of the Holocene epoch (current), about 11,700 years ago. At first, domestication was scant and spotty and took several thousand years to refine, but the outcome was revolutionary. Hunter-gatherers had to either switch roles or disappear, leaving a world that – although still fundamentally primitive – began to add social classes and technological power to a rapidly expanding sedentary population chiefly engaged in agriculture.

Plant and animal domestication occurred by trial and error, but received a boost from the auspicious climatic and environmental conditions of the Fertile Crescent, particularly Mesopotamia and Babylonia, and in parts of China, notably the Yangtze and Yellow River basins. But Diamond [14] believes that what counted most was that these locations greatly favored "those regions to which the most numerous and most valuable domesticable wild plants and animal species were native" – hence, locally handy and ready for exploitation. Starting around 8500 BC, resident planters and breeders of those "pioneer crops" formed the world's earliest centers of settlement, agriculture, and food production and then went on to spread their talents and technology elsewhere; presumably, the founders also shared their "experienced" genes to their neighbors' benefit.

In time, additional even more favorable climates than the Fertile Crescent and China were discovered – along with both new and already domesticated plants and animals – and rapidly spread to the remainder of Eurasia and parts of Africa. This progressive relocation identified east-west regions having similar temperate climatic conditions, lengths of daylight, and seasonal variations [15]. The similarities among different latitudes enhanced technological adaptation, such as irrigation and soil enrichment. Much slower spread of food production was observed in a north-south axis of Africa and another in the Americas, where hunter-gatherers and hybrid groups of semi-sedentary foragers remained active until superseded by arriving colonizers.

Rewards of Agriculture and Domestication: H. sapiens' remarkable conversion to a settled agriculture-based emphasis on farming and food production did indeed change human history forever, and in many ways. First of all, sedentary life permitted women to give birth roughly every 2 years rather than every 4 years, because once women settled down and changed to eating carbohydrate-rich diets, both their fecundity and fertility probably at least doubled, which greatly increased the population. A growing number of inhabitants generated new forms of specialized labor outside of agriculture and kindred activities, which spread to hierarchical administrative organizations, including royalty with leaders and pecking orders. These developments brought more and better goods and tools, the establishment of private property, and the development of individualized decision-making.

Downsides of Agriculture and Domestication: One little-known downside of the shift to agriculture and domestication includes the surprising fact that the nomadic life style of hunter-gatherers meant that they were physically larger and healthier than their sedentary, vitamin-deficient kinsman. Another liability, particularly in the early millenniums, was the increased prevalence of serious acute infectious diseases, which were transmitted by the domesticated animals to which Eurasian settlers were newly being exposed. A corollary consequence of thousands of years of *H. sapiens* exposure to infected animals is that the natural selection of surviving humans led to a population safeguarded by induced immunity to the prevailing bacteria and other infectious agents and other pathogens. But when unexposed indigenous populations crossed paths with those who had become immunologically protected, for example, during the Age of Discovery between the 15th and 18th centuries, some vulnerable island populations were totally exterminated, and at least 90% of several Native American populations were wiped out following contact, particularly, with immune-shielded European travelers [15].

The quintessential downside to the positive forces of agriculture and domestication, abetted by a continuously increasing population, as described later in this chapter, was the onset of warfare: the mass killing of one or more groups of human beings by other human beings. The bright side of the developing cradle of civilization has been characterized by the development of written language and by feats of human ingenuity, improving health, and rising prosperity. But the dark side created the formation of armies, the advancement of weapons, and the virtually endless practice of war and death.

Evolution of TB

TB is the largest cause of adult deaths from any single infectious disease, and ranks among the top 10 causes of death worldwide. According to the latest (2017) World Health Organization Global Tuberculosis Report, "The TB epidemic is larger than previously estimated reflecting new surveillance and survey data from India." Specifically,

In 2016 there were an estimated 10.4 million new (incident) TB cases worldwide, of which 6.2 million (59.5%) were among men, 3.2 million (30.5%) among women, and 1.0 million (10%) among children. People living with human immunodeficiency virus (HIV) accounted for 1.0 million (10%) of all new TB cases.

Furthermore,

In 2016, there were an estimated 490,000 new cases of multidrug-resistant TB and an additional 110,000 people with rifampicin-resistant TB who were also newly eligible for multidrug-resistant TB treatment.

Lastly,

there were an estimated 1.3 million TB deaths in 2016, and an additional 0.4 million deaths resulting from TB disease among people living with HIV. [16]

Early Observations
TB has traditionally been considered a disease of "antiquity." And as far back as 460 BCE, the Hippocratic Corpus included reference to TB, or whatever symptom-complex was referenced at the time; moreover, the Corpus warned physicians to avoid caring for such patients when seriously ill, because their high mortality rates were damaging to their professional reputations [17]. For centuries thereafter, arguments raged over whether TB was caused by miasmas, atmospheric imbalances, heredity constitutional defects, contagion, or even divine intervention. In 1720, an English physician, Benjamin Martin, postulated that TB was caused by "wonderfully minute living creatures," and he believed that getting too close to "consumptives" would "draw in part of the breath he emits from the lungs," which could transmit the disease [18]. But then nearly another century went by overflowing with supposition and mystery.

In the early 1800s, an important first start leading to an accurate diagnosis of TB was made by René T. H. Laennec, the "Father of Pulmonary Disease" and inventor of the stethoscope. In his studies on the pathologic findings of hundreds of autopsies, Laennec made the "inspired deduction" that the morphologic similarities among the abundant pulmonary abnormalities – including neighboring infiltrations and cavities as well as all the various extrapulmonary lesions – were caused by a single disease, which he called "phthisis" [19]. Not long afterward, Johann Schönlein of Berlin demonstrated that "the tubercle was the fundamental pathologic lesion" in all organs affected by the disease, which he therefore designated as "TB" [19]. Getting even closer to an answer, in 1865 Jean-Antoine Villemin, a French military surgeon, proved by transmitting pathologic material from victims of TB to a variety of experimental animals that TB was a communicable infectious disease [20, 21]. Villemin should have received far more attention to this seminal observation than he had hoped for, but the Franco-Prussian War intervened.

Finally, it was left for Robert Koch (Fig. 1), physician-scientist in Berlin, Germany, to author "one of the most definitive pronouncements in medical history" [22] on March 24, 1882. Like his great rival Louis Pasteur, Koch was already famous for his studies on the pathogenesis and life cycle of anthrax, a common and important disease of domestic and wild animals that occasionally strikes humans. Most accounts affirm that this was Koch's maiden exposition and he started by fumbling with his notes and was obviously nervous. But after he got going, no one cared

because slowly and methodically he convinced his spellbound audience that a bacterium, which he had invented a novel way of staining so that it could be seen under a microscope, which he had succeeded for the first time ever in growing on artificial culture medium, and which he had then used to infect laboratory animals and reproduce the identical disorder, caused the most important disease of mankind of all time – TB. [22]

Seventeen days after Koch's brilliant presentation, incredibly fast compared with current publishing norms, a seminal article announcing his discovery appeared in a major medical journal [23]. The news spread quickly. Many physicians were greatly impressed but, as expected, skeptics wanted to be certain. Koch became instantly famous, as illustrated in Figure 1. Kaiser Wilhelm I appointed him Professor and an Imperial Privy Councilor, upped his salary and research support, and added more laboratory assistants [24].

But there remained a nagging uncertainty about TB itself: was it one disease or two? Koch and other specialists knew with certainty that TB occurred in both cattle as well as humans, but no one at the time could be sure whether 2 different species of *Mycobacterium* were involved. Koch believed – wrongly – "that bovine disease posed no threat to humans" [22]. In 1896, Smith [25] showed "sharp differences" between *M. tuberculosis* and *M. bovis*, including their

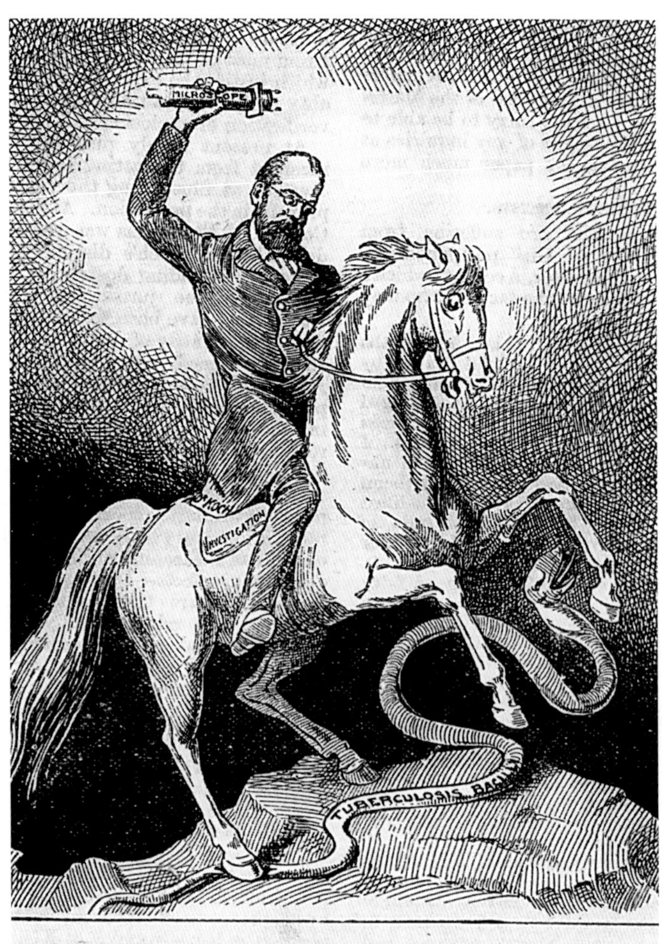

Fig. 1. An engraving depicting German Bacteriologist Robert Koch (1843–1910) as the new Saint George after he isolated the bacillus of tuberculosis. Original publication: The Review of Reviews, London. English language version of an original image published in the satirical magazine Ulk in Berlin, 1890. Photo by Hulton Archive/Getty Images, with permission.

staining characteristics, morphology, and manifestations in infants and children. Five years later (1901), Koch [26] was still trivializing the public importance of *M. bovis* as an agent of disease; he wrote, "if such a susceptibility really exists,... (it) is but a very rare occurrence."

Koch waffled about the virulence of *M. bovis*, but he triumphed once again for his discovery of *tuberculin*. Although initially he misjudged its value as treatment for TB, the subsequent use of tuberculin by skin testing as an indicator of the presence of either active disease or latent infection of both *M. tuberculosis* and *M. bovis* "led to the virtual eradication of TB-ridden cattle and other domesticated animals in industrialized countries" [27].

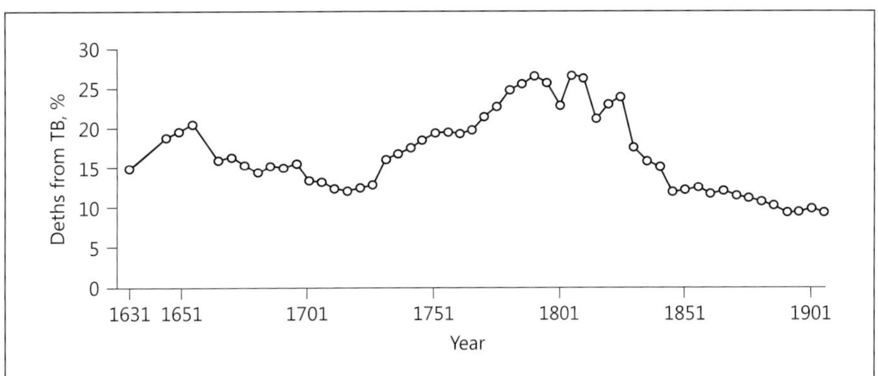

Fig. 2. Changes in mortality from presumed tuberculosis in the city of London, England, between 1631 and 1901 [54], with permission from Oxford University Press.

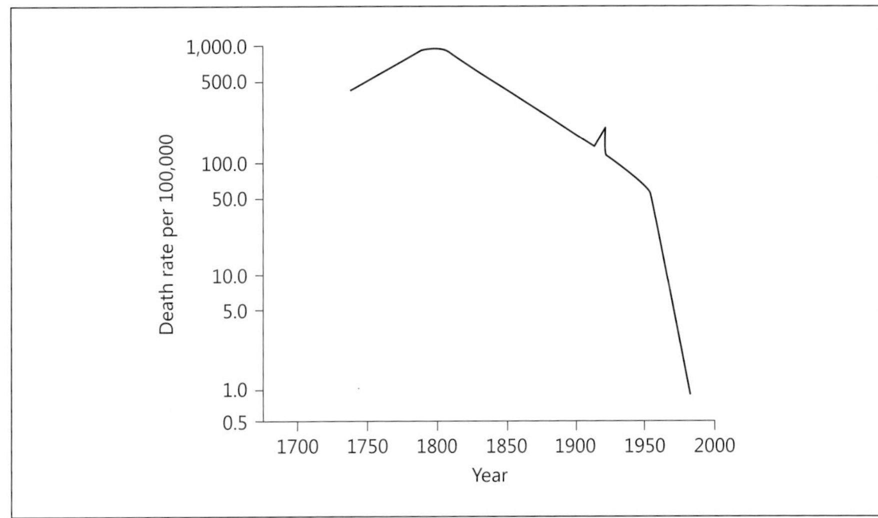

Fig. 3. Schematic model of the trend of mortality from tuberculosis in Western Europe from 1740 to 1985. Modified from [18] and using data from [57], with permission from the American Thoracic Society.

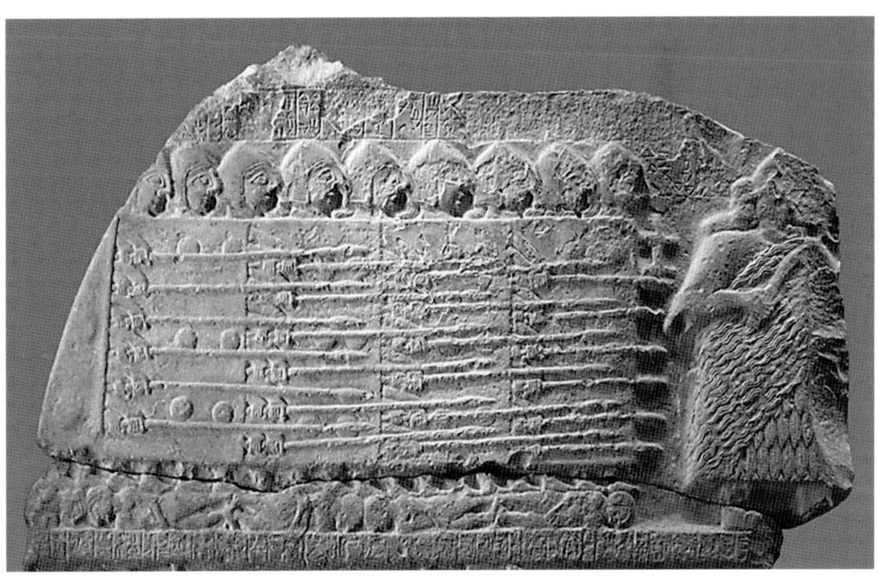

Fig. 4. Fragment from the Stele of Vultures. Victory stele of King Eannutum of Lagash over Umma, showing the first extant evidence of an ancient army equipped with helmets, shields and spears. Limestone, circa 2450 BC, Summerian archaic dynasties. Found in 1881 in Girsu (now Tello, Iraq), Mesopotamia, by Edourad de Sarzec. Currently in Louvre Museum, Paris, France. Eric Gaba, July 15, 2005, with permission from Sting.

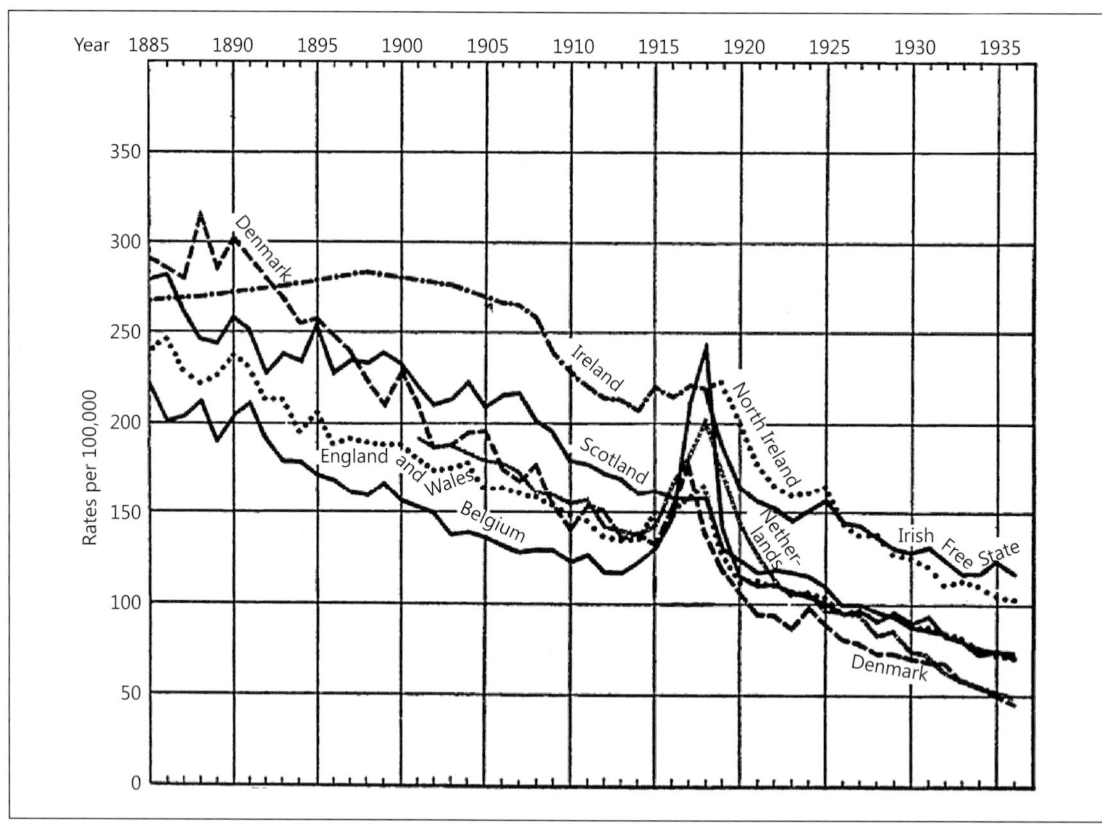

Fig. 5. Tuberculosis death rates in Great Britain, Belgium, the Netherlands, and Denmark during Fifty Year Period, 1885–1935, with permission from Sheridan Content Solutions, Sheridan, PA, on behalf of The American Public Health Association.

Population Genomics

The former prevailing, now obsolete, view of the evolutionary history of TB had long concluded that *M. bovis* was an ancient cause of the disease in cows, bison, and other bovines and that *M. tuberculosis* became a human pathogen much later during the Neolithic Demographic Transition, around 10,000 years ago: a supposition now being revisited, thanks to comparative genomic evidence. Cole et al. [28] first showed that *M. bovis* and its animal partners have a genome that is around 60,000 base pairs smaller than that of "human-adapted *M. tuberculosis*." Accordingly, it looks increasingly evident that *M. tuberculosis* and *M. bovis* both share a common ancestor, but that the ancient genomic regions present in *M. tuberculosis* predated those of *M. bovis* [29].

TB is not caused by a single bacterium but by a group of phylogenetically related bacterial cousins called the *M. tuberculosis* complex (MTBC) [30]. Human TB is most often caused by *M. tuberculosis* but *Mycobacterium africanum* is also a cause in West Africa. By far the most important animal-adapted member of the MTBC is *M. bovis*, which was previously a common cause of milk-borne TB in children before being largely controlled by pasteurization. Other MTBC species affecting animals include *Mycobacterium caprae* in sheep and goats, *Mycobacterium pinnipedii* in seals and sea lions, and *Mycobacterium microti* in voles [31]. Owing either to significant differences in communicability or to its complete absence among various human and animal contacts, MTBC species are usually found mainly in their preferred hosts. *M. microti*, for example, is not pathogenic for humans, and *M. bovis* is 6-times less virulent in humans than in cows.

Recent studies have amplified and considerably revised previous views about the origin and evolution of MTBC and its human predecessors. In 2002, for example, Brosch et al. [32] published the genomic analyses of 100 strains of MTBC, including *M. tuberculosis*, *Mycobacterium canettii*, *M. microti*, and *M. bovis* and concluded that the analysis of the regions of difference of MTBC strains can distinguish between "ancestral" and "modern" strains of human TB. In addition, all strains with TbD1 deletions appear to be derived from a single clone of human MTBC descent, which includes the major modern epidemic families, such as Beijing and Haarlem.

As reviewed at the beginning of this chapter, modern humans, *H. sapiens*, originated in Kenya and Tanzania towards the end of the Pleistocene epoch around 200,000 years ago. Descendant populations of hunter-gatherers remained small in number owing to the persistence of the last Ice Age and the accompanying lethality of its prevailing recurrent climatic changes. Survivors are thought to have collected in small bands of 25 or even fewer members, as judged from historical observations and the habits of current nomadic groups [33]. But then the climatic conditions presumably improved and humans started to migrate out of Africa: the great human expansion was underway.

In 2006, Gagneux et al. [34] and Firdessa et al. [35] first showed that human MTBC strains demonstrated a phylogeographic organization consisting of 7 different population lineages, each associated with particular geographic areas but all of which are found in Africa. Lineages 5 and 6, the most basal, often referred to as *M. africanum*, occur chiefly in West Africa. Later, Comas et al. [36] postulated that human-adapted MTBC originated in Africa and "has been infecting humans for at least the last 70,000 years," after which viable tubercle bacilli were transmitted both by and to the migrating anatomically modern humans headed toward Eurasia. Based on their model of human whole-genome variation data, Rasmussen et al. [37] determined that *H. sapiens* spread from Africa in 2 major waves: the first dispersal took place around the Indian Ocean beginning between 62,000 and 75,000 years ago, and the second dispersal occurred 25,000–38,000 years ago into Eurasia. Interestingly, one of the evolutionary models of MTBC showed that the Indo-Oceanic lineage or lineage 1 (predominant in the Indian Ocean region) split 67,000 years ago, and the lineages 2 and 4 (East Asian and Euro-American, respectively) split between 30,000 and 46,000 years ago. This evolutionary model showed a striking correlation between the human migration events and the evolutionary split of MTBC [36, 37]. Note also that the lengthy overlap in Africa of both *H. sapiens* and each of the lineages of *M. tuberculosis* has established a reciprocal evolutionary partnership in which the 2 players have been coevolving for countless millenniums.

These observations reinforce the conclusion that all MTBC species shared a common ancestral origin around 70,000 years ago, but then diversified into 7 major lineages distributed in different regions throughout the world [34, 35]. But how far back does the ancestral MTBC lineage actually extend? The recently reported 500,000-year old fossil of *H. erectus* from Turkey showing characteristic lesions of TB,

if confirmed, remarkably lengthens the historic evolution of TB [38].

The newly revised concepts that changed human history did indeed occur during the Neolithic Transition around 10,000 years ago, but not because of the arrival of human MTBC, which had been implanted many thousands of years before, but because of growing increases in population size and population density. Here again is where hunter-gatherers re-enter the picture as they began the switch from nomadic pursuits to a settled life of animal domestication and agriculture. The Neolithic Revolution took a few thousand years to implement all its dramatic changes – one of which, as emphasized in this first chapter, was the onset of warfare, a never-ending process that continues to kill and ravage today. Another derivative of the acceleration in growth of human populations and increasingly crowded surroundings with resultant multiplication of susceptible hosts was that human MTBC adapted to this stimulus by switching from a low-density infectious disease to a modern "crowd" disease; furthermore, a corollary consequence of an increasing number of potential victims unfailingly leads to higher virulence and shorter latency [36]. But crowd diseases (i.e., teeming people) caused by TB, as discussed later, do not really show up until around the 17th century.

Remember that the Holocene epoch, or current geologic period, began approximately 11,700 years ago, which is about the time humans had almost migrated from Africa into Europe, India, and China, and as Gagneux [30] correctly assumes, "human exploration, trade, and conquest" further broadened the distribution of people and increased the density of the growing populations. We are following the gospel that during the last 70,000 years humans became newly infected with *M. tuberculosis* and some must have become sick and died, but the accompanying long latency period, in theory, allowed people with hidden infection to migrate for many years and long distances before clinical signs of reactivation disease appeared; but bear in mind that the shortened human life expectancies during those hazardous years must have cut off TB latencies as well as lives. This leads to 2 important questions: when did humans migrate from Eurasia to the Americas, and did TB accompany those prehistoric migrations or did the disease recur much later through European contact?

Paulsen [39] concludes in his 1987 review that the evidence for the presence of TB in Native Americans and Alaskans in prehistoric North America remains inconclusive. And it looks like the jury is still out on that question. What remains unsettled, of course, is whether or not the heightened susceptibility of Native Americans to TB should have decimated the vulnerable inhabitants once virulent *M. tuberculosis* was brought along with the incoming migrants: which does not appear to have happened. Another Paulsen conclusion is that the evidence for the presence of TB in prehistoric South America has been "fairly well established." Both conclusions, therefore, have stood the test of time, except to advance the current South American verdict from "fairly well" to "well established."

North America: The melting of the giant ice caps of northern Canada opened up pathways to North America around 15,000 years ago. Several possible routes through or around (by boat) the remaining massive ice deposits towards the end of the Pleistocene epoch allowed humans to migrate from eastern Siberia to Alaska, then further southward. An early site at Clovis, New Mexico, for example, attracted considerable attention in the 1920s to 1930s, and is still a major reference center [40]. But several other locations have also gained archaeological importance: near Calgary, Canada, in south-central Oregon, Texas, and the Channel Islands of California. New evidence from the Wally's Beach site in Canada, using improved radiocarbon dating and supplemented by data from Clovis, New Mexico, provides a more comprehensive understanding of the contribution of the 2,000-year hunting spree by humans in the extinction of at least 6 genera of megafauna, including mammoths, mastodons, gomphotheres, sloths, horses, and camels [41]. The extinction of these giant mammals was mainly caused by dramatic changes in climate and habitat; nevertheless, even though the human population at the time was small and its weapons primitive, hunting must have played a role. First solitary then groups of animals are believed to have been hunted from roughly "15,000–13,300 years ago." But apparently no pre-Columbian European Contact with TB occurred in North America and Mexico, and throughout Mesoamerica, which comprises central Mexico south to the Central America isthmus countries that link North and South America.

Naturally, studies are underway to compare the genomes of modern Native Americans and Siberians. Findings by Dryomov et al. [42] and associates of the mitochondrial genome diversity support the hypotheses that there were "multiple streams of expansions to northern North America from northeastern Eurasia in late Pleistocene- early Holocene." More definitive information about genomic dispersal in the Americas should soon be available.

South America: An early case of TB in pre-Columbian Peru was reported in 1973 in a child 8–10 years old with radiographic features of Pott's disease plus lung, pleural and kidney disease [43]. Ziehl-Neelsen staining revealed many clumps of acid-fast bacilli and radiocarbon dating estimated death at approximately 700 A.D. Another Peruvian mummy with a radiocarbon age of 1,040 ± 4 years had pulmonary lesions with DNA unique to *M. tuberculosis*, as shown by extraction and identification techniques [44]. Another vertebral lesion was similarly identified from a pre-Columbian mummy from Arica, Chile [45]. These abnormalities provided circumstantial evidence for the presence of TB in pre-Columbian specimens, but given the lengthy differential diagnosis, definitive proof was impossible [46].

The still open question concerning the presence or absence of pre-Columbian TB seems to have been convincingly answered affirmatively in 2014 by Bos et al. [47]. Their excavations of 3 Peruvian mummies revealed mycobacterial genomes that proved that this particular and most unusual cause of human TB originated from seals and sea lions and evolved from a well-known ancient strain of non-human MTBC, which clearly differed from modern *M. tuberculosis*. All 3 specimens derived from the same period of historic Peruvian culture and had radiocarbon dates between 1028 and 1280 A.D. In addition, based on extensive genomic analyses, instead of clustering with other human strains, the Peruvian samples clustered with animal lineages, particularly *M. pinnipedii* – and provide "unequivocal evidence of human infection" by an animal – adapted strain of MTBC [47].

One possible sequence – there are not many others to go by – postulates that *M. pinnipedii-infected* seals and sea lions crossed the southern Atlantic Ocean, probably from Spain, where they colonized costal South American and (later) Australian waters. Because shore-based Peruvian and other neighboring humans had presumably been hunting and eating seals for thousands or more years, sooner or later the newly arrived seals liberated sufficient air-borne pathogen passengers to infect local humans and complete the zoonotic transfer of TB from seals to coastal humans, then from coastal humans to inland humans [47]. Previous observations have reported presumed air-borne *M. pinnipedii* transmission from seals to other mammals, including human animal keepers in a Netherland zoo [48].

Human Contact: Christopher Columbus certainly made human contact with indigenous natives in or near one of the present day Bahama Islands during his first voyage to the New World in 1492; he returned to Spain with a few gold nuggets, Indian captives, and 2 greatly unwanted gifts for the Old World: tobacco and syphilis (as many believe, but remains debatable). There is no evidence either his sailors or the aboriginal people he contacted had TB. In 1497, John Cabot landed in North America and ships from other countries soon followed. European contacts from Spain returned to South America and Mexico as conquistadores in the early 1500s, conquering and plundering the Aztec, Mayan, Toltec, Inca, and other native populations, seeking gold and other treasures. Decades later, Spanish soldiers, priests, explorers, and opportunists, whose number had increased dramatically by then, made their way north to what is now the United States. These newcomers may have brought cases of TB with them, specifically from the Euro-American lineage (the predominant lineage in North and South America), who then spread the disease to the Aboriginal populations of North America.

The arrival of European contacts from different sources harboring *M. tuberculosis*, did not lead to an instant, widespread epidemic of TB among susceptible Native Americans and Canadians: there was too much country and too few invaders. When nascent colonies started to enlarge, and Europeans began to mix with the Natives, smallpox and measles were far more frequent and deadly than TB.

An interesting study by Pepperell et al. [49] documents an unfamiliar sequence of low-level spread of TB from incoming migrants. These authors observed that a single Euro-American lineage *M. tuberculosis* – with a characteristic DS6^{Quebec} genomic deletion – was at its highest circulating frequency in both Aboriginal populations in Ontario, Saskatchewan, and Alberta, and in French Canadian residents in Quebec. In addition, substantial contact among these populations occurred during a defined historical period of fur trading from 1710 to 1870. The results of historical and genetic analyses show that for around 100 years, small, widely scattered indigenous groups became infected by *M. tuberculosis*, thanks to an infrequent number of human migrants who were infected with low numbers of tubercle bacilli. Furthermore, large-scale TB epidemics did not appear in these communities before the late 19th and 20th centuries [49].

New Observations: Knowledge about susceptibility to the development of TB after exposure to *M. tuberculosis* includes several risk factors, most of which have been recognized for decades: malnutrition, inadequate ventilation, and overcrowding; once TB infection has occurred mental and/or physical stress, and impaired immunity exacerbate the likelihood that disease will occur. To a greater or lesser extent, all of these factors are related to warfare. Much more recently, whole genome sequencing and phylogenetic analyses have demonstrated more genetic diversity of human-adapted MTBC than previously believed [50]. As already described, 7 lineages, each having a number of sublineages, have been shown to govern intrinsic bacterial forces that affect the pathogenicity of tubercle bacilli. These new factors have increasing public health importance.

The East-Asian lineage, which includes the famous Beijing strain, has spread in successive global waves during the last 200 years, first during the Industrial Revolution, later during World War I (WWI), and lastly associated with the epidemic of HIV infection [51]. According to some, Beijing strains are allegedly endowed with "selective advantages," including enhanced pathogenicity and/or virulence, and increased progression from infection to disease. Recent studies showing considerable variation among different Euro-American sublineages in the frequency of transmission of contacts to TB among index patients – from 15.7% in RD145 to 1.8% in RD219 – clearly indicate that further studies are needed to document the impact of "bacterial factors on transmissibility and pathogenicity" of human MTBC [52].

Epidemic Tuberculosis
During the 16th century, most of Europe was just beginning to recover from the devastating population losses that occurred during the 14th century pandemics of bubonic plague, which were exacerbated by local famines and wars. England's population was 2.1 million inhabitants in 1400, half the number estimated in 1348 [53]. During the next 100 years, population growth in England had resulted in 4.1 million people by 1570, and a further increase to 4.8 million in 1600. The majority of the English in the early Middle Ages were subsistence workers, farmers, and laborers, eking out life despite wretched harvests, dreadful climates, and prevalent sickness. Local magistrates took care of business on behalf of wealthy nobles and landed gentry. Workers were widely dispersed throughout the countryside; towns were small and scarce: obviously unfavorable conditions for the spread of TB. Feudal society declined, however, in the 13th and 14th centuries due in part to the rise of a thriving merchant population that established sophisticated trading networks throughout England and Europe and weekly markets and fairs that promoted greater access to commercial goods, the expansion of towns, and the development of an urban artisan population that catered to local needs. Expanded trade and communication probably hastened the spread of TB at the time.

Consequently, during the next century, agricultural practices became more efficient, requiring fewer laborers and less physical input. Food became cheaper, wages rose a trifle; industrialization advanced and towns began to increase in size and number. Meanwhile, from 60,000 to 70,000 inhabitants in 1500, London, already by far the largest city in England, kept making room for ever-increasing numbers of people, causing the population to grow to 250,000 at the end of the 17th century [54]. And to make matters worse, these indigents, often desperately poor and undernourished, had to survive packed into abysmal living conditions: London became a model of crowd diseases. So, by the year 1631, as shown in Figure 2, 15% of all deaths in the city of London that year were attributed to TB [55]; and for the next nearly 200 years, the death rate from TB in the city of London remained enormous, peaking at around 25%, and finally beginning to decline around 1830.

A schematic model showing the trend of mortality from TB in Western Europe from 1740 to 1985 is illustrated in Figure 3 [56]. Death rates from TB peaked at the astronomic value of 1,000/100,000 population in 1800, and then declined at a fairly constant rate for more than 100 years, until the abrupt upsurge that occurred during and immediately after WWI, which was in part lengthened by the Spanish influenza pandemic that lasted until around 1920. Finally, the model illustrates the arrival in 1952 of "triple therapy," which heralded the steep decline of TB mortality resulting from effective chemotherapy [56].

No one is quite sure what triggered the initial reduction in TB mortality that began around 1800. (Note that both the year and country of the decrease in death rates from TB varied from location to location, but from whatever peak was finally identified, mortality began to go down, with a few wrinkles but fairly consistently and for well over the succeeding 100 years.) In 1800 in Germany, there was no obvious cause for the decline, and it took place at least 82 years before Robert Koch discovered *M. tuberculosis*. One of the most frequently cited reasons for the reduction remains a rising standard of living, which includes better housing, improved nutrition, higher wages, and lower costs, when and if these actually occurred; public health efforts were meager at the time but may have helped somewhat; and there was the dawning realization that TB was a contagious disease that warranted isolation of sick patients.

The ups and downs of TB mortality varied considerably from one country to another during the 19th century: in Great Britain, it declined; in Ireland and Norway, it increased first; but in France mortality stayed "extremely high" the entire century [54]. During the 17th, 18th, and 19th centuries in Western Europe and then in the 18th and 19th centuries in the Eastern US, TB was by far the most important cause of death, and it remained the highest or one of the highest causes of mortality in several countries, including the US until around 1900. But once TB death rates started going down, they kept steadily decreasing until interrupted by WWI and then again by WWII.

The Industrial Revolution began in England in the mid-18th century and then spread to the rest of Western Europe. While the first and more famous phase is often dated 1760–1810, a second phase of the industrialization process based on developments in physics and chemistry and advancements in the steel and petroleum industries continued up to WWI, with Germany eventually surpassing England in industrial output. Living conditions in neighboring English mills and factories during the first phase of the broadening industrialization period were deplorable and deteriorated even further to an unprecedented extent. Five-year-old boys and girls worked dangerous 10–12 h shifts. Sanitation and personal hygiene for practical purposes vanished. Overflowing cesspools required emptying into local rivers and streams, and on a regular basis night porters emptied human excrement into the Thames River, a chief source of drinking water for London. Similar conditions existed on the continent in industrial centers, especially in the Ruhr Valley in Germany, a country that unified in 1871 and rose in power during the period of the second Industrial Revolution. Cholera was rampant and both typhus and typhoid were endemic, but as usual, TB remained the chief scourge.

Around midway, or even a little earlier during the Industrial Revolution, historically high death *rates* from TB began to go down even while the *number* of deaths continued to rise. Redeker [58] reported that TB death rates in London peaked at 950/100,000 as early as 1755. Kraus [59], however, states that mortality from "consumption," also in London, was cataloged at 1,121/100,000 during 1771–1780, after which it declined to 716/100,000 during 1801–1810. The explanation – for the decrease in death rates while the number of deaths rose – was the ongoing, striking increase in the size of the English population during that period, which included more and more new professionals, doctors, lawyers, bankers, business-men, and entrepreneurs of all sorts. "Thus was born the English middle class" [57], an increasingly important group that was much less vulnerable compared to their TB-stricken predecessors.

Two related scientific articles tackle the important question of whether there were individuals or families that stood out as being protected from TB-induced disease and death during the 17th to 19th centuries, when practically everyone was infected by tubercle bacilli and mortality from active disease hovered around 50% or even higher. Lipsitch and Sousa [60] ask whether the presence and magnitude of *natural selection* contributed to the development of resistance to TB, which had been proposed as a factor affecting the historical decline in TB, before chemotherapy was introduced. The authors concluded that natural selection by deaths from pulmonary TB cannot account for the 150-year-long ongoing reduction in TB detected in Europeans and their descendants, except during both WWI and WWII, the latter of which was recorded just before the arrival of anti-TB treatment.

Thanks to the exceptional reduction in death rates from TB chemotherapy after the mid-20th century and onwards, Stead [61] showed a significant difference in the percentage of persons who developed positive tuberculin skin test reactions following exposure to severe outbreaks of TB in white communities compared with those in African-American communities. Stead hypothesized that everyone infected by *M. tuberculosis* should develop a positive tuberculin reaction, and if an individual remained negative, it implied the presence of genetically determined innate resistance to TB in both them and their ancestors.

Both of these investigations are of interest, but fail to completely explain what actually caused the historically conspicuous and lengthy decline in TB deaths rates.

Evolution of Warfare

Wars began long before the beginning of recorded history, but the subject has been written about from every conceivable angle. After his retirement, Carl von Clausewitz [62], a Prussian veteran of Napoleonic and other wars, wrote a famous book, *On War*, in which he said, among other notable quotations, "War is merely a continuation of politics by other means – not merely a political act, but a real political instrument." Politics unquestionably played an important role in many wars, but there are additional reasons why armed men kill innocent people. Clausewitz's wars were "civilized wars," fought by officers and gentlemen who fight by rules and who are governed by military discipline and ethical principles. Keegan [63], however, adds that there have also been "non-civilized wars" that have employed atypical military techniques featuring exceptional violence and death. More than a few armies have concentrated on looting, raping, and pillaging, intensified by deliberate cruelty and excessive butchery. A legendary example was Genghis Kahn [64], who created the world's largest-ever empire in Northeast Asia in the 13th–14th centuries. Kahn specialized in annihilating Mongol tribes using a combination of advanced military tactics and merciless brutality; on one occasion, having defeated an army of Tatars along with their captured chiefs, he had all the chiefs boiled alive.

As stated earlier in this chapter, many experts agreed on the fact that "at least *H. sapiens*, and possibly earlier prehumans, possess innate, genetically programmed lethal violence." Genes may contribute, but warfare takes abundant forces, leadership, and considerable resources. Nevertheless, without that apparent, crucial genetic underpinning, it is certainly possible that wars would not be such an inviolable, practically endless feature of human existence.

Of course, the issue is debatable and controversial, but we might someday learn the correct answer. A remarkably new gene-editing technique called CRISPR allows research scientists to remove and substitute pin-pointed genes in experimental animal genomes. Ethical concerns have retarded use of the method in disordered human genomes (e.g., in sickle cell anemia, Huntington disease, and other dominant genetic disorders), but in theory it is possible. Deleting the culprit war-enhancing genes – if present – would solve the genetic role in warfare and contribute to everlasting peace.

Prehistory
Like virtually all vertebrate animals, interpersonal violence has been an integral, mostly spontaneous, component of ordinary hunter-gatherer's prehistoric life. It would be interesting to know how the group's interpersonal dynamics played out, but the band's survival must have greatly depended on all members' participation and teamwork. And it makes perfect sense. Presumably, hunter-gatherers functioned in small bands of 20–25 members and had considerable vacant space to forage in. If a hunter-gatherer band recognized that a rival gathering was in the vicinity, it seems unlikely that the 2 groups sought to kill everyone in sight; instead, they usually carefully avoided each other: that proved to be safer and healthier and, as far as we know, it probably helped everyone to stay alive and preserve the size of their bands.

Two rival hypotheses – one short and the other long – differ chiefly in the duration and intensity of late-Paleolithic, early-Holocene savagery, leading up to actual acts of warfare. But the idea of having both a short and a long incubation period leading to the buildup of warfare accommodates the fact that, first, the great majority of *H. sapiens* residing in Europe, India and surrounding countries, and throughout Asia made the successful transition during the early Holocene epoch from the foraging life of hunter-gatherers to one of farming and animal domestication – with a minimum of violence and practically no warfare [65]. And by contrast, second, several other countries – Australia, South America, North America, together with Paleoamericans and Alaskans, and New Guinea – practiced extreme violence, including the harvesting of scalps, skulls, long-bone trophies, and revenge killings, which lasted in some places until post-colonial years [66]. To summarize, each of the 2 "hypotheses" turns out to provide an apposite explanation for the different time courses of the transition from hunter-gathering to war.

Jericho

A frequently cited clue to the beginnings of warfare is ancient Jericho, one of the world's oldest cities, dated as early as 8000 BCE, which surrounded a late phase (Pre-Pottery) Neolithic settlement. Structural remnants suggest a monumental fortification, said to be built with a wall "3.0 m (10ft) thick" and "4.0 m (13ft) high", with a surrounding moat "9.1 m (30ft) wide" and "3.0 m (10ft) deep," within which was a "9.1 m (30 ft) high" tower. This impressive fortress-like structure strongly implies that it served to protect the inhabitants from invaders; others, however, claim it served as defense against floodwaters [67]. No one knows if battles actually took place or not.

A convincing finding that prehistoric warfare had definitely taken place was documented around 3500 BCE. The Syrian-American Archaeological Expedition discovered and studied the vestiges of a huge battle that destroyed Hamoukar, a remote site in northeastern Syria. In 2005, a press release from the University of Chicago proudly noted that this "discovery provides the earliest evidence of large scale organized warfare" [68]. And large scale it was. The victims, sheltered in buildings behind mud-brick walls, were besieged by assailants who bombarded the inhabitants using slings that launched inch-wide bullets; over 1,000 of which were found in the excavation, plus 120 larger clay projectiles. After destroying the old city, the attackers built a new one over the ruins.

Fast-forward another millennium to 2500 BCE to view the spectacular Stele of the Vultures [69], the few remaining fragments of limestone bas-relief now in the Louvre Museum, one of which is illustrated in Figure 4. Observe the beautifully ordered professional army, fully equipped with helmets and shields, and armed with spears. Over time, and slowly at first but then with increasing rapidity, weapons became progressively deadly. For hundreds of thousands of years, hunter-gatherers survived using a succession of flint-tipped spears and harpoons, clubs, and primitive bows and arrows in their struggle to find food. But after most of the world had settled down and begun farming, owing in large part to the impetus of warfare, new weapons were created and rapidly upgraded: metal swords, spears and axes, chariots, crossbows, catapults, battering rams, then gunpowder, guns, and bombs. In the history of the development of warfare technology, the race to annihilation has played out about as far as it can go.

Tollense War

In 1996, an amateur archeologist chanced upon a remarkable find. Protruding from the bank of the Tollense River in northern Germany was an upper arm bone with a flint arrow sticking straight out of it. Subsequently, a test excavation revealed several other bones plus a club that may have been used to pulverize the skull that was found nearby. Radiocarbon-dating indicated 1250 BCM, the year a previously unknown gigantic battle took place that may have involved up to 4,000 warriors, apparently recruited from hundreds of kilometers distance; including as far north as Scandinavia and Poland and south to Germany and Holland. Because of the results of excavations from 2009 to 2015, according to the summary by Curry [70], out goes the belief of a "peaceful" Bronze Age throughout northern Europe. Though much remains to be learned, the fierce Tollense battle "fits into a period when we have increased warfare everywhere."

Trojan War

The ancient Greeks blamed their Gods for the Trojan War and for centuries, modern historians were not sure there had actually been one. The time and location of the Trojan War remained a puzzle until 1868, when the German archaeologist, Heinrich Schliemann, became convinced that Troy existed [71]. Subsequent excavations unearthed an ancient city at Hissarlik, Turkey, which most current authorities accept as Troy. The various dates "establishing" wartime Troy have coalesced to around 1184 BCE, a Bronze Age city. Much of what we believe about the Trojan War comes from Homer's epic poems, with their own mythology and uncertain dates of origin, which reach as far back as 1200–750 BCE [72]: first the *Iliad*, which focuses on the last year of the 9-year conflict, and its sequel the *Odyssey*, which describes Odysseus' troubled return to Ithaca. Additional information comes from the *Cyclic Epics*, written between the 7th and 6th centuries BCE [73]. In addition, numerous other ancient and modern literary sources, some more accurate than others, round out the legends. Moreover, inspiration from the *Trojan War* enriched the majestic Athenian tragedies of Aeschylus, Euripides, and Sophocles, written during the 6th and 5th centuries BCE.

The Trojan War was one of the first wars to feature women. Helen, who was blamed for causing the war in the first place, was the daughter of Leda, Queen of Sparta, and consort of Zeus; Helen was celebrated as the most beautiful woman in the world. The goddesses Hera, Athena, and Aphrodite all played consequential roles. And from that time onward until the widespread development of professional armies, legions of single women and wives followed soldiers and/or hung around encampments to provide goods, services, sexual favors, and to ensure their companions got fed and had wounds attended [74].

Hundred Years' War

The Hundred Years' War actually lasted 116 years during the late Middle Ages. Traditionally, the war has been differentiated into 3 phases separated by 2 truces: first, the Edwardian Era War (1337–1360); second, the Caroline War (1369–1389); and lastly the 2-part Lancastrian War (1415–1453). Five generations of Kings, both of England and France, fought over the succession of rulers and control of large landholdings within the territory of France [75]. The events during one of the longest wars in military history led to considerable social, political, and economic turmoil. At the beginning of the war, for example, there was a switch from a major fighting role of armies of knights and nobles to the use of professional soldiers; and toward the end (1445), the first standing army since the conclusion of the Roman Empire was established in France to combat marauding militias. Weapons and strategy changed dramatically from the early utility of cavalry, to the efficacy of the longbow (English), and then artillery (French). Both countries suffered substantial population losses from intermittent warfare plus deaths from the bubonic plague [76]. Dysentery played a major role in the 1415 Battle of Agincourt. Fifty percent of the French population died during the One Hundred Years' War, including 3-quarters of the population of Normandy and two-thirds of that in Paris. England was less affected than France, because all the battles and movements of armies occurred on the continent. After the loss of its continental holdings, except for the Pale of Calais, England was reduced to an island nation, but not long afterward took advantage of its maritime proficiency to begin exploring and gaining mastery of much of the world.

Thirty Years' War

The Thirty Years' War encompassed a series of immensely destructive conflicts in Central Europe, chiefly Germany, from 1618 to 1648. Before the war, certain agreements attempted to create toleration of religious activities of both Catholics and Protestants, but in 1618, Heir-Apparent Ferdinand II, Holy Roman Emperor of Bohemia (crowned the following year), restricted religious practices among Protestants. Other Protestant states, England, the Dutch Republic, Denmark came to their brethren's support, but Ferdinand's allies, German Catholics, Spain, and the papacy were victorious, overrunning much of Protestant Germany and Denmark, with considerable help from mercenary armies [77].

In 1630, the Swedish army led by King Gustavus Adolphus and his Protestant soldiers conquered most of the German lands and kingdoms. Four years later, Spain gained ascendancy and defeated Swedish forces, but then France began to take over, reigniting the Habsburg-French rivalry. From 1636, Swedish, French, Spanish, and Austrian armies conducted ruthless "scorched earth warfare" aimed at destroying as much as possible of what remained of Germany, and left behind a landscape in which famine and starvation were equally destructive to civilians. The cost in German lives was horrific, 20% of inhabitants overall, but as high as 50% in and around Pomerania, and 8 million total. Bubonic plague caused outbreaks throughout the war; typhus and dysentery were endemic; and even scurvy caused numerous deaths during the unsuccessful siege of Nuremberg in 1632. Perhaps the only reprieve of the 30 years' war was the steadily declining role of religion, which had long been a major destabilizing influence in European politics and which led to the Peace of Westphalia, a series of treaties consummated in 1648 that effectively ended the wars of religion and established the sovereign state system [78].

World War I

Concerned Europeans knew something dreadful was going to happen and it finally did: on 28 June 1914, Archduke Franz Ferdinand, heir presumptive to the throne of Austria-Hungary, and his wife Sophie were assassinated by a Bosnian Serb terrorist. Exactly one month later, 28 July 1914, war erupted: Austria-Hungary declared war on Serbia and Russia ordered general mobilization in support of Serbia. A few days later at the beginning of August, Germany invaded neutral Luxembourg and then Belgium on its way to attack France; the next day Great Britain declared war against Germany. At the war's end, 32 countries were fighting [79].

The initial invasion by the German Army came perilously close to Paris, but the French successfully pushed back. Then, a 3-year trench-warfare stalemate occurred that resulted in relatively small back and forth shifts of occupied territory, but the repeated attacks and counter-attacks led to enormous casualties on both sides: in the early 1916 Battle of Verdun, for example, there were 700,000–975,000 dead and wounded; later the same year, there were more than one million casualties in the Battle of Somme, one of the highest numbers in a single battle ever. The Germans defeated the Russians in 1917, but after a final push by the Germans in 1918, the Central Powers were exhausted and an armistice with Germany was declared on 11 November 1918 [79].

Note that around 1780, and at greatly varying years afterwards, death rates from TB started to decline and they continued declining for well over 100 years. But then suddenly, as illustrated during the 50-year period from 1885 to 1935 (Fig. 5), 5- to 7-year-long never-before observed spikes of TB mortality rose sharply in several countries, beginning on or just before the day WWI was declared in 1914 [80]; equally remarkable was the subsequent brisk drop in mortality after hostilities and the end of the overlapping influenza pandemic were over in about 1921. After both the wartime increase and its accompanying decrease had concluded, the previous downward slope of TB mortality resumed its decline as though the war had never happened, as strikingly illustrated in Figure 5. (See also Fig. 10 in chapter 2.) These remarkable events during WWI prove without doubt the incontrovertible linkage between TB and war.

World War II
Virtually all of this book addresses the specific wartime partnerships – country by country – between TB and WWII and, thus, will be discussed only briefly in this first chapter. The deleterious influences of TB during wartime are typically exacerbated by the coexistence of several acute infectious diseases, including enteric fevers, smallpox, yellow fever, typhus, and measles, all of which served as preludes to and accompaniments of WWI and WWII [81]. In addition, as discussed later, during the majority of 19th century and later wars, there were more civilian than military casualties, an observation that is being repeated today in Syria. An introduction of what readers will find in chapters 5–19 of the book classifies countries according to one of 3 distinct patterns of TB mortality during the war years, 1939–1945: (1) countries in which there was little or no wartime rise; (2) countries in which the mortality rate rose in the first years and fell in the later years of the war; and (3) countries in which death rates rose throughout the war years to a peak after the end of the war [82, 83]. These fundamental differences explain why some wartime and post-war countries fared so much better (or worse) than others.

Biological Warfare
Biological warfare is defined as the use of both infectious agents, such as bacteria, viruses, and fungi, and/or biotoxins, with the intent to kill people, or more inclusively living organisms. The earliest practice of biological warfare, as far as is known, is documented in Hittite records of 1500–1200 BCE [84]. The strategy was simple. Victims of tularemia, presumably including Hitittes themselves, were driven into enemy territory to spread an epidemic of deadly disease. In the Trojan War, both arrow and spear tips were coated with poison; a later refinement of Scythian archers (4th century BCE), introduced tipping of arrows and spears with snake venom, blood, or feces to increase the likelihood of infection. Another early tactic was to hurl clay pots filled with poisonous snakes or scorpions on enemy ships or troops.

Corpses of bubonic plague victims have long been used as weapons. Genghis Kahn catapulted dead bodies of infected Mongol warriors to break the siege of Kaffa (Crimea), after which the defending Tartar forces retreated and the Mongols took over the city in 1346.

After more and more European settlers arrived in North America, the broadening association with Native Americans was inevitable, so was the spread of highly contagious smallpox, measles, and other infections to extremely vulnerable, immunologically naïve domestic inhabitants. Fatality rates were enormous. Spontaneously developed smallpox in the 18th century, especially, was a major cause of indigenous American depopulation; plus, there may have been instances of deliberate spread by British forces of contaminated blankets to transmit disease to Native Americans [85].

Little biological warfare occurred during WWI, chiefly by Germans who spread infectious anthrax and glanders. In 1925, the Geneva Protocol outlawed biological weapons, but research, production, and storage were unaffected. During WWII, the Japanese undertook a large-scale program to develop and use biological weapons, which engaged over 5,000 workers and "killed as many as 600 prisoners a year in human experiments" in but a single of its 26 study sites [86]. Widespread testing of pathogenic organisms on prisoners occurred, and on at least one occasion, more than 1,000 water wells were poisoned by the Japanese army in their effort to investigate outbreaks of cholera and typhus in Chinese villages. A few of the epidemics that were launched by the Japanese during the war persisted for several years after the conflict. During the Holocaust, Nazi doctors experimented on Jewish prisoners in various concentration and extermination camps [87]. These experiments often took the form of injecting prisoners with typhus as part of research projects aimed at developing a vaccine. If victims did not die during the experiments, they were killed with injections of phenol into their hearts. Because Jews were targeted for annihilation by their Nazi captors, these typhus experiments were a specific kind of biological warfare.

Beginning in 1949, the US explored the mock warfare value of experiments, studying the spread of bacterial aerosols in over 200 different sites. The author was involved in one such test in September 1950 – along with 800,000 other San Francisco Bay guinea pigs – who were exposed to a "harmless" (i.e., non-infectious) bacterial aerosol: instead of deadly anthrax [88]. In 1969, most Americans breathed easier after President Nixon terminated the weapons program, and in 1972, he signed the Biological and Toxin Weapons Convention agreement. Despite this interdiction, in 1973 the Soviet Union began operating a gigantic biological warfare research project called Biopreparat, employing over 50,000 people in several centers. Naturally, there were casualties. In the early 1970s, 3 of ten people infected with smallpox died in a Soviet biological warfare accident, and in 1979 a large outbreak of anthrax occurred following a mishap in another bioweapons factory; in this instance 66 people and numerous animals died [89]. Biological warfare research still goes on, but deeply clandestine and illegal, and poses a major threat to the US from ISIS (Islamic State of Iraq and Syria) and other terrorist groups.

Since WWII

Unfortunately, the end of WWII did not end the ongoing warfare: at last count since then, "there have been some 250 major wars" [90]. Estimates of casualties vary considerably, from 23 million to over 50 million, including both military and civilian, with more of the latter than the former plus an increasing percentage of children compared with soldiers. America is still engaged in its longest war ever – in Afghanistan – 16 years and not over yet.

Consider the period from 2011 until 2016, it appears as though the world might be beginning to pacify: wars no longer occur in over half the earth: North and South America, Europe, and Australia (Antarctica does not count). Nevertheless, civil wars remain plentiful within Asia (Middle East) and Africa, including in Iraq, Syria, Libya, and Sudan. Lesser intranational military insurgencies in Africa have involved Somalia, Mali, and other locations. The only sovereign nations still engaged in recurrent warfare are Pakistan and India (Asia).

This last word comes from the ongoing horrendous war in Syria, which metamorphosed in 2011 from peaceful demonstrations to the formation of separate rebel forces, later supplemented by units from ISIS, illustrates once again how war ignites TB that may rapidly spread to neighboring countries. From 18 March 2011 to 21 January 2015, 78,769 civilian deaths occurred in Syria, of which 77,646 took place under control of non-state armed groups compared with 1,123 in government-controlled regions [91]. Between 2010 and 2014, life expectancy of Syrians decreased 20 years. In some regions 90% of the medical and nursing staff have left; medicines of all sorts and routine medical supplies have vanished. In 2011, the prevalence of TB in Syria was 23/100,000, today in 2017 it has soared to an unknown value. Anti-TB facilities have closed and medications are no longer available. Studies of Syrian refugees in Jordan have shown a nearly 40% greater TB case detection compared with the 2012 Jordanian rate [92]. Moreover, in Lebanon, a 27% increase in TB has been identified in Syrian refugees [93]. Given the increased exposure to TB, additional injured patients, health-care workers, and other uninfected personnel are likely candidates for the disease; few cases of drug resistance are currently known but others are sure to follow.

Conclusion

This opening chapter started with an historical evolution of hominids and their multiple prehuman and near-human predecessors, beginning millions of years ago. Our direct descendants, *H. sapiens* originated toward the end of the Pleistocene epoch, roughly 200,000 years ago. Resolving ice-age obstacles finally allowed early human migration to begin around 70,000 years ago, just when humans are believed to have become infected with human and other strains of MTBC. Migrants carried *M. tuberculosis* and spread it in its chronic form until about the 17th century in England and Wales, when it took advantage of the rapidly growing population, especially in London, to become a rapidly spreading crowd disease. No one is sure when, except that it was before the advent of written language and sometime during the switch from the nomadic habits of hunter-gatherers to a settled life of farming and domesticating animals. The early years of "civilization" were accompanied by war: including the formation of armies, improvements in weapons, and the development of military strategies. TB – the largest cause of death from disease during the 17th through 20th centuries – joined forces with warfare during WWI, and as detailed in the remainder of this book, during WWII.

TB and warfare are accidental partners, not kindred spirits. When they coexist, as in WWI and WWII and later conflicts, war seems to go its separate way: certainly, the destruction of industry, infrastructure, homes and property, and including casualties, both dead and wounded, have a *raison d'etre* all their own. But then that inevitable 70,000-year-old microorganism, *M. tuberculosis*, sneaks in and profoundly worsens the human misery and grief associated with warfare. Vulnerable people already harboring latent TB infection, trapped by the debilitating effects of war-induced semi-starvation, suffering from mental and physical stress, and needing treatment for diabetes, heart disease and other illnesses are likely "to break down" and develop active TB. Every step in the chain of spread of TB – beginning with an innocent uninfected bystander to a victim of fatal disease – is greatly exacerbated by warfare.

Thanks to the development of powerful new anti-TB medications and the availability of strengthened and more efficient case finding and infection control methods, victory now seems a real but distant possibility in the 70,000-year-old battle against TB. By contrast, it seems increasingly impossible that war will ever be silenced, and that warfare will continue killing millions of men, women, and children every year. It probably no longer matters whether or not humans are genetically programmed for killing each other, because warfare has become such a constant component of daily life. Nine countries possess over 15,000 nuclear weapons, but the distribution of warheads varies greatly among various nations: the US and Russia top the list. Strong efforts to ban nuclear weapons have been put forth, but no single country is ready to give them up, cheating remains an obvious problem, and at least India, Pakistan, and North Korea are creating them as fast as resources allow. Sooner or later, some rouge nation or terrorist group is likely to explode a nuclear weapon: what, then, happens next?

Acknowledgement

The author gratefully acknowledges the major contributions of Dr. Midori Kato-Maeda of the Division of Pulmonary and Critical Care Medicine, University of California San Francisco, San Francisco, CA, USA.

References

1   Johanson DC, Edey M: Lucy: The Beginnings of Humankind. New York, Simon and Shuster, 1981.
2   Leakey M: Olduvai Gorge: My Search for Early Man, 1979.
3   Leakey LSB, Tobias PV, Napier JR: A new species of the genus *Homo* from Olduvai Gorge. Nature 1964;202:7–9.
4   Anton SC: Natural history of Homo erectus. AM J Phys Anthropol 2003;suppl 37:126–170.
5   Klein RG: Paleoanthropology. Whither the Neanderthals? Science 2003;299:1525–1527.
6   Trinkaus E: Pathology and the posture of the La Chapelle-aux-Saints Neandertal. Am J Physical Anthropol 1985;67:19–41.
7   Richter D, Grün R, Joannes-Boyau R, et al: The age of hominin fossils from Jebel Inhoud, Morocco and the origins of the Middle Stone Age. Nature 2017;546:293–296.
8   Henn BM, Cavalli-Sforza LL, Feldman MW: The great human expansion. Proc Natl Acad Sci U S A 2012;109:17758–17764.
9   Comas I, Coscolla M, Luo T, et al: Out-of-Africa migration and Neolithic coexpansion of *Mycobacterium tuberculosis* with modern humans. Nat Genet 2013;45:1176–1182.
10 Cougnac Cave Art (c.23,000 BCE) www.visual-arts-cork.com/prehistoric/cougnac-cave.htm.
11 Taçon P, Chippindale C: Australia's ancient warriors: changing depictions of fighting in the rock art of Arnhem Land, N.T. Camb Anchaeol J 1995; 4:211–248.
12 Mirazon Lahr M, Rivera F, Power RK, et al: Inter-group violence among early Holocene hunter-gatherers of West Turkana, Kenya. Nature 2016; 529:395–398.
13 Bocquet-Appel JP: When the world's population took off: the springboard of the neolithic demographic transition. Science 2011;333:560–561.
14 Diamond J: Evolution, consequences and future of plant and animal domestication. Nature 2002;418: 700–707.
15 Diamond J: Guns, Germs, and Steel: The Fates of Human Societies. WW Norton, New York, 1997.
16 World Health Organization: Global Tuberculosis Report 2017. World Health Organization, Geneva, Switzerland, 2017.
17 Hippocrates: The "Greek Miracle" in Medicine. www.ucl.ac.uk/-ucgajpd/medicineantigua/sa-hip-pint.html.
18 Koehler CW: Consumption, the Great Killer. http://pubs.acs.org/subscribe/archive/mdd/v05/htm/02/html/02timeline.
19 Murray JF: The white plague: down and out, or up and coming? J. Burns Amberson Lecture. Am Rev Respir Dis 1989;140:1788–1795.
20 Daniel TM: Jean-Antoine Villemin and the infectious nature of tuberculosis. Int J Tuberc Lung Dis 2015;19:267–268.
21 Rieder HL: Jean-Antoine Villemin: ending an alpine divide. Int J Tuberc Lung Dis 2015;19:253.
22 Murray JF: *Mycobacterium tuberculosis* and the cause of consumption: from discovery to fact. Am J Respir Crit Care Med 2004;169:1086–1088.
23 Koch R: Die Aetiologie der Tuberkulose: Berlin Klin Wschr 1882;19:221–230: translation by Pinner B, Pinner M. Am Rev Tuberc 1932;25:298–323.
24 Brock TD: Robert Koch: A Life in Medicine and Bacteriology. Madison, Science Tech Publishers, 1988.
25 Smith T: Two varieties of the tubercle bacillus from mammals. Trans Assoc Am Physicians 1896; 11:75–95.
26 Koch R: An address on the fight against tuberculosis in the light of the experience that has been gained in the successful combat of other infectious diseases. Br Med J 1901;2:189–193.
27 Murray JF, Rieder HL, Finley-Croswhite A: The king's evil and the royal touch: the medical history of scrofula. Int J Tuberc Lung Dis 2016;20:713–716.
28 Cole ST, Brosch R, Parkhill J, et al: Deciphering the biology of *Mycobacterium tuberculosis* from the complete genome sequence. Nature 1998;393: 537–544.
29 Garnier T, Eiglmeier K, Camus JC, et al: The complete genome sequence of *Mycobacterium bovis*. Proc Natl Acad Sci U S A 2003;100:7877–7882.
30 Gagneux S: Host-pathogen coevolution in human tuberculosis. Philos Trans R Soc Lond B Biol Sci 2012;367:850–859.
31 Smith NH, Kremer K, Inwald J, et al: Ecotypes of the *Mycobacterium tuberculosis* complex. J Theor Biol 2006;239:220–225.
32 Brosch R, Gordon SV, Marmmiesse M, et al: A new evolutionary scenario for the *Mycobacterium tuberculosis* complex. Proc Natl Acad Sci U S A 2002;99:3684–3689.
33 Hamilton MJ, Milne BT, Walker RS, et al: The complex structure of hunter-gatherer social networks. Proc Biol Sci 2007;274:2195–2202.
34 Gagneux S, DeRiemer K, Van T, et al: Variable host-pathogen compatibility in *Mycobacterium tuberculosis*. Proc Natl Acad Sci U S A 2006;103: 2869–2873.
35 Firdessa R, Berg S, Hailu E, et al: Mycobacterial lineages causing pulmonary and extrapulmonary tuberculosis, Ethiopia. Emerg Infect Dis 2013;19: 460–463.
36 Comas I, Coscolla M, Luo T, et al: Out-of-Africa migration and Neolithic coexpansion of *Mycobacterium tuberculosis* with modern humans. Nat Genet 2013;45:1176–1182.
37 Rasmussen M, Guo X, Wang Y, et al: An Aboriginal Australian genome reveals separate human dispersals into Asia. Science 2011;334:94–98.
38 Roberts CA, Pfister LA, Mays S: Letter to the editor: was tuberculosis present in *Homo erectus* in Turkey? Am J Phys Anthropol 2009;139:442–444.
39 Paulsen HJ: Tuberculosis in the native American: indigenous or introduced? Rev Infect Dis 1987;9: 1180–1186.
40 Curry A: Coming to America. Nature 2012;485: 30–32.
41 Waters MR, Stafford TW Jr, Kooyman B, Hills LV: Late Pleistocene horse and camel hunting at the southern margin of the ice-free corridor: reassessing the age of Wally's Beach, Canada. Proc Natl Acad Sci U S A 2015;112:4263–4267.

42 Dryomov SV, Nazhminenova AM, Shalaurova SA, et al: Mitochondrial genome diversity at the Bering Strait area highlights prehistoric human migrations from Siberia to northern North America. Europ J Human Genet 2015;23:1399–1404.

43 Allison MJ, Mendoza D, Pezzia A: Documentation of a case of tuberculosis in pre-Columbian America. Am Rev Respir Dis 1973;107:985–991.

44 Salo WL, Aufderheide AC, Buikstra J, Holcomb TA: Identification of *Mycobacterium tuberculosis* DNA in a pre-Columbian Peruvian mummy. Proc Natl Acad Sci U S A 1994;91:2091–2094.

45 Arriaza BT, SaloW, Aufderheide AC, Holcomb TA: Pre-Columbian tuberculosis in northern Chile: molecular and skeletal evidence. Am J Phys Anthropol 1995;98:37–45.

46 Mackowiak PA, Bios VT, Aguilar M, Buikstra JA: On the origin of American tuberculosis. Clin Infect Dis 2095;41:515–518.

47 Bos KI, Harkins KM, Herbig A, et al: Pre-Columbian mycobacterial genomes reveal seals as a source of New World human tuberculosis. Nature 2014;514:494–497.

48 Kiers A, Klarenbeek A, Mendelts B, et al: Transmission of *Mycobacterium pinnipedii* to humans in a zoo with marine mammals. Int J Tuberc Lung Dis 2008;12:1469–1473.

49 Pepperell CS, Granka JM, Alexander DC, et al: Dispersal of *Mycobacterium tuberculosis* via the Canadian fur trade. Proc Natl Acad Sci U S A 2011;108:6526–6531.

50 Kato-Maeda M, Shanley CA, Ackart D, et al: Beijing sublineages of *Mycobacterium tuberculosis* differ in pathogenicity in the guinea pig. Clin Vaccine Immunol 2012;19:1227–1237.

51 Merker M, Blin C, Mona S, et al: Evolutionary history and global spread of the *Mycobacterium tuberculosis* Beijing lineage. Nat Genet 2015;47:242–249.

52 Feng JY, Jarisberg LG, Rose J, et al: Impact of Euro-American sublineages of *Mycobacterium tuberculosis* on new infections among named contacts. Int J Tuberc Lung Dis 2017;21:509–516.

53 Lee S. Aspects of European History, 1494–1789. New York, Routledge, 1984.

54 The Emergence of Modern Europe, 1500–1648. Economy and society. htt s://www.britannica.com/to Euro e-1500-1648.

55 Wilson LG: Commentary: Medicine, population, and tuberculosis. Int J Epidem 2001;34:521–524.

56 Murray JF: A century of tuberculosis. Am J Respir Crit Care Med 2004;169:1181–1186.

57 Murray JF: The Industrial Revolution and the decline in death rates from tuberculosis. Int J Tuberc Lung Dis 2015;19:502–503.

58 Redeker F: Epidemiologie und Statistik der Tuberkulose; in Hein J, Kleinschmidt H, Uehlinger R (eds): Handbuch der Tuberkulose. Georg Thieme, Stuttgart, Germany,1958, Vol 1, pp 407–498.

59 Kraus AK: Tuberculosis and public health. Am Rev Tuberc 1928;18:271–322.

60 Lipsitch M, Sousa AO: Historical intensity of natural selection for resistance to tuberculosis. Genetics 2002;161:1599–1607.

61 Stead WW: Variation in vulnerability to tuberculosis in America today: random, or legacies of different ancestral epidemics? Int J Tuberc Lung Dis 2001;5:807–814.

62 von Clausewitz C: On War. Translation by Howard M, Paret P. Princeton University Press, 1974/84.

63 Keegan J: A History of War. First Vintage Books Edition: Alfred A. Knopf, Inc. New York, 1993.

64 Genghis Khan. Biography. Warrior, Military Leader (c 1162–1227). www.biography.com/people/genghiskhan-9308634#the-universal-ruler.

65 Fry DP, Soderberg P: Lethal aggression in mobile forager bands and implications for the origins of war. Science 2013;341:270–273.

66 Allen MW, Jones TL (eds): Violence and Warfare Among Hunter-Gatherers. New York, Routledge, 2014.

67 The Wall of Jericho. https://en.wikipedia.org/wiki/Wall of Jericho.

68 University of Chicago: University of Chicago-Syrian team finds first evidence of warfare in ancient Mesopotamia. http://www- news.uchicago.edu/releases/05/051216.hamoukar.shtml.

69 Stele of the Vultures. Victory stele of Eannatum, King of Lagash. Early Dynastic period, c. 2450 BC. Louvre Museum. Paris, France.

70 Curry A: Slaughter at the bridge. Grisly find suggests Bronze Age northern Europe was more organized-and violent-than thought. Science 2016;351:1384–1389.

71 Bryce T: The Trojans and their Neighbors. New York, Routledge, 2006.

72 Wood M: In Search of the Trojan War (ed 2). Berkeley, University of California Press, 1985.

73 Burgess JS: The Tradition of the Trojan War in Homer and the Epic Cycle. Baltimore, The Johns Hopkins University Press, 2001.

74 Finley-Croswhite A: Engendering the wars of religion: female agency during the catholic league in dijon. Fr Hist Stud 1997;20:127–154.

75 Green D: The Hundred Years' War: A People's History. New Haven, Yale University Press, 2014.

76 Neillands R: The Hundred Years' War. Revised Edition. London, Routledge, 2001.

78 Cowley R, Parker G (eds): The Reader's Companion to Military History, Houghton Mifflin Harcourt Publishing Co, 1996.

78 Parker G (ed): The Thirty Years' War. London, Routledge, 1997.

79 Murray JF: Tuberculosis and World War I. Am J Respir Crit Care Med 2015;192:411–414.

80 Drolet GJ: World War I and tuberculosis. A statistical summary and review. Am J Public Health Nations Health 1945;35:689–697.

81 Smallman-Raynor M, Cliff AD: War and disease: some perspectives on the spatial and temporal occurrence of tuberculosis in wartime. Chapter 4; in Gandy M, Zumia A (eds): The Return of the White Plague: Global Poverty and the "New" Tuberculosis: New York, Verso, 2003.

82 Daniels M: Tuberculosis in Europe during and after the Second World War. Br Med J 1949;2:1135–1072.

83 Daniels M: Tuberculosis in Europe during and after the Second World War. Br Med J 1949;2:1065–1140.

84 Trevisanato Sl: The 'Hittite plague', an epidemic of tularemia and the first record of biological warfare. Med Hypotheses 2007;69:1371–1374.

85 Boot M: War Made New: Technology, Warfare and the Course of History. 1500 to Today. New York, Gotham, 2007.

86 Frischknecht F: The history of biological warfare. Human experimentation, modern nightmares and lone madmen in the twentieth century. EMBO Rep 2003;4(spec no):S47–S52.

87 Lifton RJ: The Nazi Doctors: Medical Killing and the Psychology of Genocide. New York, Basic Books, 1986.

88 Secret Testing in the United States: The Living Weapon. http://www.pbs.org/wgbh/americanexperience/features/general-article/weapon- secret-testing/.

89 Biopreparat: A huge Soviet Union biological warfare research center. https://fas.org/nuke/guide/russia/agency/bw.htm.

90 War and Peace. www.ppu.org.uk llearn/infodocs/st-war-peace.html.

91 Sahloul MZ, Monla-Hassan J, Sankari A, et al: War is the enemy of health. Pulmonary, critical care, and sleep medicine in war-torn Syria. Ann Am Thorac Soc 2016;13:147–155.

92 Cookson ST, Abaza H, Clarke KR, et al: "Impact of and response to increased tuberculosis prevalence among Syrian refugees compared with Jordanian tuberculosis prevalence: case study of a tuberculosis public health strategy". Confl Health 2015;9:18.

93 Cousins S: Experts sound alarm as Syrian crisis fuels spread of tuberculosis. BMJ 2014;349:g7397.

John F. Murray, MD, Professor Emeritus of Medicine
University of California San Francisco
P.O. Box 0841
San Francisco, CA 94143-0841 (USA)
E-Mail johnfmurr4@aol.com

Murray JF, Loddenkemper R (eds): Tuberculosis and War. Lessons Learned from World War II.
Prog Respir Res. Basel, Karger, 2018, vol 43, pp 20–32 (DOI: 10.1159/000481472)

Challenges in the Assessment of Tuberculosis Epidemiology during Wartime

Hans L. Rieder[a, b] · Robert Loddenkemper[c]

[a]Epidemiology, Biostatistics and Prevention Institute, University of Zurich, Zurich, and [b]Tuberculosis Consultant Services, Kirchlindach, Switzerland; [c]German Central Committee against Tuberculosis, Berlin, Germany

Abstract

The natural history of tuberculosis (TB) provides an intuitively clear pattern for the understanding of its epidemiology: exposure to the etiologic agent may result in latent infection with *Mycobacterium tuberculosis* without evidence of disease. Latent infection may then progress to overt clinical TB, and those afflicted may succumb to it. This sequence reflects a series of conditional probabilities in a cascade of events, each step hinging on the presence of its precedent step, for example, only a person infected with tubercle bacilli may develop TB, and only a person who is ill from TB can die from TB. These sequential probabilities vary by time, place, and person, resulting in observable temporally aligned metrics (infection, morbidity, mortality) defining the epidemic. These metrics are subject to measurement errors. As epidemiology bases its line of argumentation on comparisons, it uses relative measurements such as ratios, proportions, and rates. These depend on numerators (persons with or events of the condition sought) and denominators (the population from within which the persons come from or the events arise). Accurately enumerating events and counting populations is difficult, and these difficulties are compounded during wartime. This chapter focuses on identifying such challenges using examples from different settings during wartime.

© 2018 S. Karger AG, Basel

When discussing the epidemiology of tuberculosis (TB), it would be appropriate to refer back to the classification of TB proposed by the American Thoracic Society [1]. It follows the pathogenetic sequence and separates exposure (no evidence for latent infection), latent infection with *Mycobacterium tuberculosis* complex (without evidence of disease), TB (the disease), and death from *M. tuberculosis*. TB (the disease) has been subdivided into potentially transmissible forms (such as TB of the respiratory tract) and non-transmissible manifestations (such as most extrapulmonary forms; Fig. 1) [2, 3]. Conditional probabilities for progression from one step to the next in the chain of events are determined by various risk factors, both exogenous (such as exposure and acquisition of infection) and endogenous (such as progression from latent infection to overt clinical disease) [4].

This model will guide the following discussion on the challenges and difficulties in obtaining an accurate picture of the epidemiologic situation of TB during warfare using selected examples to illustrate attempts in ascertaining transmission of *M. tuberculosis*, TB, and death from *M. tuberculosis*, addressing both numerator and denominator issues that are always present in epidemiology, but become accentuated during wartime.

Transmission of Tubercle Bacilli

The extent to which *M. tuberculosis* is transmitted during a given period of time – the incidence of infection with *M. tuberculosis* – determines the subsequent incidence of TB (the disease). The latter determines TB fatality (the magnitude modified by chemotherapy) in the individual and thus TB

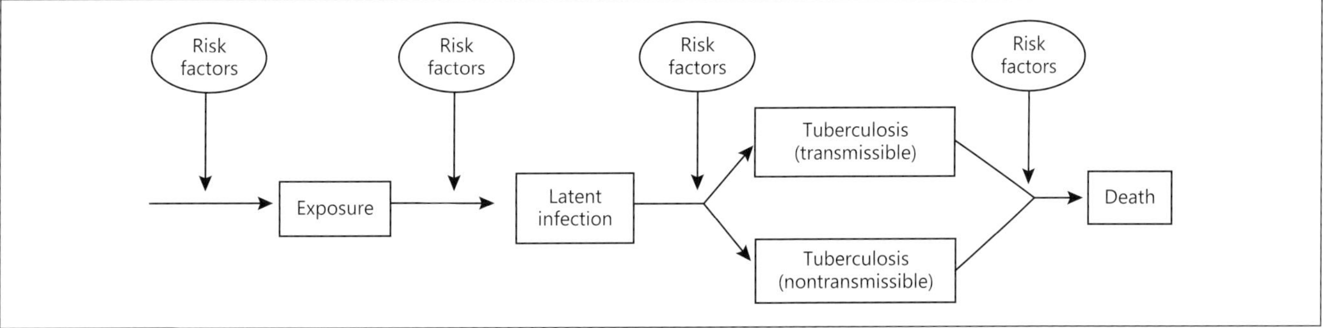

Fig. 1. Model used in the discussion of the epidemiology of tuberculosis, based on the classification of tuberculosis by the American Thoracic Association and the Centers for Disease Control and Prevention. Adapted from [2, 3].

mortality in the population. Because TB has no defined incubation period, the extent of transmission during a specified period of time also has long-term consequences as latent infection may progress to TB many years, even decades, after acquisition of infection. This is demonstrated in studies among untreated contacts (placebo-recipients in a preventive therapy trial) of newly diagnosed TB patients in the United States [5, 6]. The risk of progression was highest during the first 2 years following infection, and dropped to about one tenth of the initial annual risk in the subsequent years, but it never became zero as is the case with diseases that are characterized by a well-defined incubation period. Thus, the extent of transmission that occurs has both immediate and long-term implications for expected TB morbidity subsequent to acquisition of infection with *M. tuberculosis*.

Tuberculin Skin Test

The tool to measure infection with *M. tuberculosis* has long been the tuberculin skin test, but currently is gradually being replaced by the introduction of interferon-gamma release assays [7]. Various methods of applying tuberculin have been developed, mostly in the first decade of the 20th century, chiefly percutaneous [8] and intracutaneous testing [9, 10]. Infection with *M. tuberculosis* results in a cell-mediated immunologic response that can be elicited by a tuberculin skin test. Like any test, the tuberculin skin test has the intrinsic operating characteristics of sensitivity and specificity. Lack of sensitivity (i.e., the proportion with a false-negative result) is determined by the immune status of the person tested and is also reduced by faulty tuberculin reagents and technical errors [11–13]. The most prominent causes for lack of specificity (i.e., the proportion with a false-positive result) are cross-reactions attributable to infection with other mycobacteria, notably several types of environmental mycobacteria and the Bacille Calmette-Guérin (BCG) vaccine strain *M. bovis* BCG. The predictive value of a positive test diminishes rapidly with decreasing prevalence of the sought-after condition if the operating characteristics remain unchanged.

The estimated annual incidence of *M. tuberculosis* infection has dropped below 10% in industrialized countries by about 1910, and became even substantially lower by the time of World War II (WWII) [3]. In other words, a relatively small and increasingly smaller problem would require at least 2 sequential tuberculin surveys 1 year apart to determine the annual incidence of transmission of infection by *M. tuberculosis*. During World War I (WWI), BCG was not yet in use anywhere, but by WWII, most European countries – with the notable exceptions of Germany [14], the Netherlands [15], and the United Kingdom [16] – had begun introducing BCG vaccination nationally in a systematic manner. Thus, prior BCG vaccination adversely affected the tuberculin test specificity, and thus the predictive value of a positive test result in a large number of countries in Europe. Of lesser importance among younger population groups, repeat tuberculin testing can boost the response and falsely suggest incident infection [17]. To solve the problem of extracting incidence information from serial prevalence measurements [18, 19], the incidence of infection was approximated by the calculation of an average annual risk of infection, algebraically derived from single or repeat tuberculin skin test prevalence surveys [20, 21]. Whereas this approach ingeniously circumvents these difficulties, it has an intrinsic problem that it calculates an average over the lifetime of a person (Fig. 2). A tuberculin skin test survey is conducted among persons born in year b at calendar time $b + a$, where a is the age of the birth cohort under consideration. The annual risk of the observed prevalence of infection with *M. tuberculosis* is the algebraically derived average (using a compound interest calculation approach) of the probability

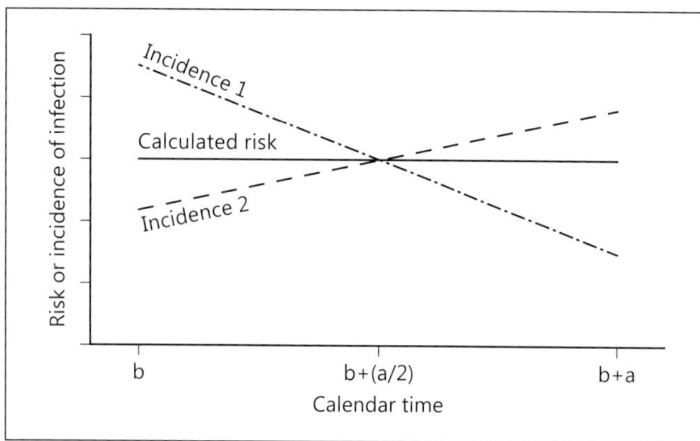

Fig. 2. Difference between calculated average annual risk of infection and actual incidence of infection with *M. tuberculosis*.

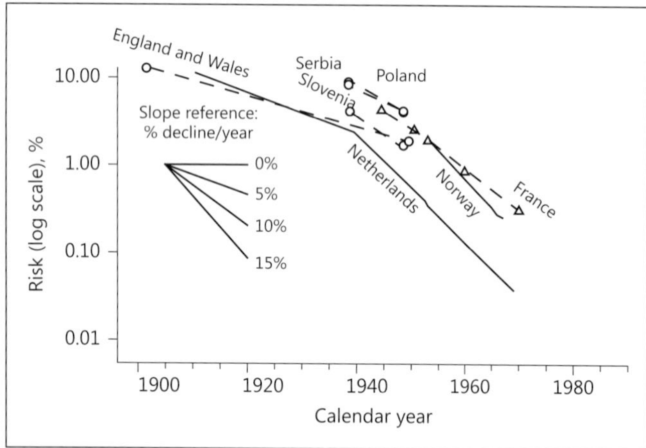

Fig. 3. Secular trend in the average annual risk of infection with *M. tuberculosis* in selected European countries. Adapted from data given in [20, 23–27]. A straight line (The Netherlands, Norway) is only shown if there were annual data. If only occasional surveys were available, this is denoted by a dashed line (almost overlapping for Serbia and Poland) and a hollow circle (triangle for France) to denote the time points for which the annual risk of infection could be calculated. A slope reference is shown as an inlet to allow visual estimation of the average annual decline in the annual risk of infection: for instance, the average annual decline for The Netherlands after 1940 is roughly between 10 and 15%.

of becoming infected (or reinfected) during the course of 1 year. By convention [22], it is put on the calendar time in between the years of birth and survey conducted as a pragmatic approximation. The actual incidence of infection, however, may have decreased or increased over the life span of the tested individual, or even taken a more complex course, and there is no way to actually know its precise current level. It follows that the younger the tested population, the closer the calculated annual risk of infection approxi-

mates to the actual incidence of infection, while conversely, the older the population tested, the less certain one can be about the actual magnitude of current transmission. Thus, a recent increase in infection incidence will show up only with a substantial delay and is averaged out to a much-diluted value.

Tuberculin surveys also take substantial resources and are rarely carried out annually. The secular trend in the average annual risk of infection with *M. tuberculosis* in selected European countries is shown in Figure 3, which is adapted from [3] with data from [20, 23–27]. It summarizes analyses from a multitude of tuberculin skin test surveys conducted in Europe (largely but not exclusively in Western Europe) during the 20th century, converting the prevalence measurements into a series of annual risks of infection with *M. tuberculosis* from which the secular trend was derived. First of all, the overall picture demonstrates that all examined countries show a substantial reduction in the annual risk of infection. Second, while the absolute level at any given point in time may differ between countries, the speed of decline is remarkably similar everywhere. Among the seven countries depicted, only the Netherlands had annual prevalence data covering every WWII year, from which a series of annual risks could be calculated. After 1947, the surveys were performed yearly among military recruits, but from 1926 to 1947 the information was obtained from prevalence surveys among children up to age 13 years. Thus, in contrast to surveys among recruits, the age of children allowed calculation of an average risk of infection that must have approximated the actual incidence relatively closely.

No increase was noted at any time during the war years in both England and Wales and in the Netherlands, but there was an abrupt change in 1940 when the continuity of the downward trend in the risk of infection accelerated substantially. The authors report, however, difficulties with the interpretation of these data from Amsterdam [20]. First, the surveys were not conducted every year. Second, the von Pirquet (percutaneous) testing method that was used was difficult to quantify. Third, the original data were lost and data were read from graphs. Finally, the proportion of reactors among children under the age of 2 years was much larger than would have been expected from older children. A possible interpretation postulates that this might have been attributable to infection from *M. bovis* as mandatory pasteurization of milk did not begin in the Netherlands until 1940. The introduction of obligatory pasteurization of milk appears to coincide temporally with the acceleration in the decline of the risk of infection. However, such an interpretation is highly questionable if one considers that a delay must be expected between the time point a change in infection incidence occurs and the time this change becomes reflected in a change in the calculated average annual infection risk. There is no such delay here – the change is abrupt and occurs in 1940. Thus, the temporal coincidence between measures against bovine tubercle bacilli and the change in the risk of infection may not be entirely causal.

Rist reported on 2 comparative tuberculin skin test surveys carried out in about 12,000 French students annually (von Pirquet method) in 1938 and 1943, respectively [28]. Among the 19-year-olds, the prevalence of positive results was 56 versus 50% in 1939 and 1943, respectively. The respective percentages among the 20-year-olds were 59 and 56% and among the 21-year-olds 62 and 54%. The author noted that morbidity decreased in parallel while mortality increased. He hypothesized that the decrease in infection prevalence might have been attributable to accelerated and increased deaths resulting in higher mortality, thereby diminishing the opportunity for transmission. As discussed before, the early life experience of the tested cohorts of a diminishing risk of infection was so substantial over the first 15 years after birth that even a relative increase in the risk of infection over the most recent 5 years did not translate into a measurable effect in the calculated average. We note thereby (as shown in Fig. 3) that the average annual decline between 1900 and the end of WWII had already been in the order of close to 5%. Rist confirmed this by using data from a hospital for sick children in Paris, where the prevalence of infection among 5-year-old children declined from 54 to 35% between 1919 and 1925, a 6% average annual decline, and in addition declined on average by 5.4% among 10-year-old children [28].

Tuberculin skin test survey data were available among school children aged 7–11 years in some villages in the Akkar district of north Lebanon [29]. The first survey data were obtained from 1980 to 1984, and the second data set was obtained in 1990 from the same villages. In the initial survey, the prevalence of infection was 3.8% (16 of 421 children reacting positively), and in the second 10.0% (28 of 281 children). There was no evidence for an increase in BCG vaccination coverage. The civil war in Lebanon lasted from 1975 to 1990; accordingly, the majority of children in the first and all children in the second survey were born during war years. Contemporaneously, the number of new TB cases attending a clinic in Tripoli, also in north Lebanon, reported a fairly constant number of around 30 cases annually from 1980 through 1985, when TB cases started to increase to over 400 in 1990 [29, 30].

One may conclude that as far as transmission of *M. tuberculosis* is concerned, there are no data from WWI, and those from WWII are sketchy at best. Surveys from children in Amsterdam in the Netherlands and from young adults and a selected group of children in France are difficult to interpret, but they do not suggest that there was an excess of transmission of *M. tuberculosis* to children during WWII years. This might be due to problems in interpreting tuberculin skin test prevalence data that typically lag in showing effects of changing transmission incidence. Alternatively or in combination, it might indeed be that while the incidence of infectious TB may have increased, case fatality was accelerated, shortening the average duration of infectiousness. The latter hypothesis will be examined more closely in the following sections. In contrast, when comparative repeat tuberculin test surveys were available from young children, case notification data showed in parallel a tenfold increase in TB; moreover, the prevalence of tuberculin positivity in the children during the civil war in Lebanon more than doubled. The conclusion, therefore, is inescapable that transmission to the youngest generation increased as a result of a massively deteriorating TB situation temporally correlated with the war.

Tuberculosis Morbidity

To quantify the magnitude of TB in any given area, a functional surveillance system for newly diagnosed cases must be in place. The public health interest in reporting cases was often met with fierce opposition from physicians who were reluctant to disclose to the government who among their patients had TB [31], an issue that persists in certain countries even today [32, 33]. At the British Congress on Tuberculosis in London in 1901, Koch made a strong plea for mandatory notification of TB [34]; in his presentation he referred to the success of notification, first voluntary, then mandatory in New York City. Beginning in 1899, Biggs of the New York City Health Department proposed a systematic approach to the control of TB [35]. The first and most important element was mandatory notification of TB. In 1907, Biggs defined the strategy more precisely in what he called "the administrative control of TB" and presented data about TB mortality in New York City [31]. There were no morbidity data in his report, but he proposed practical ways of approaching morbidity surveillance. One reason why it was easier to obtain information on death than disease was

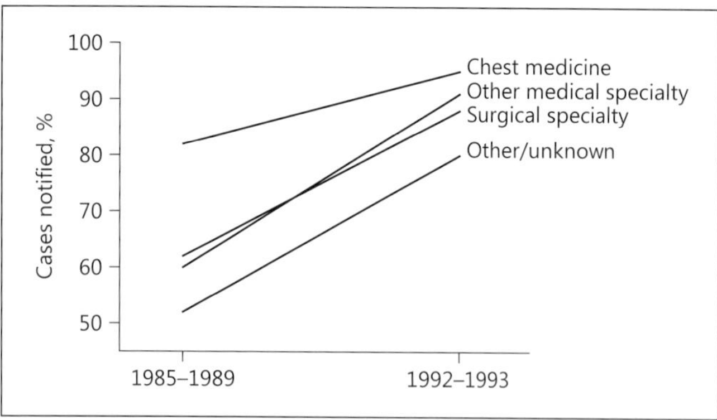

Fig. 4. Notification of tuberculosis in 2 hospitals in London by medical specialty in the period 1985–1989 compared to 1992–1993. Data reproduced from [49], with permission from BMJ Publishing Group Ltd.

the attitude of practicing clinicians who suspected hardship for their patients when disclosing their condition to the authorities, while after death this obstacle was obviated. Interestingly, Biggs recounts a talk with Koch who told him that in Germany a notification system similar to the one implemented in New York City could only be possible when the current generation of professionals now in control would have passed away. Elsewhere in Germany, however, Saxony claims to have been the first to introduce legislation mandating notification of TB cases in 1900 [36], while Prussia prepared legislation for mandatory notification of TB cases considered to be transmissible (defined as pulmonary or laryngeal) in 1903 [37]. In 1901, Norway became another of the early countries in Europe to introduce national mandatory notification of TB cases [38, 39]. In Denmark, legislation for mandatory notification of transmissible cases came into parliament in 1904 [40, 41]. Other European countries and jurisdictions followed suit in the first decade of the 20th century, but it remained voluntary for many years in some administrations [42].

Reliable notification of TB cases remained difficult to implement. In the United States, uniform national reporting was introduced only in 1953 [43]. A 1993 analysis of case notification systems in 14 Western European countries showed the dismal state of surveillance, in some as recently as between 1974 and 1991 [44]. As a disease with a slowly changing epidemiology, it is contrary to its nature to exhibit large annual changes at the country level. Changes of more than 10% in either direction from 1 year to another are epidemiologically decidedly unusual, and more likely reflect inconsistencies, inaccuracies, and blatant errors in the surveillance system. While in most of the examined 14 countries, the amplitude was constrained to realistic values, it was

definitively not so in some others. Of course, even where there is consistency (smaller year-to-year amplitudes) in reporting, this view of the data cannot reveal the extent of underreporting. Nevertheless, it underlines the fact that where there is not at least a minimum consistency and instead huge year-to-year amplitudes are reported, the data are not trustworthy. We note that these data are not from the times of war but in a peaceful period when Western Europe was moving to ever-greater prosperity. Subsequent to this rather embarrassing assessment, a consensus was reached in Europe to base its TB case surveillance system on a uniform and more rigorous base by taking recourse at its core to mandatory notification, not just by physicians but notably as well by laboratories that isolate and identify *M. tuberculosis* complex [45]. In 1996, a Europe-wide "EuroTB" program for the surveillance of TB was set up to collect, analyze, and disseminate data on TB cases notified in the World Health Organization (WHO) European region, which began to produce annual reports from 1998 onwards [46]. The project was funded by the European Union through 1997, and the last annual report appeared in 2008 [47]. Subsequently, the responsibility was transferred to the European Centre for Disease Prevention and Control and the WHO Regional Office for Europe [48].

The impediment to early attempts to implement surveillance resulting from the reluctance of physicians to report cases of TB among their patients has already been mentioned. That such reluctance was nevertheless not necessarily the only or even main problem in case notifications are exemplified in a study from 2 London hospitals (Fig. 4) [49]. The same 2 hospitals were visited in 2 periods and their records examined for newly diagnosed TB cases, and the results were then compared to the actually notified cases. Chest physicians reported only four of five diagnosed cases, surgeons only 3 of 5, and other specialties only half of the known cases. Reluctance to report is likely to have been a minor issue in hospitals in this period in the United Kingdom. More likely is forgetfulness or preoccupation with care of patients rather than administrative public health tasks. That this is actually the case is suggested by the improvement in notifications when the same hospitals were visited again a few years later. Apparently, the first visit had sensitized the hospital staff about the necessity to report. Based on these considerations, the European recommendations for surveillance emphasized a certain need for both physicians and microbiologic laboratories to notify bacteriologically confirmed cases of TB [45]: there are fewer laboratories than physicians and for them the administrative procedures for reporting can easily be automated.

Most countries in the world probably have at least a mandatory legal notification system of cases. Nevertheless, it is quite remarkable that India – the highest burden country in the world – legally mandated notification of TB only as recently as May 2012. This long overdue edict resulted in about a 30% increase of notified cases from 2013 to 2014 [50], which rose to 34% from 2013 to 2015 [51].

Thus, in the last quarter of the 20th century, even in prosperous Western Europe, surveillance of TB cases was in a deplorable state in some countries and has only slowly been improving. Globally, some of the highest burden countries have started only recently to address issues with their sometimes inefficient surveillance systems [52, 53]. For these reasons, one must be prepared to have a critical mind when judging morbidity data from countries at earlier times and when their situation was in turmoil due to war, such as often prevailed during WWII.

So far, this chapter has addressed only numerator data, that is, actual TB case counts. To allow comparison across populations or over time, the magnitude of a problem is commonly expressed in rates; in other words, case counts are divided by the population from which the cases arose and by the observation time, usually 1 year of surveillance. Population data are obtained by a census that is repeated ever so often and then interpolated for intercensal years. Demography has a long history, and methods have been developed on whom to count and how to avoid losing targeted people in the count, which is a non-trivial task. The problem is compounded when jurisdictions change through political decisions, but may also be heavily affected by population movements. In wartime, movements are introduced through mobilization of population segments, most notably young men, into the military, imposing challenges on how and where to count such people. This might be relatively easily accomplished during a census, but the difficulties for health departments can be substantial between census years. It must be feasible to define the jurisdiction in which the cases occur and the correct population count for that jurisdiction, else correct rates cannot be calculated. This may require requesting information from one of more other authorities which may or may not be willing to share population information.

As an example, a fairly complex picture emerges for the population of Berlin from 1910 through 1946, as shown in Figure 5. Between 1910 and 1920, there were 4 censuses, an unusually high frequency for taking a census. The extrapolations from one census to the next have thus high credibility. The first complexity starts after the census in October 1919 and the next census taken in June 1925. On October 1, 1920,

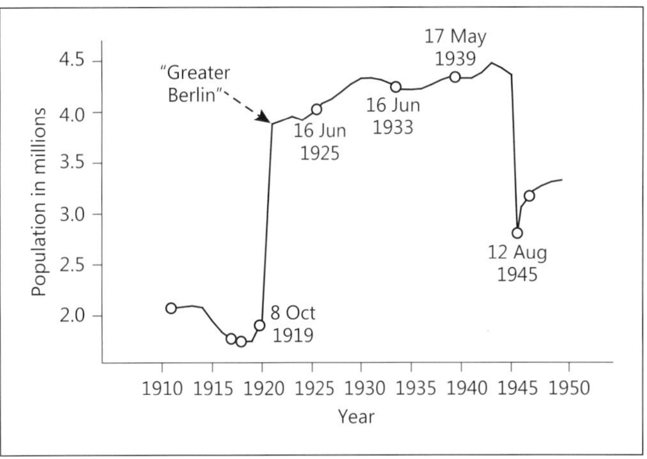

Fig. 5. Population data for Berlin, 1910–1946, obtained from census data (indicated by hollow circles) and extrapolated for intercensal years. The dashed line shows the political decision to expand the city of Berlin to "Greater Berlin" in 1920 [81].

the population size doubled when the surface of the newly designated city of Greater Berlin increased more than tenfold. This raises the question of how one might appropriately calculate a rate for the year 1920 when both the numerator and denominator changed during the year in a complex manner. Even if both the numerator (cases) and denominator (population) were correct, the appropriate technical approach is not easy to decide upon. The population characteristics of the old and new parts of the city are likely to be substantially different, probably more urban versus relatively less rural, judging from the population density (i.e., the same population size in less than a tenth of the surface in the old compared to more than 90% of the greatly expanded new city surface). The changed city definition was also likely to affect TB case rates, which often disproportionally affected urban dwellings. Thus, even if all numbers and calculations were correct, a decrease in the rates in the same city might result from a calculation from 1 year to the next, even if the problems remain unchanged. During the entire period of WWII, no census was taken in Berlin. Whether the population really increased during the war years, as graphically suggested here, and then actually dropped by more than one third at some time in 1945 before the August 1945 census may be anyone's best guess. While there are good reasons to construct the estimates in this way, they remain estimates rather than measures. If the postulated mass exodus that led to this drop occurred, then how would the TB case rate have been determined; in other words, how would the numerator data (case numbers) have been obtained?

The entire war period for Berlin poses almost insurmountable problems in obtaining both credible numerator and denominator data. While in other parts of Germany the changes might have been less abrupt than for the capital, a correct enumeration of both the incident TB cases and the population from which they arose likely created substantial problems throughout most of Germany. A large proportion of the male population was in the military service, and the military is often assumed or known to have a tendency to be rather discreet about the magnitude of the TB problem among its rank and file [54].

Heaf reports on pulmonary TB cases that were "notified or otherwise known to local health authorities" for England and Wales from 1938 to 1941 [55]; he showed a decrease of 6.1% from 1938 to 1939 that was followed by an increase of 4.9% the following year, and of 8.7% from 1940 to 1941, which coincided with attacks by Germany towards the end of June 1940 and onwards. Otherwise reported morbidity data from the United Kingdom remain scarce in Tubercle, its main easily accessible publication. Heaf himself does not put much trust in notifications of TB cases: "until the incidence is found out by a comprehensive survey in various groups of the community, we can only rely on mortality figures as a guide to the rise or fall of the incidence in the general population" [55].

Morbidity data are scarce during much of WWII, but these considerations about the calculation of rates also apply to mortality. This will be addressed in more detail in the next chapter on ascertainment of TB deaths.

Death from *M. tuberculosis*

Case fatality designates the proportion of people with TB who succumb to it: thus, the numerator is deaths, and the denominator is TB cases among whom the deaths occurred. Tuberculosis mortality has the same numerator as fatality, but the denominator is the entire population (rather than just TB cases) from which the TB cases arose and it has an observation time (usually 1 year). These 3 components make the definition of a "rate" [56].

Tuberculosis case fatality from untreated sputum smear-positive TB was large in the pre-chemotherapy era. One of the earliest long-term observations from a sanatorium in Switzerland showed a cumulative fatality of 70% after 17 years of follow-up (Fig. 6) [57]. What was designated "open tuberculosis" are patients excreting tubercle bacilli, and is thus largely synonymous with sputum smear-positive TB, because cultures were rarely used in routine testing at that

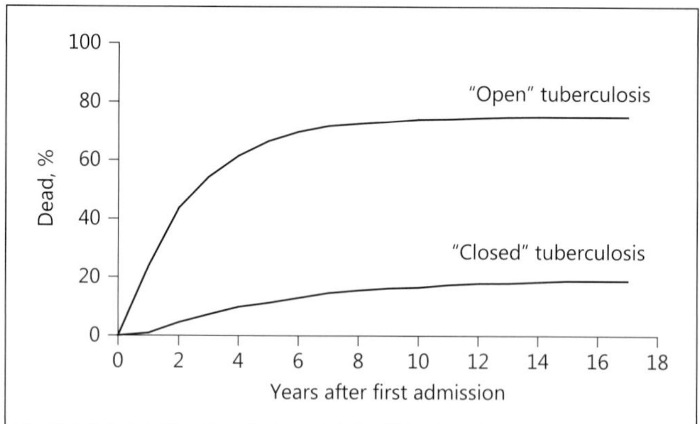

Fig. 6. Fate of untreated pulmonary tuberculosis, long-term follow-up, Barmelweid Sanatorium, Switzerland, reproduced by permission from Springer [57].

time. By contrast, "closed tuberculosis" referred to any other form of TB (both pulmonary and extrapulmonary). "Sputum" is also almost uniformly "direct," which means spontaneously produced rather than induced or via bronchoscopy. Clearly, the "closed" form with 18% fatality was substantially less deadly than "open" (pulmonary) TB. Similarly, high fatality ratios were determined in Denmark (68% after 10 years) [58], in Sweden (84% after 18 years) [59], and in the United Kingdom (86% after 11 years) [60]. A meta-analysis put the weighted mean after 10 years at 70% [61]. To obtain a reasonable estimate of case fatality, a longer observation period improves the estimate, but it is not required. For instance, it is perfectly justified to have only an approximate observation time for each case in treatment outcome analysis. Therefore, it suffices to state that a certain number of all patients who should have completed treatment died prematurely from *M. tuberculosis*. According to the WHO/Union definition, those who died of other causes are added to this numerator. Without observation time, we then get a simple proportion rather than a rate.

The variation in case fatality at the end of long observation time is relatively large: 68–86% in the four pre-chemotherapy studies mentioned here. For better comparability of these studies, the observation end point was fixed at ten years as in the meta-analysis. The median is then very narrow: between 1.2 and 1.7 years (Fig. 7) [57–60]. In other words, about half of the deaths occur within the first 1.5 years, while the other half occurs over the next 8.5 years. As the final cumulative fatality is so high, it cannot get much higher under the influence of an adverse situation, such as wartime. What could change substantially was the speed at which patients died, as suspected by Rist [28]. Whether this

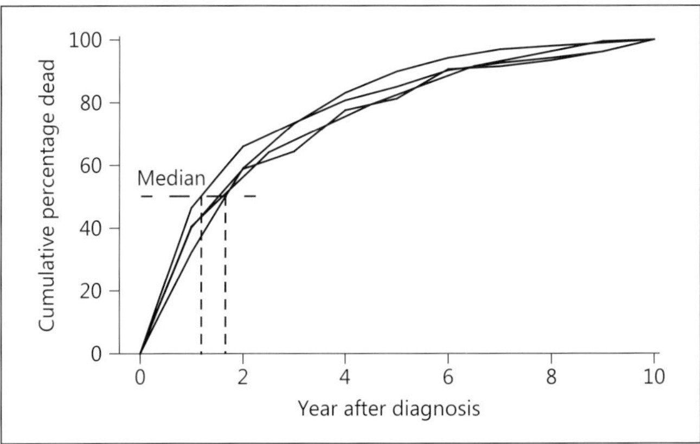

Fig. 7. Cumulative case fatality from untreated sputum smear-positive tuberculosis in four studies from Denmark [58], Sweden [59], Switzerland [57], and the United Kingdom [60], with permission from Elsevier.

hypothesis can be confirmed or has to be refuted will be examined shortly.

The determination of case fatality poses no problems with the denominator (patients with TB) as the cases are known and all that is needed is to learn about their outcome (e.g., the number of deaths among the cases). In contrast, the determination of mortality can be complex as it requires knowledge of both the correct numerator and denominator, that is, the accurate enumeration of deaths (numerator) and population (denominator) from which the cases arose as discussed above.

The famous compilation of data by Redeker about mortality in Germany (Fig. 4 in chapter 1), includes the years 1892–1940 [62]. In many ways, these are the most remarkable data. For one, there is a huge spike commencing shortly after the beginning of WWI in 1914, then rapidly accelerating to a peak lasting from 1917 to 1919, then precipitously falling to less than pre-war levels by 1921; the second smaller peak denotes the period of hyperinflation in 1923. It is difficult to reconcile what actually happened. One must always consider the succinct possibility of errors in the numerator and denominator, as discussed above. The last pre-war census was held in 1910, enumerating a population of 65 million. Two wartime censuses were held in 1916 and 1917, both covering a population of around 62 million. A census in 1919 reported a population of 61 million and the next regular census of 1925 counted 62 million inhabitants (https://en.wikipedia.org/wiki/Census_in_Germany). During this 15-year interval, the population appeared to have been much too stable to account for a gross denominator error in the calculation of the mortality rates. Potentially more biased might

have been the numerator data, obtained by counting deaths from *M. tuberculosis*, particularly among males. The Spanish influenza pandemic beginning in early 1918 cost millions of lives and could have contributed to misattributing influenza deaths to TB or actually be co-responsible for causing TB deaths [63, 64] or that indeed the H1N1 1918 influenza epidemic removed TB sources of transmission [65]. Tuberculosis mortality in Germany had actually peaked in 1917, one year before the influenza pandemic, thus this type of misclassification could not account for the observation in that year, but influenza could have accounted at least partially for the subsequent decline in TB mortality. If one removes the years 1915 through 1923 and regresses linearly on the remaining data, the regression line suggests that the pre-war secular trend resumed its projection from 1924 onwards, as if the 10-year epidemic surge had had no influence whatsoever.

If we recall the discussion of the epidemiologic transitions in the model discussed at the beginning of this chapter, it suggests probably only one rational explanation: the decline in the transmission of *M. tuberculosis* at the core of the TB epidemic continued uninterrupted throughout the period of WWI and afterward. There was no ratchet effect in that a declining trend was resumed at a higher level after the 10-year epidemic was over: it continued as if the epidemic had never happened. This may imply that in the final analysis, any excess sources of infection that might have arisen as a result of the war, influenza, and post-war miseries did not contribute equally to the excess transmission as one would normally have expected. As morbidity data are unavailable for Germany during this period, one must thus conclude that either there was no excess morbidity, only excess fatality (as Rist implied [28]) or that both "usual" plus excess cases all died at an accelerated speed. The latter hypothesis is considerably more likely as the untreated case fatality of 70% [61] can simply not double, which would have to be postulated in the former case.

Case-to Death Ratio

To take the potential uncertainty about the correct denominator out of the equation, we can examine only numerators where they exist. For example, we can examine either the ratio of TB cases to TB deaths or the ratio of the respective rates, as both likely used the same denominator, and thus cancel out the influence of potentially faulty denominators. One problem with this is that for simplicity we have to use incident cases from a given year and deaths from the same year. Yet, patients dying from *M. tuberculosis* were incident cases not just in the current but also in earlier years as we know from the survival curves discussed earlier.

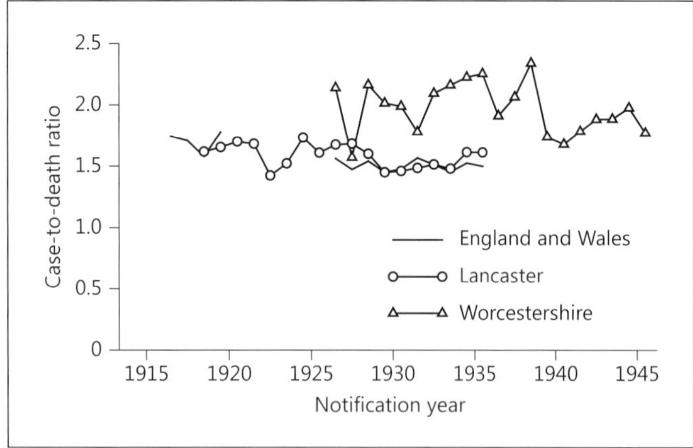
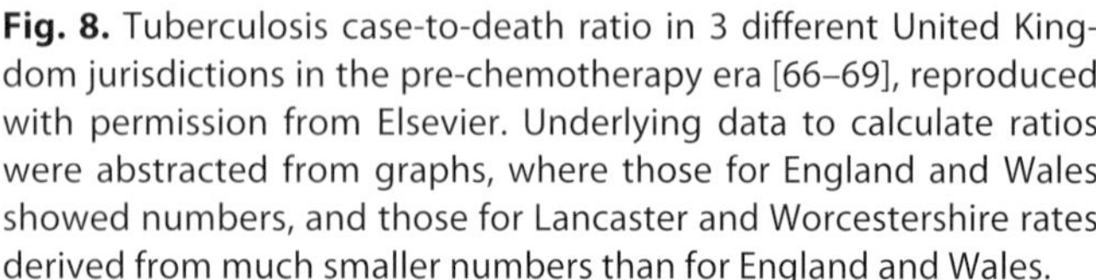

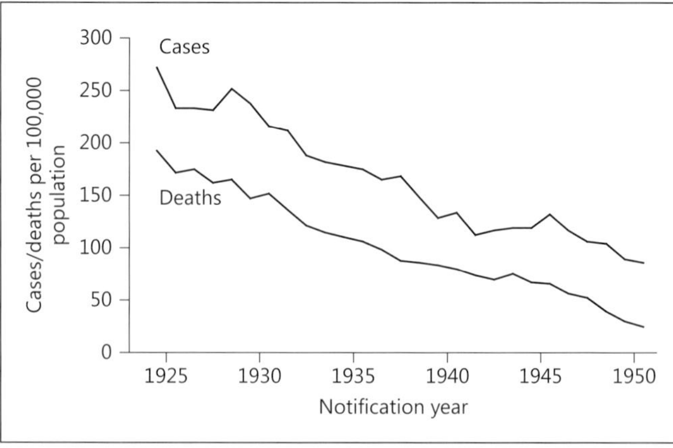

Fig. 8. Tuberculosis case-to-death ratio in 3 different United Kingdom jurisdictions in the pre-chemotherapy era [66–69], reproduced with permission from Elsevier. Underlying data to calculate ratios were abstracted from graphs, where those for England and Wales showed numbers, and those for Lancaster and Worcestershire rates derived from much smaller numbers than for England and Wales.

Fig. 9. Reported notifications of cases of infectious tuberculosis and tuberculosis deaths (all forms) per 100,000 population, Norway, 1924–1950. Data to reproduce figures were abstracted from graph in [71], reproduced with the permission of the European Respiratory Society.

While morbidity data are available only for some countries in their entirety, some sub-country jurisdictions have notifications of both pulmonary TB cases and deaths for multiple sequential years. Three jurisdictions with such data were chosen from the United Kingdom to exemplify the use of case-to-death ratios. These were England and Wales over 2 time periods [66, 67], Lancaster [68], and Worcestershire [69]. None of the 3 studies revealed a marked change during the war years as far as they were included (Fig. 8). The data from England and Wales are based on large case numbers (60,000–70,000 per year), whereas the data from Lancaster and Worcestershire yielded rates based on much smaller case and population numbers (cities as opposed to 2 entire regions of the United Kingdom). The case-to-death ratio is remarkably constant over all the observation years with an average of about 1.6 for England and Wales, and Lancaster. The ratio in Worcester is higher at approximately 2.0 on average, but it also fluctuates much more as might be expected for the smallest among the 3 jurisdictions. This example demonstrates that in the pre-chemotherapy era, the case-to-death ratio – an approximation to the reciprocal of case fatality – was fairly constant in the inter-war years and was similar during wartime when TB, in Worcester for instance, did not increase [69].

Lewis-Faning examined specifically the interval between TB notification and death from *M. tuberculosis* and the effect of WWII on it, but could not find any difference, suggesting an effect of the war on acceleration of progression to death in Middlesex County, United Kingdom [70]. Rist not-

ed that TB case notifications in Paris continued to decline during WWII, yet reported that the number of deaths increased in parallel [28]. Unfortunately, he did not provide the numbers to define this relationship more precisely.

Norway, as mentioned earlier, is one of the few countries that has collected comprehensive TB morbidity data since the beginning of the 20th century. Figure 9 shows national notification rates of infectious respiratory TB and TB mortality rates (all forms) from 1924 through 1950 [71]. Tuberculosis cases declined to a nadir in 1941, then increased slowly to a peak in 1945, subsequently to resume the pre-war decline. The increase in cases during war years was a relatively modest 17.5%. A similar increase is not discernible for mortality. Calculating the case-to-death ratio from these data (Fig. 10) [71] shows a fairly flat course hovering around an average of about 1.6 from 1920 through 1943. Subsequently, the ratio gradually increases to 3.5 in 1950 in the wake of the progressively successive introduction of chemotherapy that reduced case fatality. The data from Norway do not confirm Rist's hypothesis of accelerated progression from disease to death, which might be attributable to the relatively small effect the war seems to have had on TB in Norway.

Like Norway, Denmark introduced systematic notification of TB cases early on [72]. Figure 11 shows the comparison of notified pulmonary TB cases and TB deaths from 1921 through 1957 [72]. The first nadir of cases was reached in 1940, then increased to a peak in 1946, resulting in an increase of 53.4%; in other words, a much larger increase than report-

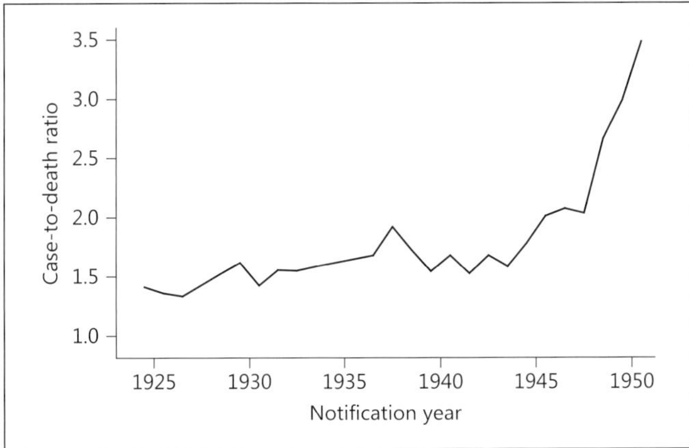

Fig. 10. Case-to-death ratio of notified infectious respiratory tuberculosis case rates to tuberculosis mortality (all forms) rates, Norway, 1924–1950. Underlying data to calculate ratios were abstracted from the graph in [71].

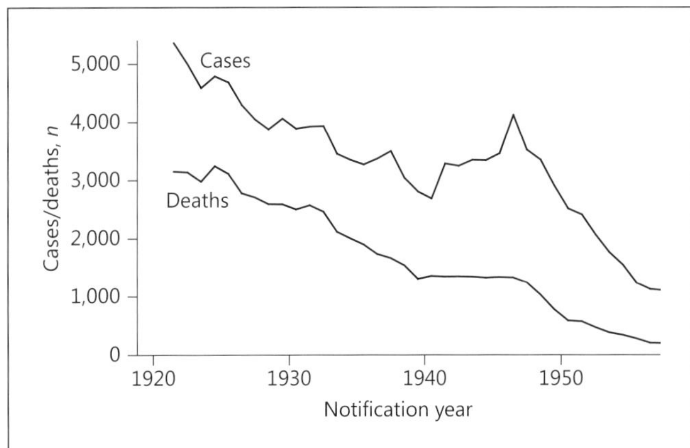

Fig. 11. Reported notifications of pulmonary tuberculosis cases and tuberculosis deaths (all forms), Denmark, 1921–1957. Data to draw graph were abstracted from [72], reproduced with the permission of the World Health Organization.

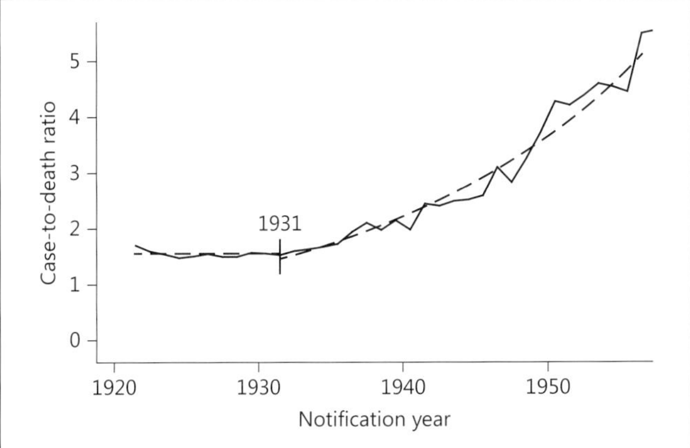

Fig. 12. Case-to-death ratio of notified pulmonary tuberculosis cases to tuberculosis deaths (all forms), Denmark, 1921–1957. Data to calculate ratios were abstracted from graph in [72], reproduced with the permission of the World Health Organization. The dashed line to the left of the 1931 vertical line is the average ratio during that period, the line to the right the regression from that year onwards through the end of the observation period.

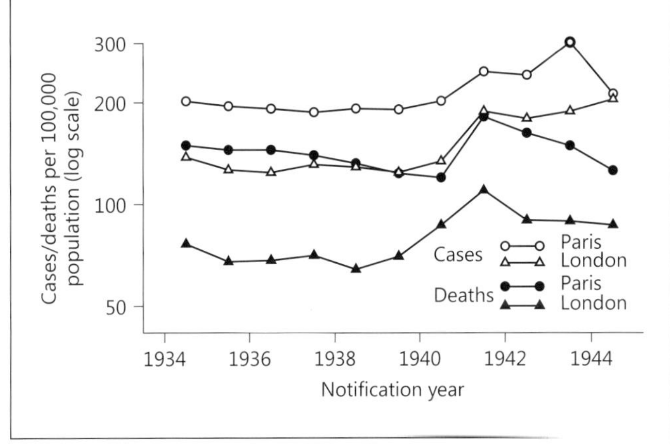

Fig. 13. Reported cases and deaths from pulmonary tuberculosis, per 100,000 population, London and Paris, 1934–1944. Data to reproduce graph were abstracted from [73], reproduced with permission from Elsevier. For better proportional comparison, data are shown semi-logarithmically.

ed from Norway during the war years. Over the same period, the number of deaths remained essentially unchanged. Calculating the case-to-death ratio, the ratio hovers around an average of slightly over 1.5 during the 11 years from 1921 through 1931. Subsequently, there is a regular, virtually exponential increase in the ratio by an average 5.2% annual increase until the end of the observation period (Fig. 12). The ratio had substantially increased to 3.1 in 1946 when the peak morbidity was reported. By the end of the observation period, the ratio had risen to over 5.5, testifying the power of chemo-

therapy in saving lives. In the period from 1940 to 1946, when cases increased, the ratio also increased. This is quite the opposite of what would be expected if Rist's hypothesis for France holds good. In other words, there is no evidence in Denmark that cases of TB succumbed at an accelerated pace during the war years; in fact, it was just the reverse.

Finally, we turn to Paris and London for which comparative rates for pulmonary cases and deaths are available for the period 1934 through 1944 (Fig. 13) [73]. The reported burden is larger in Paris than in London, and the course is

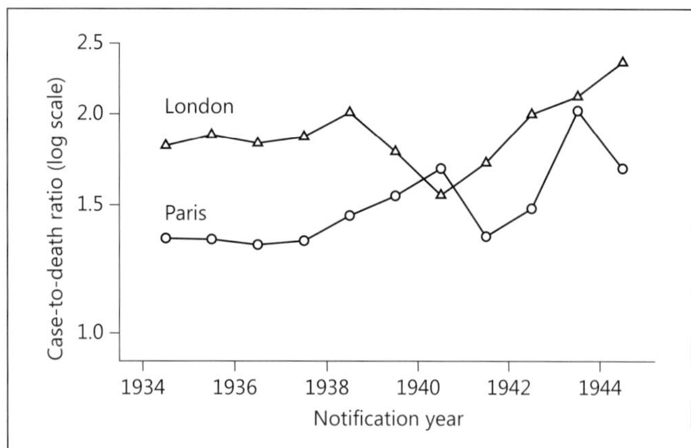

Fig. 14. Case-to-death ratio of notified pulmonary tuberculosis cases and deaths, per 100,000 population, London and Paris, 1934–1944. Underlying data to calculate ratios were abstracted from graph in [73], reproduced with permission from Elsevier. For better proportional comparison, data are shown semi-logarithmically.

parallel for the observation period, except that in the final year of observation TB cases in Paris declined while in London they continued to increase. The case-to-death ratio (Fig. 14) is generally higher in London than in Paris, but there are major fluctuations in the ratio over the observation period. However, there seems to be no indication in either city that, while there are fluctuations, the ratio is getting systematically smaller during the war years compared to the pre-war years. On the contrary, should one like to construe an interpretation, if anything, the ratio may tend to get larger with time. Again this does not suggest accelerated progression to death during WWII.

In summary, the examination of comparative morbidity and mortality data in various settings does not give any indication that TB tends to progress faster to death at times when TB morbidity increases during wartime. The data examined here were almost exclusively from Western European countries of the inter-war years and WWII, because morbidity data from WWI seem to be rarely available. Tuberculosis epidemiology during and in the aftermath of WWII is, however, not at all comparable with that during and after WWI. The reported excess peak in mortality in Germany reported in WWII was not anywhere nearly as large as that reported for WWI. Second, the period after WWII brought chemotherapy, which had a substantial impact on the duration of infectiousness of cases and case fatality. The 2 post-war situations cannot thus possibly be compared. The phenomenon reported by Redeker [62] of a seeming resumption of the pre-war (WWI) secular trend without a ratchet effect after the hyperinflation period

(Fig. 4 chapter 1) stands out as a unique puzzle. A similar phenomenon has been reported for some countries, but few had actually a sufficiently long observation period before WWI and/or did collect data during the war years [74, 75]. Among those countries with longer series of mortality data before and during WWI, there are indications, however, that in countries with particularly large mortality spikes (such as Belgium, Denmark or The Netherlands), a similar phenomenon [76, 77] as that reported by Redeker for Germany [62] is discernible. The "Rist hypothesis" – formulated on unfortunately sketchily reported observations of an accelerated progression from disease to death – has still the greatest appeal, at least for WWI, even if there is scarce if any evidence for it that could be found in other settings and other times. That such a shortening of lifespan could take place in the pre-chemotherapy era was reported from Chemnitz, Germany [78]. Deaths occurring in the years 1938 to 1943 were taken, and the average number of years elapsed since diagnosis were calculated (Fig. 6 in chapter 3). The regression on years surviving and death year then shows a substantial average decrease in survival years of 7.5% annually. Because these are averages and the events cover both pre-war and war years, it remains impossible to tease out the actual role of the war years on the observed accelerated case fatality. It also points to some of the difficulties discussed in this chapter in the epidemiologic assessment as diagnosis of incident cases and their ultimate death do not occur in the same calendar year. Perhaps the hypothesis that the influenza pandemic of 1918 contributed to hastening the decline of TB [65] not just in the United States will deserve further scrutiny.

Concluding Reflections and Remarks

M. tuberculosis is mainly transmitted by the airborne route and remains the chief mycobacterial pathogen; *M. bovis* seems to have played a very minor role in wartime-associated TB resurgences. *M. tuberculosis* is most likely transmitted where population density is high and thus opportunity for exposure is increased. Transmission is much more likely to occur indoors than outdoors where tubercle bacilli are rapidly dispersed in the ambient air. Thus, where the climate is cold, people collect indoors, and poverty forces crowded living conditions that facilitate transmission. The latter situations are typically enhanced during wartime, and the tuberculin skin test surveys among children in Lebanon during the civil war discussed above may thus make a case in point. Airborne transmission of *M. tuberculosis* takes center stage in the pathogenetic sequence of TB (Fig. 1). Because increased transmission has long-term implications due to the open-ended incubation period of TB, it provides a key to better understand the epidemiology of TB in general and during wartime specifically. However, there are serious methodological barriers to ascertain transmission and there is scarcity of information about it.

We have alluded to factors that may increase the risk of progression from latent infection with *M. tuberculosis* to TB, yet have refrained from a comprehensive discussion that has been the focus of more general discussions of the epidemiologic basis of TB control [3, 79, 80]. Risk factors for progression from latent infection with *M. tuberculosis* to TB as they pertain in particular to periods of war will be addressed in chapter 3. We have at length tried to determine whether case fatality or faster speed at which untreated TB progresses to death is changed during war times, but have not been able to determine this in a satisfactory manner.

Finally, at the outset we have put the importance of data accuracy above all. It is always difficult to be sure about the numerator and the denominator, and this is particularly compounded during civil strife, armed conflict, and war. Data reported during such times will thus always have to be viewed with great reservation.

References

1 Diagnostic standards and classification of tuberculosis in adults and children. This official statement of the American Thoracic Society and the Centers for Disease Control and Prevention was adopted by the ATS Board of Directors, July 1999. This statement was endorsed by the Council of the Infectious Disease Society of America, September 1999. Am J Respir Crit Care Med 2000;161:1376–1395.

2 Rieder HL: Opportunity for exposure and risk of infection: the fuel for the tuberculosis pandemic. Infection 1995;23:1–3.

3 Rieder HL: Epidemiologic basis of tuberculosis control, ed 1. Paris, International Union against Tuberculosis and Lung Disease, 1999.

4 Rieder HL, Cauthen GM, Comstock GW, Snider DE Jr: Epidemiology of tuberculosis in the United States. Epidemiol Rev 1989;11:79–98.

5 Ferebee SH, Mount FW: Tuberculosis morbidity in a controlled trial of the prophylactic use of isoniazid among household contacts. Am Rev Respir Dis 1962;85:490–521.

6 Ferebee SH: Controlled chemoprophylaxis trials in tuberculosis. A general review. Adv Tuberc Res 1970;17:28–106.

7 Pollock JM, Andersen P: The potential of the ESAT-6 antigen secreted by virulent mycobacteria for specific diagnosis of tuberculosis. J Infect Dis 1997;175:1251–1254.

8 von Pirquet C: Der diagnostische Wert der kutanen Tuberkulinreaktion bei der Tuberkulose des Kindesalters auf Grund von 100 Sektionen. Wien Klin Wochenschr 1907;(No. 88):1123–1128.

9 Mendel F: Die von Pirquetsche Hautreaktion und die intravenöse Tuberkulinbehandlung. Med Klin 1908;(No. 12):402–404.

10 Mantoux C: L'intradermo-réaction à la tuberculine et son interprétation clinique. Presse Méd 1910;(No. 2):10–13.

11 Margolis ML, Van Uitert BL: Anergy in tuberculosis. Biomed Pharmacother 1985;39:292–298.

12 Chaparas SD, Vandiviere HM, Melvin I, et al: Tuberculin test. Variability with the Mantoux procedure. Am Rev Respir Dis 1985;132:175–177.

13 Snider DE Jr: The tuberculin skin test. Am Rev Respir Dis 1982;125:108–118.

14 Auersbach K: Zur Einführung der Calmette-Impfung in Deutschland. Ärztl Wschr 1946;1:314–317.

15 van Geuns HA: BCG vaccination in school-leavers? Selected Papers 1987;23:25–50.

16 Anonymous: BCG vaccination. A memorandum from the Ministry of Health. Tubercle 1949;30:183.

17 Snider DE Jr, Cauthen GM: Tuberculin skin testing of hospital employees: infection, "boosting," and two-step testing. Am J Infect Control 1984;12:305–311.

18 Narain R, Nair SS, Chandrasekhar P, Rao GR: Problems connected with estimating the incidence of tuberculosis infection. Indian J Tuberc 1965;13:5–23.

19 Liard R, Tazir M, Boulahbal F, Perdrizet S: Use of two methods of analysis to estimate the annual rate of tuberculosis infection in Southern Algeria. Tuber Lung Dis 1996;76:207–214.

20 Stýblo K, Meijer J, Sutherland I: Tuberculosis surveillance research unit report No. 1: the transmission of tubercle bacilli; its trend in a human population. Bull Int Union Tuberc 1969;42:1–104.

21 Sutherland I: Recent studies in the epidemiology of tuberculosis, based on the risk of being infected with tubercle bacilli. Adv Tuberc Res 1976;19:1–63.

22 Cauthen GM, Pio A, ten Dam HG: Annual risk of tuberculous infection. 1988. Bull World Health Organ 2002;80:503–511.

23 Sutherland I, Stýblo K, Sampalík M, Bleiker MA: [Annual risks of tuberculosis infection in 14 countries according to the results of tuberculosis surveys from 1948 to 1952]. Bull Int Union Tuberc 1971;45:80–122.

24 Lotte A, Uzan J: Evolution of the rates of tuberculous infection in France and calculation of the annual risk by means of mathematical model. Int J Epidemiol 1973;2:265–282.

25 Waaler H, Galtung O, Mordal K: The risk of tuberculous infection in Norway. Bull Int Union Tuberc 1975;50:5–61.

26 Sutherland I, Bleiker MA, Meijer J, Stýblo K: The risk of tuberculous infection in the Netherlands from 1967 to 1979. Tubercle 1983;64:241–253.

27 Vynnycky E, Fine PE: The annual risk of infection with *Mycobacterium tuberculosis* in England and Wales since 1901. Int J Tuberc Lung Dis 1997;1:389–396.

28 Rist E: Tuberculosis in France during the war. Tubercle 1946;27:13–18.

29 Bahr G, Costello AM, Alahdab Y, Stanford J: Epidemic tuberculosis in north Lebanon. Lancet 1991;337:983–984.

30 Bahr GM, Stanford JL, Costello AM: Bad news from north Lebanon. Tubercle 1991;72:73–74.

31 Biggs HM: The administrative control of tuberculosis. New York City, Department of Health, City of New York, Sixth Avenue and Fifty-fifth Street, 1907.

32 Swallow J, Sbarbaro JA: Analysis of tuberculosis casefinding in Denver, Colorado, 1965–70. Health Serv Rep 1972;87:375–384.

33 Jelastopulu E, Alexopoulos EC, Venieri D, et al: Substantial underreporting of tuberculosis in west Greece: implications for local and national surveillance. Euro Surveill 2009;14. pii:19152.

34 Koch R: An address on the fight against tuberculosis in the light of the experience that has been gained in the successful combat of other infectious diseases. Br Med J 1901;2:189–193.

35 Frieden TR, Lerner BH, Rutherford BR: Lessons from the 1800s: tuberculosis control in the new millennium. Lancet 2000;355:1085–1092.

36 Renk: Die Anzeigepflicht bei Tuberkulose im Königreich Sachsen. Tuberculosis (Berlin) 1905;4:32–41.

37 Anonymous: Die Regelung der Anzeigepflicht bei Tuberkulose in Preussen. Tuberculosis (Berlin) 1903;2:68–77.

38 Dewez: La lutte contre la tuberculose en Norwège. Tuberculosis (Berlin) 1904;3:504–514.

39 Holmboe M: Die Anzeigepflicht in Norwegen in 1902. Tuberculosis (Berlin) 1905;4:28–32.

40 Anonymous: Die dänischen Gesetzentwürfe zur Bekämpfung der Tuberkulose. Tuberculosis (Berlin) 1905;4:41–47.

41 Anonymous: Die dänischen Gesetzentwürfe zur Bekämpfung der Tuberkulose. Tuberculosis (Berlin) 1905;4:100–106.

42 Newsholme A, Lecky HC: An account of the system of voluntary notification of phthisis in Brighton, and of the treatment and training of patients in its isolation hospital. Tuberculosis (London) 1907;4:226–242.

43 Centers for Disease Control and Prevention. Epidemiologic notes and reports. Expanded tuberculosis surveillance and tuberculosis morbidity – United States, 1993. Morb Mortal Wkly Rep 1994; 43:362–367.

44 Raviglione MC, Sudre P, Rieder HL, et al: Secular trends of tuberculosis in Western Europe. Bull World Health Organ 1993;71:297–306.

45 Rieder HL, Watson JM, Raviglione MC, et al: Surveillance of tuberculosis in Europe. Working Group of the World Health Organization (WHO) and the European Region of the International Union Against Tuberculosis and Lung Disease (IUATLD) for uniform reporting on tuberculosis cases. Eur Respir J 1996;9:1097–1104.

46 EuroTB (CESES/KNCV) and the national coordinators for tuberculosis surveillance in the WHO European Region. Surveillance of tuberculosis in Europe. Report on tuberculosis cases notified in 1996. EuroTB 1998:1–95.

47 EuroTB and the national coordinators for tuberculosis surveillance in the WHO European Region. Surveillance of tuberculosis in Europe. Report on tuberculosis cases notified in 2006. EuroTB 2008: 1–115.

48 European Centre for Disease Prevention and Control, WHO Regional Office for Europe. Tuberculosis surveillance in Europe 2008. Copenhagen, European Centre for Disease Prevention and Control, 2010.

49 Brown JS, Wells F, Duckworth G, et al: Improving notification rates for tuberculosis. BMJ 1995;310: 974.

50 World Health Organization. Global tuberculosis report 2015. World Health Organization Document 2015;WHO/HTM/TB/2015.22:1–192.

51 World Health Organization. Global tuberculosis report 2016. World Health Organization Document 2016;WHO/HTM/TB/2016.13:1–201.

52 Wang L, Liu J, Chin DP: Progress in tuberculosis control and the evolving public-health system in China. Lancet 2007;369:691–696.

53 Central TB Division. TB India 2014. Revised National TB Control Programme Annual Status Report. Reach the unreached – find, treat, cure TB, save lives. New Delhi, Ministry of Health and Family Welfare, 2014.

54 Dupuis J: Tuberculose et armée. Tuberculosis (Berlin) 1905;4:297–311.

55 Heaf F, Rusby L: A further review of tuberculosis in wartime. Tubercle 1942;23:107–130.

56 Elandt-Johnson RC: Definition of rates: some remarks on their use and misuse. Am J Epidemiol 1975;102:267–271.

57 Krebs W: Die Fälle von Lungentuberkulose in der aargauischen Heilstätte Barmelweid aus den Jahren 1912–1927. Beitr Klin Tuberk 1930;74: 345–379.

58 Buhl K, Nyboe J: Epidemiological basis of tuberculosis eradication. 9. Changes in the mortality of Danish tuberculosis patients since 1925. Bull World Health Organ 1967;37:907–925.

59 Berg G: The prognosis of open pulmonary tuberculosis. A clinical-statistical analysis, ed 1. Lund, Sweden, Håkan Ohlson, 1939.

60 Thompson BC: Survival rates in pulmonary tuberculosis. Br Med J 1943;2:721–721.

61 Tiemersma EW, van der Werf MJ, Borgdorff MW, et al: Natural history of tuberculosis: duration and fatality of untreated pulmonary tuberculosis in HIV negative patients: a systematic review. PLoS One 2011;6:e17601.

62 Redeker F: Epidemiologie und Statistik der Tuberkulose; in Hein J, Kleinschmidt H, Uehlinger E (eds): Handbuch der Tuberkulose, Vol I of IV, ed 1. Stuttgart, Georg Thieme, 1958, pp 407–498.

63 Oei W, Nishiura H: The relationship between tuberculosis and influenza death during the influenza (H1N1) pandemic from 1918–19. Comput Math Methods Med 2012;2012:124861.

64 Zürcher K, Zwahlen M, Ballif M, et al: Influenza pandemics and tuberculosis mortality in 1889 and 1918: analysis of historical data from Switzerland. PLoS One 2016;11:e0162575.

65 Noymer A: The 1918 influenza pandemic hastened the decline of tuberculosis in the United States: an age, period, cohort analysis. Vaccine 2011;29(suppl 2):B38–B41.

66 Anonymous: Tuberculosis statistics. Tubercle 1921;2:274.

67 Anonymous: Tuberculosis statistics. England and Wales. Mortality and new cases contrasted, 1926 to 1935. Tubercle 1937;18:503.

68 Anonymous: Tuberculosis statistics. The trend of tuberculosis during recent years in the administrative county of Lancaster. Tubercle 1937;18:458.

69 Anonymous: Annual reports. Tubercle 1947;28: 171–175.

70 Lewis-Faning E: Respiratory tuberculosis. Effect of the war on the length of the interval between notification and death. Br Med J 1943;2:684–685.

71 Bjartveit K: The tuberculosis situation in Norway. Scand J Respir Dis 1978;Suppl 102:28–35.

72 Groth-Petersen E, Knudsen J, Wilbek E: Epidemiological basis of tuberculosis eradication in an advanced country. Bull World Health Organ 1959; 21:5–49.

73 Anonymous: Statistics. Tubercle 1947;28:56–57.

74 Anonymous: Tuberculosis statistics. Mortality from tuberculosis (all forms) in certain European countries not engaged in the great war. Tubercle 1936;17:308.

75 Anonymous: Tuberculosis statistics. Mortality from tuberculosis (all forms) during recent years in certain European countries engaged in the great war. Tubercle 1936;18:70.

76 Drolet GJ: World War I and tuberculosis. Am J Public Health 1945;35:689–697.

77 Murray JF: Tuberculosis and World War I. (Occasional essay). Am J Respir Crit Care Med 2015; 192:411–414.

78 Klesse M: Beitrag zum quantitativ-exogenen Tuberkuloseproblem und Wege zur Feststellung des wirklichen Tuberkuloseverlaufs im zweiten Weltkrieg. Dtsch Gesundheitswesen 1946;1:688–695.

79 Styblo K: Epidemiology of tuberculosis; in Meissner G (ed): Infektionskrankheiten und ihre Erreger. Jena, VEB Gustav Fischer Verlag, 1984, pp 77–161.

80 Styblo K: Epidemiology of tuberculosis, ed 2. The Hague, Royal Netherlands Tuberculosis Association, 1991.

81 Wikipedia: https://de.wikipedia.org/wiki/Einwohnerentwicklung_von_Berlin (accessed March 16, 2017).

Hans L. Rieder, MD, MPH
Tuberculosis Consultant Services
Jetzikofenstrasse 12
CH–3038 Kirchlindach (Switzerland)
E-Mail TBRieder@tbrieder.org

Murray JF, Loddenkemper R (eds): Tuberculosis and War. Lessons Learned from World War II.
Prog Respir Res. Basel, Karger, 2018, vol 43, pp 33–43 (DOI: 10.1159/000481473)

Risk Factors for the Increase of Tuberculosis during Wartime

Robert Loddenkemper[a] · Hans L. Rieder[b, c]

[a]German Central Committee against Tuberculosis, Berlin, Germany; [b]Tuberculosis Consultant Services, Kirchlindach, and
[c]Epidemiology, Biostatistics and Prevention Institute, University of Zurich, Zurich, Switzerland

Abstract

During wartime, in most cases, both environmental and host factors are likely to be co-responsible for commonly observed increases in tuberculosis (TB). The 2 most important risk factors are indoor overcrowding, which increases the risk of transmission, and malnutrition, which weakens the immune defenses of the host. Together, these and other factors increase the prevalence of latent infection and the subsequent risk of progression to active disease, respectively, thereby resulting in an increase in morbidity, and in consequence also mortality. As a result of this increased morbidity, transmission is likely to increase further because of the excess prevalence of transmissible TB and the greater opportunity for person-to-person spread due to overcrowding. In this chapter, multiple factors will be analyzed that may explain the variations observed in different countries. In addition, various TB control measures are addressed which existed before the war and which evolved during and after World War II as a response to the deterioration of the TB situation. © 2018 S. Karger AG, Basel

World War II (WWII) involved almost the whole world. With an estimated more than 50 million fatalities in both military and civilian populations, it was the deadliest conflict in human history. According to Daniels [1, 2], tuberculosis (TB) was the major health disaster of this war; he emphasized that "the number of additional deaths from TB during the war must run into many hundreds of thousands, and the number of surviving sufferers must number between 5 and 10 million." All countries – both Axis and Allies – were affected by TB as a consequence of the war, albeit with distinctly different patterns as outlined in chapter 1: countries in which there was little or no wartime rise; countries in which the mortality rate rose in the first years and fell in the later years of the war; and countries in which death rates rose throughout the war years to a peak at the end of the war [3, 4]. Even non-belligerent countries observed an increase in TB, whereas only a few belligerent countries saw a fall in the numbers of TB cases (Bulgaria, Denmark, and England and Wales) [5].

As discussed in chapter 2, several problems impede the retrieval of reliable epidemiological data during wartime. They include destruction of public health infrastructure, redeployment, transfer or elimination of health resources and personnel, collapse of communication systems, lack of diagnostic capabilities and also censorship, propaganda, and the intentional falsification of information [5]. However, it is likely that at least the observed trends delineated in detail in chapters 5–19 are germane and plausible.

In this chapter, factors that may explain the variations observed in the situation from one country to another during wartime will be analyzed. Both environmental and host-dependent factors that may increase the risk of infection with tubercle bacilli and the risk of progression from latent TB infection to overt clinical TB and finally to death from the disease will be discussed. During wartime, in most cases, both environmental and host factors are likely to be responsible; of these, the 2 most important ones are: first, overcrowding in small dwellings, which increases the risk of transmission through the inhalation of *Mycobacterium tuberculosis* (*M. tuberculosis*) containing droplet nuclei, and second, malnutrition, which weakens the immune defenses of the host. Together, these factors increase the risk of progression to active disease among the prevalent latently infected individuals, thereby resulting in a short-term increase in morbidity and mortality. In addition, environmental transmission increases because of the higher prevalence of active disease and greater opportunity for person-to-person spread due to overcrowding. New infections resulting from this increase in community transmission may develop into cases of active disease, months or years later [6].

Environmental Risk Factors

Infection with *M. tuberculosis* is in the overwhelming majority of cases acquired through the inhalation of bacilli-containing droplet nuclei. The risk of infection following TB exposure is primarily governed by exogenous factors that are determined by an intrinsic combination of the infectiousness of the source case, duration of exposure to tubercle bacilli-containing ambient air and, as mentioned below, social and behavioral risk factors including living hygiene, and possibly smoking, alcohol, and indoor air pollution [7]. In settings with increased likelihood of social mixing (together with overcrowding), transmission will be high. Conditions that prolong the length of exposure to an infectious patient include health system-related factors such as delay in diagnosis or faulty treatment.

Crowding
Crowded living favors increased transmission of tubercle bacilli [8]. Such conditions unfold during wartime among the civilian population and are inherent in military encampments. Typical examples during WWII include the destruction of the housing infrastructure by bombing as seen in London and other cities in the UK, and in Berlin and other large German cities. According to Sartwell et al. [9], "density of population 1.5–2.5 persons per room" and "a large number of [infectious] cases living at home" due to "the fact that before the close of hostilities patients with open TB had been generally permitted to work in factories and other industrial plants". Similarly, owing to the dense congregation in bunkers, Long stated "In one bunker-type shelter in Mannheim (Germany), it is said that 18,000 people congregated during raids" [10] and in cellars during air raids, aggravated by loss of sleep and interference with meals [11].

Other examples include the close crowding in concentration and prison camps, in refugee camps, in the billeting and close-quarter accommodations, and in facilities such as military assembly and training camps.

Crowding was often aggravated by the influx of diseased prisoners of war (POWs) or of foreign (slave) workers from high TB incidence countries. Large population movements and the many displaced persons with communicable TB worsened the situation further at the end of WWII, especially in Germany and the formerly occupied countries. Another example that increased the spread of TB was the absconding of fugitives with TB from Europe to Britain and to some non-belligerent countries (Ireland, Spain) during WWII [5].

Patients with infectious TB have often been discharged from institutional care too early, because TB hospitals and sanatoria were occupied by injured or otherwise incapacitated military personnel. Accordingly, these factors increased the risk of transmission to the civilian population considerably. In Germany, thousands of injured civilians crowded the hospitals after large bombing raids, contributing to the shortage in hospital beds [9]. Furthermore, in Germany due to the increasing requirement to augment the labor force, TB patients were forced to work, thereby reducing any chance of recovery and accelerating their path to a fatal outcome. With only a few limitations, even patients with contagious TB were considered capable to work. Other inhumane measures of accelerating death included purposefully starving moribund patients and shortening the lives of so-called anti-social cases in selected TB hospitals, which often were combined with those for patients with psychiatric disorders [12].

Interestingly, the significant rise in TB mortality between 1937 and 1947 in Bavaria, which is illustrated in Figure 1, was almost completely due to pulmonary TB; by contrast there was only a small increase in extrapulmonary TB (Fig. 2), possibly due in part to unavailable or insufficient diagnostic methods. This phenomenon was also seen in other German provinces: pulmonary TB ranging from 91% of all TB deaths in Berlin down to 82% in Hesse in 1947. In the U.S. Zone, 85% of the mortality was ascribed to pulmonary TB and 15% to TB of other organs. These proportions are identical with the figures for all of Germany over the 3-year period, 1935–1937 [9]. That the rise of TB deaths was caused mainly by pulmonary TB was also observed in other countries (see chapters 6–19).

The data from Bavaria confirm that the TB mortality during wartime and at the end of the WWII was generally larger in the cities than in the rural districts, as shown on Figure 2.

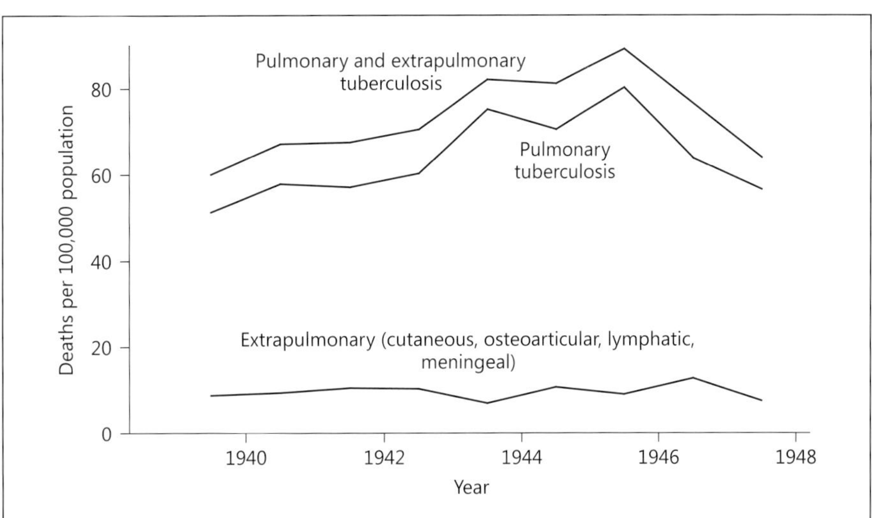

Fig. 1. Tuberculosis mortality in Bavaria, Germany, 1937–1947, adapted from [13], with permission of Springer.

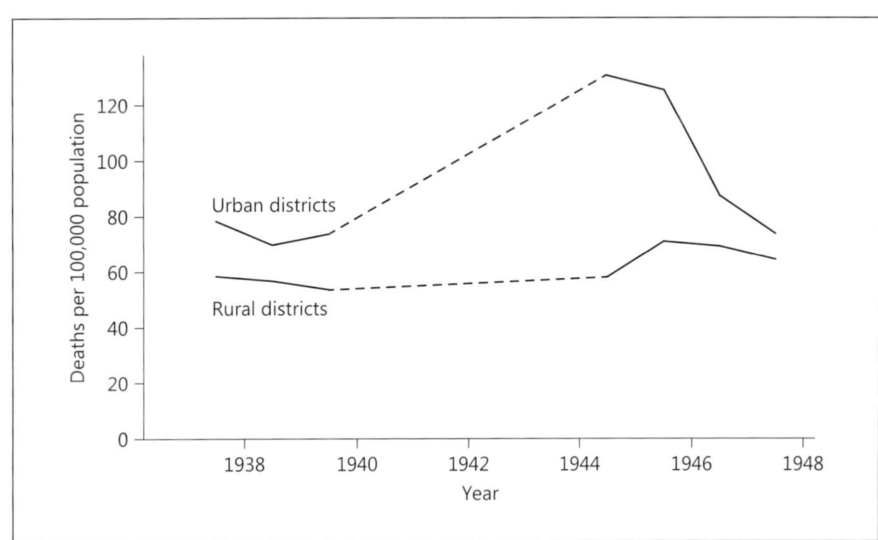

Fig. 2. Increase of TB mortality in Bavaria, Germany, at the end of WWII, mainly in cities compared to rural districts, adapted from Ref. [13], with permission of Springer.

One of the reasons for higher TB mortality rates in large cities (Fig. 3) may be owing to either the prevailing insufficient food supply (or to the better provision of food in rural areas). In Berlin, for example, food shortages were presumably enhanced because of the difficulty in procuring food from the surrounding farmland [14]. A further reason was presumably that living conditions were less crowded in rural areas [9]. An additional reason for the exacerbation of the prevalence of TB in big cities such as Berlin was the considerable loss of housing accommodations by massive allied bombing raids after 1943. Meyer mentions that in the different districts of Berlin between 25 and 50% of houses had been destroyed, heaviest in industrial districts where the lower social classes lived [14]. Virtually the same pattern of destruction occurred in England where industrial cities were the main target of German bomb and V2 attacks.

Rich versus Poor

Using available data from different parts of the city, Klesse [15] infers a steeper increase in TB mortality from 1939 to 1944 within Berlin districts predominantly inhabited by working class people compared to those where the more affluent preferred living. For instance, in the whole of Greater Berlin, TB mortality increased by 53% during this period, whereas in the Neukölln district it rose by 68%. Moreover, Neukölln was not among the poorer city areas; in fact, it was rather by averaging richer and poorer dis-

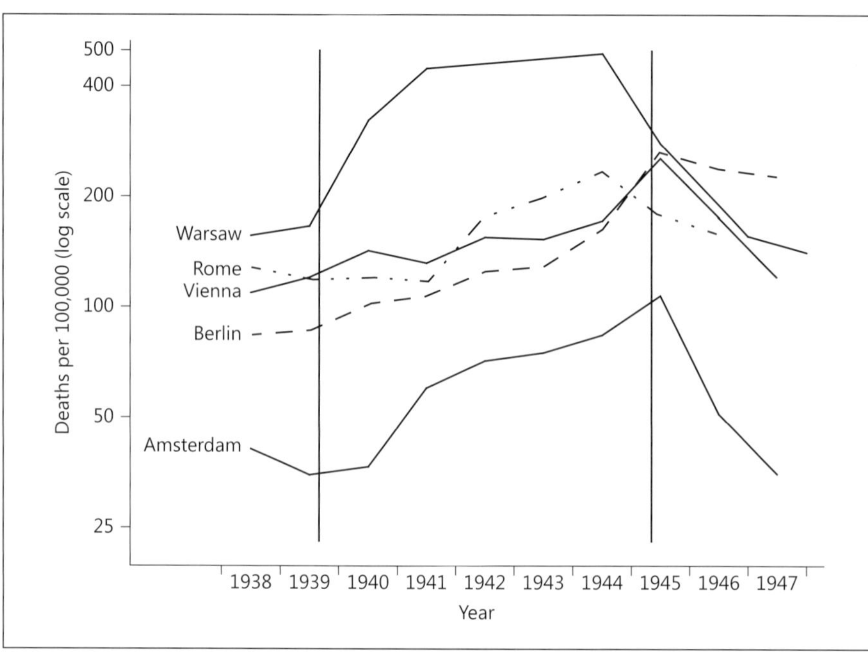

Fig. 3. TB mortality in selected European cities, 1938–1947, adapted from Ref. [3].

tricts that Klesse concluded that some poorer districts had more TB than other more affluent ones. The same was true for Vienna, as mentioned by Daniels [3], where the highest TB mortality was in the working class boroughs (up to 322 per 100,000 inhabitants).

An interesting explanation for the faster elimination of infectious sources in the Soviet zone (GDR) during the first years after WWII in comparison with the western zones of Germany (FRG; Fig. 7 at the end of chapter 5 has been presented by Ferlinz et al.: the twofold higher TB mortality of infectious sources after the war – presumably due to the lack of TB drugs and the worse economic situation – reduced the spread of the TB bacilli to the population. Additional factors were the less favorable conditions in the FRG due to the substantially larger proportion of foreigners (immigrants as well as asylum seekers) from countries with high TB incidence [16].

Host-Dependent Risk Factors

Host-dependent factors are important conditions that weaken the immune defense system of the body. The defense mechanisms against *M. tuberculosis* are complex, a variety of factors are involved, from innate and adaptive cellular to humoral immune responses. If these are impaired, it increases TB morbidity, chiefly through increased progression from already present latent infection to active disease with accompanying mortality. Impaired immune defenses are an increasing cause of TB disease and death in developed as well as in underdeveloped countries.

While the risk of becoming infected with *M. tuberculosis* is largely exogenous in nature as described above, the risk subsequent to acquisition of latent infection with *M. tuberculosis* is largely endogenous [17]. Thus, crowded congregate settings are conducive to increase the probability of successful transmission of tubercle bacilli. While infection with *M. tuberculosis* is the necessary or initiating cause, some reduction in the body's resistance, probably decreased cellular immunity, is undoubtedly the sufficient or promoting cause [18]. What we refer to here as host-dependent factors broadly circumscribes a multitude of factors that increase the risk of progression from latent infection with *M. tuberculosis* to overt clinical disease by putatively undermining cellular immune defenses [19]. Many of these factors are well established, leaving little doubt about their causal role in increasing the risk of progression to TB (such as diabetes mellitus, silicosis, immunosuppressive therapy with certain drug classes, etc.), while the relationship is causally less certain in others (such as gastrectomy, certain blood groups). One factor of major global implication because of its shear population magnitude is malnutrition or, more precisely, protein energy malnutrition.

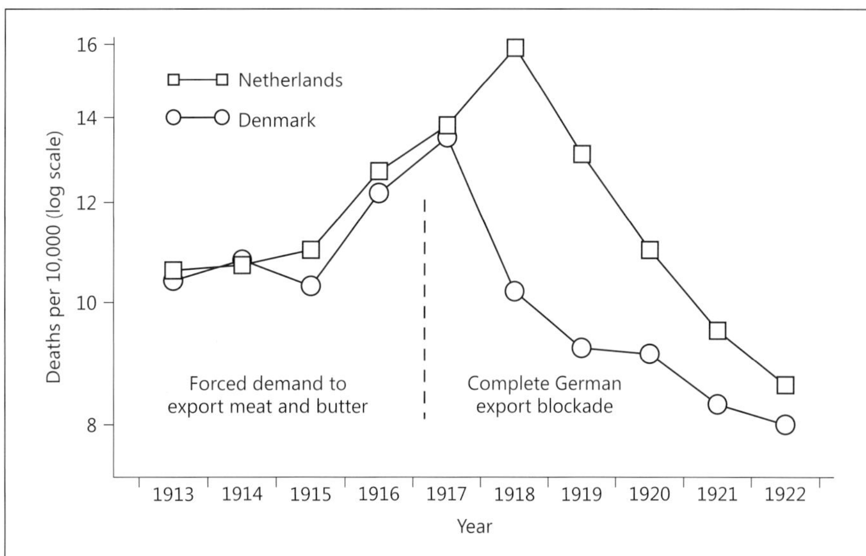

Fig. 4. Tuberculosis mortality comparatively shown for Denmark and The Netherlands, 1913–1922, with the time indicated for an abrupt change in nutrition for the Danish population as a result of policy change imposed by the warring countries, data from [28].

Malnutrition

It is well established that malnutrition adversely affects the functioning of the immune system, both innate and acquired, in its defense mechanisms against a broad range of infectious diseases [20]. Whether malnutrition actually increases the risk of TB among individuals infected with *M. tuberculosis* has been subject to substantial discourse. The most authoritative review to-date is that by Cegielski and McMurray [21] who conclude that malnutrition is an important risk factor for TB. Under this premise, the role of malnutrition on TB incidence in wartime is discussed in the following.

Malnutrition with hypovitaminoses and hypoproteinemia remain prevalent in some low-income countries [22] and are postulated to be a major cause of the rise in TB during wartime. Deficiencies usually result from the disruption of agricultural production or food supply lines, imposition of food rationing and distribution controls. Extreme examples are Nazi-governed concentration camps and the famine, near-starvation 900-day-long siege of Leningrad [23].

Apart from these extremes, malnutrition is most often mentioned in the war literature as one of the main reasons for the deteriorating TB situation, but how such assertions are arrived is questionable [24]. A major review on malnutrition as a risk factor for latent infection progressing to active TB has noted how thin the evidence actually is and how much anecdotal sources cloud the subject [21]. Nevertheless, as mentioned above, the authors do conclude that malnutrition might indeed account for a substantial population attributable risk. There have been attempts to determine a relationship between TB mortality and dietary constituents; for instance in England and Wales during WWII [25] or in Denmark during the WWI [26], but remain subject to vivid discussions about fact and fiction [27]. Faber has provided a comprehensive review about nutrition during WWI and TB mortality [28]. A summary of one of his major findings is shown in Figure 4.

In 1917, mortality in the Netherlands and in Denmark was about the same. But by 1918, mortality had continued rising to a peak in the Netherlands, while it had substantially declined in Denmark. Faber recalls that Denmark's principal occupation then was producing animal foodstuffs, such as beef, pork, butter, milk, and eggs, while it imported feed for the animals and cereals for human and animal consumption. Both Great Britain and Germany consumed a heavy share of these products, as reflected in the country's exports and imports from 1913 to 1917. In February 1917, this changed drastically when Germany declared unrestricted marine welfare and imposed a complete blockade for food exports by Denmark. This had a significant impact on food availability: bread for instance had to be rationed, while butter was now available in abundance: while before it had been the other way around. As a result of the changes and diligent rationing, the earlier food crisis ceased in 1918. Most notably, fish and meat consumption rose to unprecedented levels, and margarine was replaced by butter, etc. The association between the change in nutrition and the reversal of the TB mortality is striking to say the least. Causality cannot necessarily be inferred from this association. The enthusiasm of Faber for animal proteins and fat could not of

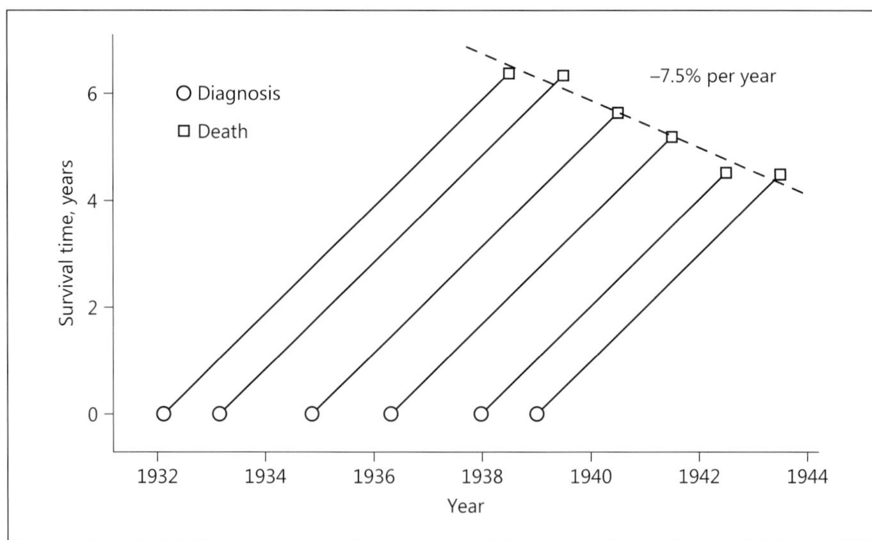

Fig. 5. Time from year of death elapsed since average time of diagnosis, back-calculated for Chemnitz, Germany, unpublished data from Fröhlich, reported by Klesse [15].

course remain undisputed [29]. Malmros used the example of Norway to show that a moderately reduced calorie supply – as was the case throughout the war – does not lead necessarily to substantially increased TB morbidity (see also Fig. 9, [30]), provided the conditions are otherwise favorable.

Tuberculosis fatality increased in Berlin stepwise during WWII from 19.0 in 1939 to 49.5% in 1945 when almost half of all TB patients died from the disease, most probably, as Meyer assumes, due to the lowered resistance to the disease caused by undernourishment, in particular protein deficiency [14].

The observation that TB became a more acute disease during wartime is underlined by data from the Moselle region in Germany, in which the survival time from diagnosis to death became much shorter during the war period 1940–1945 than in comparable periods before and after [31]. This was also observed by Fröhlich in Chemnitz/Saxony [15], as shown in Figure 5.

In 1946, Leyton reported that Russian POWs had more severe TB than British POWs and that there were large differences in the frequency of TB between British and Russian POWs. He also assumed that malnutrition stood out as the only causative factor among the Russians [24].

Brozek et al. [23] observed a more acute and severe course of TB in their report on the health consequences of semi-starvation in the Leningrad siege, one of the longest and most destructive sieges in history and possibly the costliest in terms of casualties: "The increase in the incidence of TB was gradual, a few cases appearing December 1941, the peak being in May and June 1942. Much TB was seen, but remarkable was the fulminating character of the TB with hemorrhagic pleural effusion, widespread pulmonary disease and damage, miliary spread, and early death."

Daniels describes for France that in regions with ample supply of animal food and milk (Normandy, Brittany, Eastern France), where there had always been a high TB mortality, the rate declined throughout the war in contrast to regions with severe food shortages which showed a substantial rise, most prominently in Paris from 155 in 1938 to 215 per 100,000 population in 1941 [3].

Other Host-Dependent Factors

Stress

Severe physical and mental stress (which may also weaken the immunologic resistance to TB [5]) was incurred during wartime in both civilian workers and those occupied in ammunition production or in military service. Innes, for example, explains the higher percentage of female deaths compared with pre-war years in the county of Rochdale (near Manchester/England), with the more extensive employment of women in the heavy industries for longer hours with less time and energy to devote to housekeeping [11].

Age and Sex

It is well-known that TB frequency may differ substantially by age and sex. During wartime, the epidemiology in this respect may change considerably, as illustrated in Figure 6 in Bavaria.

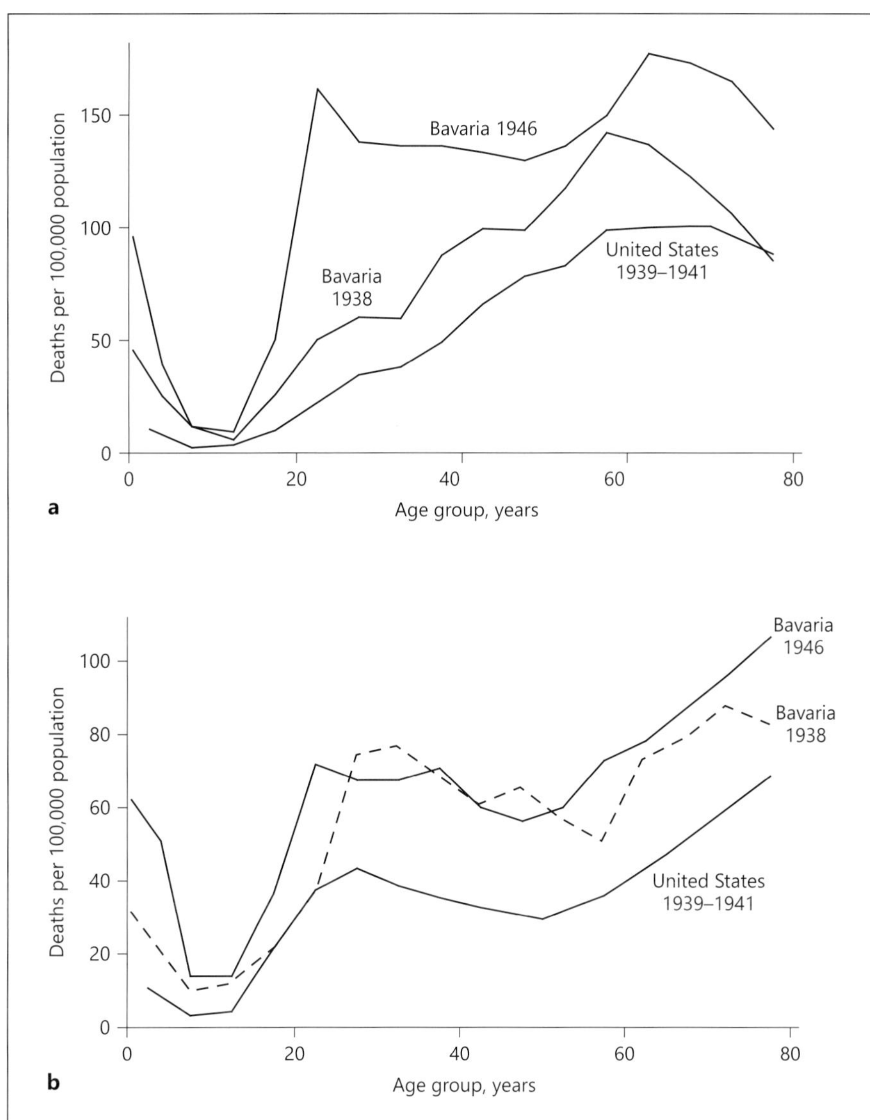

Fig. 6. Mortality rates for all forms of tuberculosis by sex and age for Bavaria (1938 and 1946) and United States of America (1939–1941). **a** Males, **b** females. Fig. 2 from [9].

Age-specific rates for each sex for the years 1938–1946 were compared with the corresponding rates for the white population of the United States averaged for 1939–1941 [9]. "In 1938, Bavaria's age distribution of mortality in both sexes was roughly parallel to, although somewhat higher than that in the United States. In 1946 the TB mortality for males in Bavaria was greatly increased in infancy and in all adult age groups (Fig. 6a). The most marked excess was in the 20–34 year age span and it was assumed that the excessive mortality among repatriated prisoners has contributed to this high rate. Roentgen surveys of such groups have revealed a high prevalence of significant TB. Among females, on the contrary, the only population groups showing an increase in 1946 as compared with 1938 were infants and young chil-

dren, among whom a rise similar to the male rise was recorded (Fig. 6b). There was practically no difference between prewar and postwar mortality in adult females. Presumably had there been no war, the 1946 rates would have shown a decrease, but at least there was no rise. The increase in infant mortality from TB in both sexes suggests that, at least in this age group, the frequency of infection was greater in 1946 than before the war." One reason may have been the imperfect or absent pasteurization of the milk [32].

As an additional explanation, it was assumed that there was a sex selection process during the war among the civilian population. Healthy males were drafted to the army, were killed or returned sick – in particular, after war captivity – whereas the non-drafted males had prevalent TB [14].

Tobacco Smoking

A potentially large population-attributable fraction of TB might be related to smoking. However, smoking cannot be clearly established as a risk factor for TB because of the multitude of potentially confounding factors (notably socio-economic ones which are co-shaping the TB epidemic, independent of smoking habits) that tend to interfere with a clean etiologic analysis. An early case-control study nested into the large British cohort study on smoking examined the relationship between smoking and TB and found a dose-relationship, a finding that always enhances the credibility of and strengthens the case for postulating causality [33]. Since this early study, a multitude of cohort studies have added to the evidence base and established increasingly the veracity of establishing smoking as an independent risk factor for the progression from latent infection with *M. tuberculosis* to TB. The potential of increased smoking burden contributing to increased TB incidence is thus discussed in the following. However, it should be kept in mind that the overall differential population-attributable fraction might have been fairly modest.

Tobacco smoking is a risk factor for both pulmonary and extrapulmonary TB [34, 35]. Several pathogenetic mechanisms have been discussed, though the main cause is most likely the suppression of the immune defense against *M. tuberculosis* [36]. Cigarette consumption increased considerably during WWI and even more so in WWII, in particular in the military [37, 38]. Thus, it is possible that active and passive cigarette smoking played an additional role in the TB epidemic during WWII, although this is not mentioned specifically in the literature.

Indoor Air Pollution

Indoor air pollution may be a further risk factor for TB and, although often linked with passive smoking, emerges as an independent risk factor in some epidemiological studies [39]. However, in a recent systematic review and meta-analysis, the level of evidence for the association between domestic use of solid fuels and TB was found to be very low [40]. Authors from India observed that using solid cooking fuel was associated with a 1.8 higher risk for bacteriologically positive pulmonary TB [41]. Although this again is not mentioned specifically in the literature, it can be assumed that indoor air pollution in limited settings may have played an additional role in the TB exacerbation during WWII.

Alcohol Consumption

A further, difficult to quantify, potential risk factor for TB is alcohol abuse. The epidemiologic difficulties are similar to those of smoking, that is, the direct and indirect potential confounding with socio-economic factors. Such factors and specific behaviors of substance abusers in general may put them at an increased risk of acquisition of infection with tubercle bacilli rather than at an increased risk of progression to TB subsequent to infection. Experimental animal studies seem to establish alcohol as a risk factor for the latter mechanism, although animal experiments with substance abuse are to be viewed particularly critical: most animals quite in contrast to humans – albeit with some notable exceptions – have little "natural" inclination for intoxication. In this context, alcohol abuse is also discussed in the following. Again, the overall differential population-attributable fraction must be fairly small as a substantial quantitative change in massive alcohol abuse at the population level is much less likely and widespread than for instance famine and protein energy malnutrition.

The association of alcohol abuse with TB is well known [42]. However, again an increased consumption of alcohol is not described as a specific risk factor for TB during WWII, but may have been an additional one. Daniels mentions that a fall in alcohol consumption in France due to the introduction of rationing wines and spirits during the war may have been responsible in part for the decline in TB mortality. He underlines this assumption by adding "a marked fall in morbidity and mortality from diseases attributable to alcoholism, a fall not paralleled in any disease other than TB" [3].

Other Factors

Some other factors that increase the risk of progression from latent infection to TB disease are immune deficiencies from any medical cause including diabetes mellitus and immunosuppressive therapy, plus other medical conditions such as chronic renal failure, silicosis, and gastrectomy [7]. Whether these factors played an additional role in the epidemiology of TB during WWII is not specifically mentioned in the literature.

Human Immunodeficiency Virus

Human immunodeficiency virus (HIV) was not yet known during WWII, but the link between TB and HIV is now well established: "The risk of active TB doubles in the first year of HIV co-infection, and the risk of developing active disease in those who have LTBI is on average 10% per year in the course of an untreated HIV infection, HIV-TB co-infected individuals have reduced survival and are at higher risk for subsequent opportunistic infections. In overcrowded and poor living conditions, the combined effect of the 2 epidemics is magnified" [34], and, thus, HIV could have a major impact on the TB epidemiology in current and future wars. This is confirmed in the comprehensive review of Kimbrough and associates on the burden of TB in crisis-affected populations, where the risk of excess mortality among HIV-positive individuals was substantially enlarged [6]. However, most of the studies were done before the era of widespread access to antiretroviral medicines that most likely will reduce the excess risk due to HIV in ongoing and forth coming crises.

The World Health Organization (WHO) postulates that more resources should be directed to screening, diagnosis, and treatment of HIV and TB drug resistance, monitoring early indicators of resistance and integrating HIV and TB prevention and intervention [43]. Kerridge et al. [44] regard these recommendations as even more critical in conflict-affected states with weakened public health infrastructure in which antiretroviral therapy programs can be destabilized, and treatment and supply chains interrupted.

TB Control Measures

The TB situation in the years before WWII varied considerably throughout the world. There were countries with a far developed TB control program and others with a poor program. Details are given in the country-specific chapters 5–19 in which the pre-war TB situation and its development during and after the war are described. Here we will list the various potential measures which existed before the war and which evolved during and after WWII as a response to the deterioration of the TB situation.

Pre-War Control Measures
The epidemiologic assessment of the TB situation is based mainly on mortality data. The notification of active TB cases for the assessment of TB morbidity was not yet commonly introduced.

TB control measures mainly aimed at preventing the transmission of the TB bacilli from infectious patients to their contacts. An important step for the isolation of infectious patients was to admit them to a TB sanatorium. Many TB sanatoria had been opened already in most countries. There, bed rest, provision of high-caloric food, and sunlight were the leading therapeutic approach; in selected cases treatment modalities such as artificial pneumothorax or more invasive surgical procedures were performed [46]. Compulsory isolation of "difficult" patients was allowed in Germany. Most countries had already introduced an ambulatory structure with dispensaries for special TB care, usually run under the responsibility of the local or national government.

The main diagnostic method was the microscopic examination of the expectorated sputum in suspicious cases. Radiography or fluoroscopy for diagnostic purposes had been introduced in the 1920s, but were not used for routine screening of the general population. X-ray screening was applied, however, in the military service of some countries. Tuberculin skin tests were usually not performed as a routine screening method, but sometimes for diagnosis of cases suspected of having TB.

The pasteurization of milk and the culling of infected (tuberculin-positive) cattle to prevent the transmission of bovine TB was not generally introduced. Only in few countries, BCG vaccination was established on a broad basis.

TB Control during War
During the war, medical services for the general population were frequently reduced or disrupted. In particular, a shortage of experienced TB personnel did result, many doctors and also nurses were drafted into the military service. TB sanatoria and hospitals were used for wounded soldiers, thus often substantially reducing the number of beds for TB patients. Patients had to be discharged, thus facilitating the spreading of the TB bacilli into the population. Transportation became difficult and was doubly injurious to TB care, preventing patients from going to clinics or dispensaries for diagnosis and treatment, and impeding TB nurses to visit the homes of patients to give advice and provide home care.

The governments often instituted committees composed of TB specialists who developed strategies to maintain TB services and to improve the condition of TB patients. Special attention – as far as possible – was devoted to providing adequate nutrition and accommodation. Educational information on precaution against TB was provided to the public, guidelines for doctors were developed, and teaching of TB in medical schools intensified. Directives against the spread of TB in schools, kindergarten, and similar institutions were decreed. In countries suffering from air raids, shelter conditions were improved to prevent droplet infection. If possible, separate bunkers and/or masks for TB patients were provided. Children (and TB patients) were evacuated from the cities to the countryside. For patients with an artificial pneumothorax, the refilling with air was ensured.

As often a shortage of workers developed during the war, even patients with active TB were used by the industry. This could have a negative impact on the course of the disease and limited the provision of medical care to the patients. In the Soviet Union, to secure care for patients, night sanatoria were established in which the patient received special supervision and treatment after finishing work.

Post-War TB Control

After the war, an almost catastrophic TB situation was present in many countries. The TB control programs were often almost completely disrupted, in particular in the most affected countries. Thus, it was necessary to restore or restructure the TB services.

In 1943, the United Nations Relief and Rehabilitation Administration (UNRRA) was founded, which became part of the United Nations in 1945. Its purpose was to "plan, co-ordinate, administer or arrange for the administration of measures for the relief of victims of war in any area under the control of any of the United Nations through the provision of food, fuel, clothing, shelter and other basic necessities, medical and other essential services." UNRRA cooperated closely with dozens of volunteer charitable organizations, today called non-governmental organizations (NGOs). In Germany and Austria, these tasks were mainly organized by the military governments of the Allies.

One of the main and most urgent problems was the shortage of food. If possible, food supplements were provided to TB patients. The number of hospital and sanatorium beds for TB patients had to be substantially increased, and technical equipment for diagnostic and therapeutic purposes had to be supplied as radiographs, fluoroscopes, microscopes, pneumothorax apparatus, thoracoscopes, and other surgical instruments; doctors and nurses had to be trained, and case finding and case supervision by the local public health organizations had to be intensified to get reliable epidemiological statistics. Repeat mass radiography screening and tuberculin testing were introduced in some countries to find infected and diseased TB cases as was – for prevention – a BCG vaccination program (in some European countries with the help of Danish and Swedish Red Cross); the housing accommodation had to be improved; the pasteurization of milk and the culling of infected cattle was started or enhanced.

The International Union against Tuberculosis (IUAT) resumed its activities in 1946 [45], and became – after the founding of the WHO in 1946 – the first NGO to be officially recognised by WHO. National TB organizations and societies enhanced their activities, too, and improved international co-operation. Research in TB diagnostics, therapy, and prevention was essentially stimulated by the discovery of anti-tuberculosis agents. Almost simultaneously at the end of 1944 – only 3 weeks apart – the first para-aminosalicyclic acid was used successfully in Sweden and thereafter streptomycin in the USA for the treatment of active TB in each one patient [46]. Other cases with successful treatment soon followed, which started a new era in the fight against TB and contributed substantially to the further success of TB control after WWII. But, as is well known, the hope expressed by Daniels in 1949 that TB "should be almost eradicated before this century is out" has not been fulfilled [4].

References

1 Daniels M: Tuberculosis in post-war Europe; an international problem. Tubercle 1947;28:201.

2 Daniels M: Tuberculosis in post-war Europe an international problem. Tubercle 1947;28:233–238.

3 Daniels M: Tuberculosis in Europe during and after the second world war. Br Med J 1949;2:1065–1072.

4 Daniels M: Tuberculosis in Europe during and after the second world war. Br Med J 1949;2:1135–1140.

5 Smallman-Raynor M, Cliff AD: War and disease: some perspectives on the spatial and temporal occurence of tuberculosis in wartime. Chapter 4 in Gandy M, Zumia A (eds): The Return of the White Plague: Global Poverty and the "New" Tuberculosis New York, Verso, 2003, pp 70–92.

6 Kimbrough W, Saliba V, Dahab M, et al: The burden of tuberculosis in crisis-affected populations: a systematic review. Lancet Infect Dis 2012;12:950–965.

7 Diel R, Loddenkemper R, Zellweger JP, et al: Old ideas to innovate tuberculosis control: preventive treatment to achieve elimination. Eur Respir J 2013;42:785–801.

8 Beggs CB, Noakes CJ, Sleigh PA, et al: The transmission of tuberculosis in confined spaces: an analytical review of alternative epidemiological models. Int J Tuberc Lung Dis 2003;7:1015–1026.

9 Sartwell PE, Moseley CH, Long ER: Tuberculosis in the German population, United States Zone of Germany. Am Rev Tuberc 1949;59:481–493.

10 Long ER: Tuberculosis in Germany. Proc Natl Acad Sci U S A 1948;34:271–277.

11 Innes J: Pulmonary tuberculosis in wartime. Med Off 1946;75:61.

12 Wolters C: Tuberkulose und Menschenversuche im Nationalsozialismus. Das Netzwerk hinter den Tbc-Experimenten im Konzentrationslager Sachsenhausen [Tuberculosis and human experiments in national socialism. The network behind TB experiments in the concentration camp Sachsenhausen]. Stuttgart, Franz Steiner Verlag, 2011.

13 Lydtin K: Übersicht über das Tuberkulosegeschehen in Deutschland während des 2. Weltkrieges und in der Nachkriegszeit [the development of tuberculosis during war and post-war]. Munch Med Wochenschr 1950;92:62–71.

14 Meyer C: Die Entwicklung der Tuberkulose in Berlin [The development of tuberculosis in Berlin]. Beitr Klin Tuberk Spezif Tuberkuloseforsch 1951;105:408–428.

15 Klesse M: Beitrag zum quantitativ-exogenen Tuberkuloseproblem und Wege zur Feststellung des wirklichen Tuberkuloseverlaufs im zweiten Weltkrieg [contribution to the quantitative-exogeneous tuberculosis problem and ways to the appraisal of the real tuberculosis development in the Second World War]. Dtsch Gesh Wes 1946;22:688–695.

16 Ferlinz R, Schicketanz KH, Ferlinz C: Die Tuberkuloseentwicklung in Deutschland. Ein Vergleich zwischen der ehemaligen Bundesrepublik und der ehemaligen DDR[Development of tuberculosis in Germany – a comparison between former West and East Germany]. Pneumologie 1994;48:160–163.

17 Rieder HL, Cauthen GM, Comstock GW, Snider DE Jr: Epidemiology of tuberculosis in the United States. Epidemiol Rev 1989;11:79–98.

18 Comstock GW: Tuberculosis – a bridge to chronic disease epidemiology. Am J Epidemiol 1986;124:1–16.

19 Rieder HL: Epidemiologic Basis of Tuberculosis Control. Paris, International Union against Tuberculosis and Lung Disease, 1999.

20 Schaible UE, Kaufmann SH: Malnutrition and infection: complex mechanisms and global impacts. PLoS Med 2007;4:e115.

21 Cegielski JP, McMurray DN: The relationship between malnutrition and tuberculosis: evidence from studies in humans and experimental animals. Int J Tuberc Lung Dis 2004;8:286–298.

22 Bhargava A, Chatterjee M, Jain Y, et al: Nutritional status of adult patients with pulmonary tuberculosis in rural central India and its association with mortality. PLoS One 2013;8:e77979.

23 Brozek J, Wells S, Keys A: Medical aspects of semistravation in Leningrad (siege 1941–1942). Am Rev Sov Med 1946;4:70–86.

24 Leyton GB: Effects of slow starvation. Lancet 1946;2:73–79.

25 Anonymous: Statistical page. The war, tuberculosis and food. Tubercle 1945;26:58–59.

26 Hindhede M: The effect of food restriction during war on mortality in Copenhagen. JAMA 1920;74:381–389.

27 Christiansen J: Nutrition of Denmark during the war (Correspondence). BMJ 1938;1:1174.

28 Faber K: Tuberculosis and nutrition. Acta Tuberc Scand 1938;12:287–335.

29 Malmros H: The relation of nutrition to health; a statistical study of the effect of the war-time on arteriosclerosis, cardiosclerosis, tuberculosis and diabetes. Acta Med Scand Suppl 1950;246:137–153.

30 Bjartveit K: The tuberculosis situation in Norway. Scand J Respir Dis Suppl 1978;102:28–35.

31 Federhen L: Die Lungentuberkulösen eines Bevölkerungsgebietes von 350,000 Einwohnern während eines Zeitraumes von 1928–1951 [Pulmonary tuberculosis in a district with 350, 000 inhabitants during a period of time from 1928–51]. Beitr Klin Tuberk Spezif Tuberkuloseforsch 1955;114:110–120.

32 Kröger E, Reuter H: Entwicklung und gegenwärtiger Stand der Tuberkulose in deutschen und anderen Ländern [Development and present status of tuberculosis in Germany and other countries]. Dtsch Med Wochenschr 1949;74:721–725.

33 Edwards JH: Contribution of cigarette smoking to respiratory disease. Br J Prev Soc Med 1957;11:10–21.

34 van Zyl Smit RN, Pai M, Yew WW, et al: Global lung health: the colliding epidemics of tuberculosis, tobacco smoking, HIV and COPD. Eur Respir J 2010;35:27–33.

35 Murray JF, Buist AS: Respiratory disorders related to smoking tobacco; in Loddenkemper R, Kreuter M (eds): The Tobacco Epidemic, revised and extended ed 2. Basel, Karger, 2015, pp 72–84.

36 O'Leary SM, Coleman MM, Chew WM, et al: Cigarette smoking impairs human pulmonary immunity to *Mycobacterium tuberculosis*. Am J Respir Crit Care Med 2014;190:1430–1436.

37 Proctor RN: Chapter 3: War likes tobacco, tobacco likes war. Golden holocaust: origins of the cigarette catastrophe and the case for abolition. Berkeley and Los Angeles, University of California Press, 2011, pp 44–48.

38 Hanafin J, Clancy L: History of tobacco production and use; in Loddenkemper R, Kreuter M (eds): The Tobacco Epidemic, ed 2. rev. and ext. Prog Respir Res, Basel, Karger 2015;42:1–18.

39 Lin HH, Ezzati M, Murray M: Tobacco smoke, indoor air pollution and tuberculosis: a systematic review and meta-analysis. PLoS Med 2007;4:e20.

40 Lin HH, Suk CW, Lo HL, et al: Indoor air pollution from solid fuel and tuberculosis: a systematic review and meta-analysis. Int J Tuberc Lung Dis 2014;18:613–621.

41 Dhanaraj B, Papanna MK, Adinarayanan S, et al: Prevalence and risk factors for adult pulmonary tuberculosis in a metropolitan city of South India. PLoS One 2015;10:e0124260.

42 Rehm J, Samokhvalov AV, Neuman MG, et al: The association between alcohol use, alcohol use disorders and tuberculosis (TB). A systematic review. BMC Public Health 2009;9:450.

43 World Health Organization: Priority Research Questions for TB/HIV in HIV-Prevalent and Resource-Limited Settings. Geneva, World Health Organization, 2010.

44 Kerridge BT, Saha TD, Hasin DS: Armed conflict, substance use and HIV: a global analysis. AIDS Behav 2016;20:473–483.

45 Enarson DA, Rouillon A: History of the IUATLD. CDC TB Notes 2000;(No. 1):33–37.

46 Murray JF, Schraufnagel DE, Hopewell PC: Treatment of tuberculosis. A historical perspective. Ann Am Thorac Soc 2015;12:1749–1759.

Robert Loddenkemper
German Central Committee against Tuberculosis
Hertastrasse 3
DE–14169 Berlin (Germany)
E-Mail robert.loddenkemper@pneumologie.de

Murray JF, Loddenkemper R (eds): Tuberculosis and War. Lessons Learned from World War II.
Prog Respir Res. Basel, Karger, 2018, vol 43, pp 44–62 (DOI: 10.1159/000481474)

Nazi Medicine, Tuberculosis, and Genocide

Annette Finley-Croswhite[a] · Alfred Munzer[b]

[a]Old Dominion University, Norfolk, VA, and [b]Washington Adventist Hospital, Takoma Park, MD, USA

Abstract

This chapter explores the connections between Nazi medicine, tuberculosis (TB), and genocide. TB was deeply enmeshed in Nazi ideology of racial purity and viewed as a marker of genetic inferiority. In Germany in the 1930s, people with TB were stigmatized, prohibited from marrying, forced to undergo sterilization, and eventually euthanized in the so-called "mercy-killings." Once the war began, the Nazis used TB as a form of biological warfare. Nazi doctors euthanized TB sufferers throughout Germany and the eastern occupied lands or used TB as a convenient excuse to kill those they deemed "life unworthy of life," such as the Jews, whether they actually had TB or not. They conducted torturous medical experiments on children and adults in ill-conceived attempts to find a TB vaccine or effective TB medications. The Nazi state also stimulated TB epidemics. Crowded living conditions in the ghettos and camps, poor sanitation, and near starvation diets contributed to the spread of the infectious disease. When the Allies liberated the camps in Germany and Austria at the end of the war, TB was the most serious infectious disease they faced. This chapter argues that the Nazi state used TB as a justification for murder and targeted disease by eradicating people.

Disruptions caused by war and civil unrest led to an increased prevalence of communicable diseases during World War II (WWII), including tuberculosis (TB). The Third Reich diverted resources required for war that in peacetime might have been allocated to public health systems and used for diagnosis and treatment. The picture of TB in wartime was further complicated because the disease was deeply en-meshed, metaphorically and literally, in the Nazi ideology of racial purity. Adolf Hitler equated the Jews with bacilli and referred to them as the "racial TB of the nations" [1]. TB thus served as a metaphor for the "Jewish problem" that suggested aggressive means as a "solution." In *Mein Kampf*, Hitler expounded on this metaphor:

> It is no accident that man mastered the plague more easily than TB. The one comes in terrible waves of death that shake humanity to the foundations, the other slowly and stealthily; the one leads to terrible fear, the other to gradual indifference. The consequence is that man opposed the one with all the ruthlessness of his energy, while he controls the other with feeble means. Thus he mastered the plague, while TB masters him. [2]

The "aggressive means" led to the mass incarceration of Jews, Roma, Sinti (Gypsies), and other "undesirables" in ghettos and camps where crowded conditions, malnutrition and a lack of hygiene and medical care promoted the progression and transmission of TB and other infectious diseases. Death resulted from lack of treatment, starvation, and/or murder. Nazi ideology incorporated the eugenics movement with its focus on racial hygiene as central to public health and thus promoted TB as a marker of genetic inferiority legitimating stigmatization, sterilization, and even euthanasia of people afflicted by the disease. Nazi doctors and nurses also endorsed cruel medical experiments on human subjects including adults and children. Some of the experiments targeted TB using study subjects that the Nazis deemed undesirable such as the Jews and Roma or others considered genetically inferior as the result of physical or mental disabilities.

This chapter explores the connections between Nazi medicine, TB, and genocide, stressing that without WWII, the extermination of those the Nazis identified as *"lebensunwertes Leben"* or "life unworthy of life," would not have been possible because the war masked Nazi medical crimes and created subterfuge around sites where experimentation and death occurred [3]. The place of TB in the history of the Holocaust and WWII is also explored since German doctors and public health officials used the disease as a form of biological warfare. They justified victim experimentation and extermination as both public health research and disease control even while their racist beliefs and failed ethics stimulated TB epidemics in the ghettos and camps. The history of the medical application of TB to genocidal practices in WWII is not well integrated into Holocaust scholarship, however. Greater emphasis on disease and Holocaust has been given to typhus even though the literature on Nazi medicine and TB is substantial but usually focused on specific examples or included in generalized discussions of infectious disease in the ghettos and camps. This chapter broadens the historical understanding of TB and medical genocide by focusing on the interaction between perpetrators, victims, and liberators in the context of the disease, exposing the major impact TB had on the mass extermination practices of the Third Reich [4].

Nazi View of Medicine and Murder

Euthanasia and Racial Hygiene
In July 1933, barely 6 months after Hitler became Chancellor, the Law for the Prevention of Genetically Diseased Offspring was promulgated. It called for the forced sterilization of people with diseases and conditions ranging from mental retardation and physical deformity to schizophrenia and alcoholism. Between 1934 and 1939, an estimated 400,000 Germans were sterilized under the law, some without knowledge of what had been done to them [5]. In 1935, the Law for the Protection of the Genetic Health of the German People was passed that prevented individuals from marrying if they suffered from a variety of diseases deemed to be "genetic," including TB, despite evidence to the contrary. These laws were directed at what Hitler termed the Aryan population as a means of improving the overall health of the nation based on the principles of eugenics. Linking biology and heredity, the goal rendered those identified as "unfit" from passing on their defects via marriage and reproduction, thus regulating the Aryan gene pool and engineering what Hitler conceived as the ideal Nordic race [6].

While the measures in Germany went to extremes not contemplated elsewhere, the eugenics movement in the United States fostered similar beliefs in the role of heredity in diseases [7]. Early in the 20th century, American scientists correctly identified Huntington's chorea, pre-senile cataract and chronic familial jaundice as hereditary diseases. An additional group of diseases including epilepsy, manic depressive disorder, alcoholism, and cleft palate were felt to have their origins when a defective gene in one "normal" parent was combined with a similar defective gene from the other "normal parent" [7]. Soon the focus of the eugenics movement moved to "socially defective individuals" like the insane and mentally retarded, criminals, paupers, and the chronically ill, including those afflicted with TB. While Robert Koch's discovery of the *Mycobacterium tuberculosis* in 1882 had established that TB was an infectious disease that led to the modern public health movement with education as the principal means of controlling its spread, there continued to be a belief in the medical community that heredity played a major role in the transmission of TB. A respected TB specialist, S. Adolphus Knopf, for example, stated that TB parents transmitted a "physiological poverty to their offspring" [8]. Physicians were urged to advise their patients with TB not to marry. Some states refused marriage licenses to patients with TB. And starting in the 1920s, adherents of the eugenics movement in the United States advocated forced sterilization as a means of controlling the spread of TB. Joseph Spencer DeJarnette, the superintendent of Western State Hospital in Virginia, was one of the most powerful advocates for forced sterilization and was instrumental in the passage of the Virginia Sterilization Act of 1924, which served as a model for thirty other states, resulting in an estimated 60,000 forced sterilizations between 1924 and 1960 for a variety of conditions including TB [9]. The American example may well have influenced Nazi medicine in the 1930s.

Convinced that TB was propagated within families and weakened the German nation, Nazi Germany hijacked the public health system to screen the population for the disease by means of X-rays [10]. During the mid-1930's, pulmonary TB was the most prevalent infectious disease in Germany [11]. It was second only to cardiac and circulatory causes of death and was more common than cancer. The slow progression of the disease and the economic drain on families and society made it one of the most feared diagnoses one could receive. As early as the mid-1920s, a central radiologic registry was considered as a measure to detect early TB and prevent transmission of the disease. Registration of TB became mandatory in 1934 as part of the centralization of health care under the Third Reich. German doctors used mass screening for TB as an essential tool for the detection and control of the disease. Control did not mean treatment, however, but rather labeling patients with TB as genetically inferior. Patients with TB were stigmatized as socially unfit and burdens to society. Many were sent to psychiatric hospitals along with the mentally ill and the disabled, where beginning in the late 1930's, they were killed by starvation and neglect [4–6, 11].

An even more sinister motive for the mass screening of TB was to collect personal information to serve as a means for racial classification. Professor Hans Holfelder of the University of Frankfurt, for example, re-organized the *SS-Sanitätssturmbann* (SS Medical Service Unit), in 1939 to include the *SS Röntgensturmbann*, a comprehensive radiology battalion with X-ray equipment housed in buses for mobile mass screening. The official purpose of the battalion was the early detection and control of TB. The actual and more nefarious purpose, however, was to "to register the German *Volk* and other peoples by way of serial X-ray examinations in accordance with Prof. Dr. Holfelder's system" [12]. The screenings identified tubercular persons and further aimed to eradicate them by use of Nazi racial medicine. Using the ruse of a signature over illegibly small print, the SS devised the program to identify healthy young men who showed no signs of TB and who might otherwise have been drafted into the army but were instead recruited into their own ranks [12].

The popularity of the eugenics movement in Nazi Germany was tied in part to the fact that the medical profession embraced it and the Nazi party. Racial hygiene theory was already well established before Hitler's rise to power, but the creation of the Nazi state made the application of eugenics and its focus on racial medicine more acceptable. German doctors played a critical role in the initiation, administration, and execution of Nazi public health incorporating eugenics into health care policy. Physicians joined the Nazi party in greater numbers than any other profession; between 45 and 50% were members [13]. Stephen Post states, "Doctors were not unwitting victims, but rather active and responsible agents committed to hygienic theories that legitimized Nazi racial ideology" [14]. The April 13, 1933 issue of the *Deutsches Ärzteblatt*, the news organ of the German Medical Association, laid out Hitler's intentions "for cleansing of the nation and particularly the intellectual elite from foreign influence and contamination by alien races" [13]. Hitler stated, "What we have to do today is build a firm

foundation for the genetic development of the nation. German physicians are called upon to participate in this work through their scientific research, through their far-reaching education of the population, and through their practical assistance" (cited in [15]). Nazi physicians received special training in genetic pathology and eventually adopted the idea that euthanasia was the best means to rid the population of those considered "non-contributive mouths to feed," especially in times of war.

The euthanasia program began in 1939 prior to the war, first targeting severely handicapped children and transferring them to clinics where they were starved to death or killed by lethal injection. Known by the codename, "T-4," for the address in Berlin where the program's headquarters were housed, Tiergartenstrasse 4, it was headed by Karl Brandt, Hitler's personal physician and Philipp Bouhler, Head of the Führer's Chancellery and administered by Bouhler's subordinate, Viktor Brack. Brandt and Bouhler recruited numerous doctors and other medical personnel and nursing support staff into the program designed to use so-called "mercy-killings" as a way of creating more space in German hospitals and asylums for wounded soldiers [6].

No euthanasia law was passed, but Hitler issued a statement on his personal stationary endowing certain doctors in the Reich with the power to euthanize their patients. The process was done in secret because it involved murdering German citizens, although knowledge of the killings eventually leaked out. Doctors also signed forged death certificates, falsifying the causes of death [16]. When parents received notification of the death of their children, the reason given was often "TB" [17]. By October of 1939, the program had been extended to include adults as well, and special killing centers were designed at Brandenburg, Grafeneck, Bernberg, Sonnenstein, and Hadamar in Germany and Hartheim in Austria to ensure secrecy; some used carbon monoxide to kill patients, the first use of gas to exterminate victims in specially designed transport buses or gas chambers. While the assault on the Soviet Union was initially successful in June of 1941, it also drained resources and increased the need to free up hospital space, thus advancing euthanasia practices [4]. The expansion of the war also spread the practice of euthanasia into the German occupied lands. In June and July of 1941, for example, 583 patients from Slovenia were killed at Hartheim after being transferred from a psychiatric hospital in Novo Celje [18].

Public outcry eventually halted the euthanasia program briefly in August of 1941, but it resumed in 1942 and continued for the duration of the war based largely on the

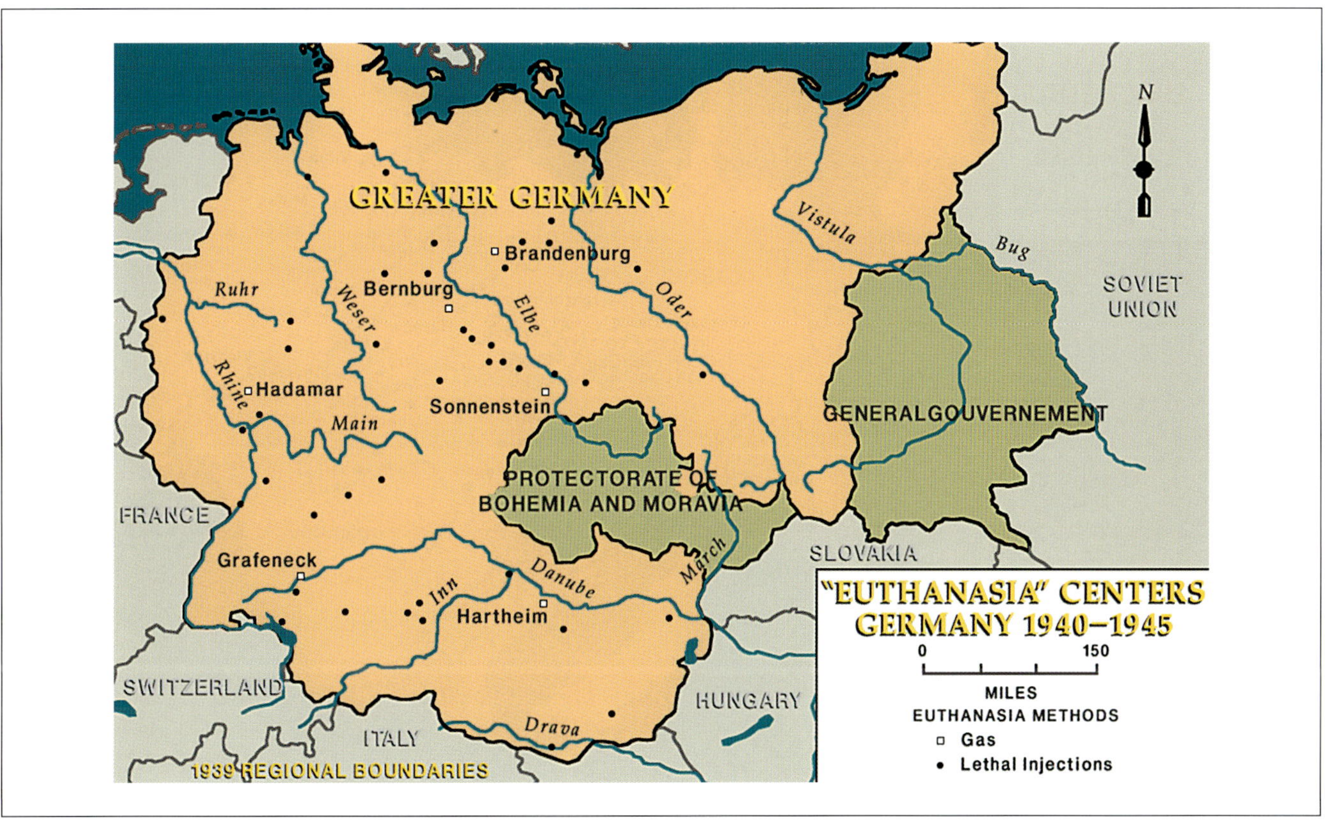

Fig. 1. Euthanasia centers in Germany, 1940–1945, courtesy of United States Holocaust Memorial Museum.

power bestowed on Nazi doctors to determine who to starve, poison or gas [4]. These unrestricted killings are often referred to in the scholarly literature as "wild euthanasia" when medical murder occurred in numerous institutions throughout the Reich (see Fig. 1), such as at Meseritz-Obrawalde in Prussia, where over 10,000 persons were euthanized by lethal injections after 1942 [19]. Following doctors' orders, it was the nursing staff at Meseritz-Obrawalde who administered the injections that killed these victims. In this period of "wild euthanasia," the support staff in many institutions murdered their patients or at the very least prepared the solutions the doctors injected. As the Germans moved into Poland and the Soviet Union, euthanasia was used on Polish and Russian asylum patients as well. In May of 1942, Arthur Greiser, Gauleiter of the German occupied Warthegau in western Poland, wrote to Himmler to ask permission to euthanize Poles with incurable TB [17].

The most notorious example of Nazi medicalized killing of people supposedly suffering from TB occurred at the Hadamar euthanasia center in Hesse between June of 1944 and March of 1945. Until that point only German nationals had been euthanized at Hadamar, a psychiatric clinic for the mentally ill that also included a "mixed-race" ward where forty-one half-Jewish German children were euthanized during the war [20]. Towards the end of the war, however, during a time when German manufacturing relied extensively on slave labor, 476 Polish and Russian prisoners including 16 children were sent to Hadamar probably from factories and workhouses in the surrounding area. All of them were euthanized by hospital staff a day or 2 after arrival, killed with injections of morphine or scopolamine and buried in mass graves behind the clinic. Their death certificates indicated they had died of TB, although it was later revealed that no physical examination of the victims had been made [21]. As part of the investigation surrounding the post-war Hadamar trial, US Army pathologist, Major Herman Bolker, examined the bodies of 6 of the victims exhumed for discovery purposes. In each case, Bolker found the victim to have been in relative good health before death. He determined they all died from lethal injection, and in only one body did he find what would have been active TB.

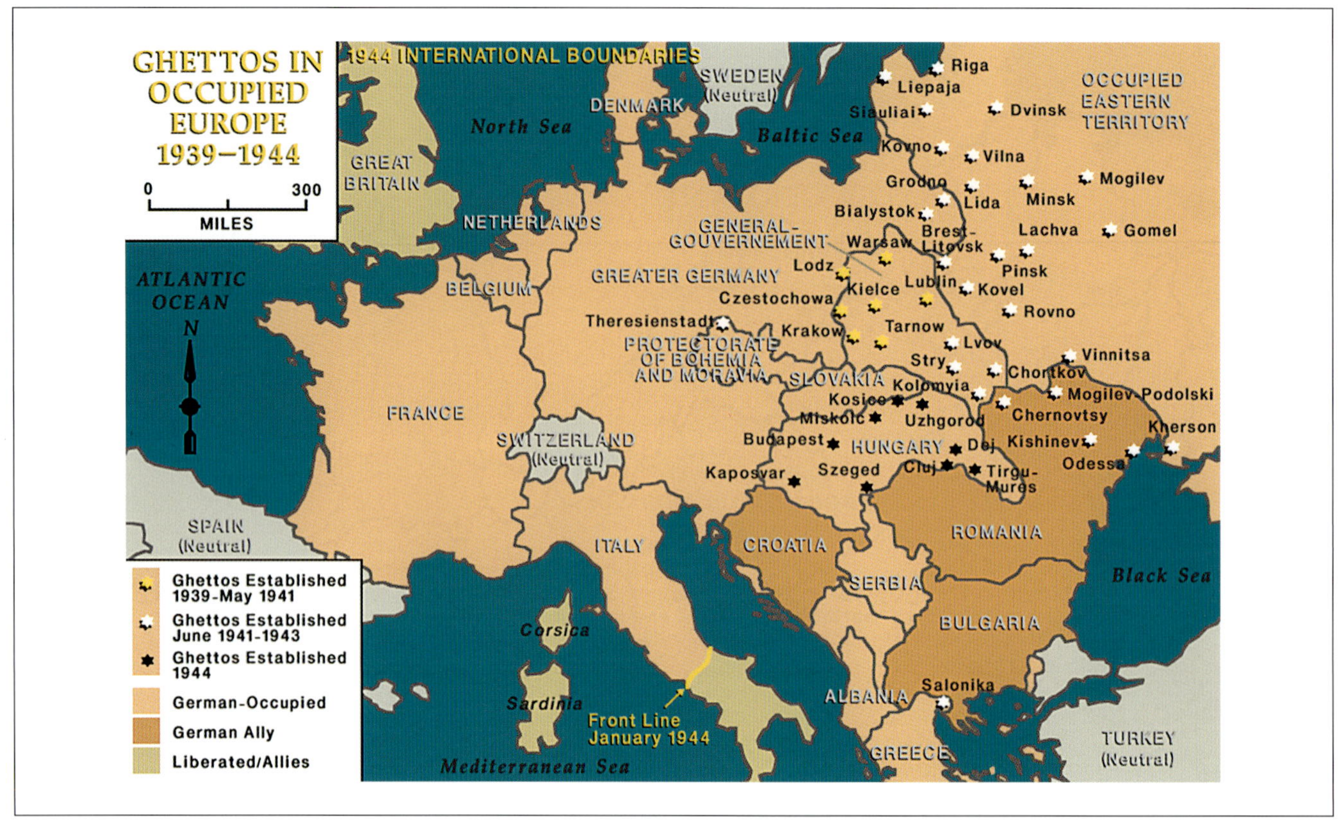

Fig. 2. Major ghettos in occupied Europe, 1939–1944, courtesy of United States Holocaust Memorial Museum.

As least 15,000 people were euthanized at Hadamar. The institution's reputation for killing was so well known that even the local children referred to the transports bringing victims to the clinic as the "murder vans" [22]. Evidence at the Hadamar trial revealed that the medical staff celebrated the extermination of their 10,000th victim with a small beer party, toasting their success over the deceased's body [6, 17, 21, 23].

T-4 doctors and planners also incorporated medical experimentation into the euthanasia program. Some of the most repugnant TB experiments were trials of the Bacillus Calmette Guérin (BCG) vaccine carried out on German mentally and physically disabled infants and children removed from their parents' homes under the guise of being sent to special treatment centers but actually destined for euthanasia. The BCG vaccine was developed in France by Drs. Albert Calmette and Camille Guerin from bovine TB weakened by 230 sequential subcultures and first tested on humans in 1921. A disastrous trial of the vaccine in Lübeck in 1930 in which a virulent TB strain was accidentally substituted for the attenuated strain resulting in the death of 72 of 251 immunized children led to a ban on the further use of the BCG vaccine in Germany [24–26]. In late 1941, however, the ban was partially lifted to permit Dr. Elmar Türk to conduct 2 series of experiments initiated by the Vienna University Pediatric Clinic and conducted at the Spiegelgrund children's euthanasia facility on 5 victims all under the age of 5 [24]. At first, Türk vaccinated one girl with BCG and then infected her and 2 other children with a virulent strain of *M. tuberculosis*. Three months later, the doctor repeated the experiment on 2 other children. One of the victims, a deformed infant named Günther Pernegger, was only 6 weeks old when the experiments began and survived only a few weeks of torture [27]. Türk subjected all of the children to painful procedures, euthanizing them afterwards by lethal injection, starvation or exposure so that he could proclaim the effectiveness of the vaccine from post-mortem examinations. He and pathologist Barbara Uiberrak extracted the brains and spinal cords of the victims to use in future research. Similar experiments on TB were conducted on sick or disabled children at pediatric centers in Berlin and elsewhere [28].

Ghettos and Segregation

Waystations to Genocide

When the Germans invaded Poland on September 1, 1939 and began WWII, they had not yet crafted a plan for the mass destruction of the Jewish population living in eastern Europe. Three weeks later Reinhard Heydrich, head of the *Reichssicherheitshauptamt* or the Reich Security Main Office, issued a directive implementing the movement of Jews living in small towns and villages in Poland to larger population centers in demarcated urban areas called "ghettos." Even so, Heydrich crafted no specific policy for ghettoization and as a result, their creation in Poland occurred for different reasons at different locations (see Fig. 2) [29]. Nazi officials battled over policy issues as some "productionists" favored profiting off cheap ghetto labor while radical "attritionists" pushed for more extreme measures to destroy the Jewish population through disease and starvation [30]. In short, the ghettos in Poland were not initially conceived as a logical step towards genocide, especially during the early days of the war when the Germans discussed not killing the Jews but resettling them somewhere, perhaps in Madagascar, an island off the coast of Africa.

In the summer of 1941, with the German assault on the Soviet Union in Operation Barbarossa, ghettoization procedures changed. The Germans created ghettos for the Jews in the Soviet Union who managed to escape the mass executions that occurred in the wake of the initial invasion as *Einsatzgruppen* or mobile killing units followed the German army and enacted "Holocaust by bullets" on over 1.5 million Jews [31]. In this context, the Nazis established ghettos in the newly occupied Soviet territories and the Baltic States as temporary solutions to planned mass extermination, and as a result these ghettos had a more limited existence, rarely exhibiting some of the common problems associated with those in Poland with longer histories. Nevertheless, the creation and swift liquidation of ghettos in the Soviet Union established a precedent for what became known as the "Final Solution of the Jewish Question" with the more radicalized policy of extermination, and thus led to the liquidation of ghettos in Poland as well. The Polish ghettos were then transformed into staging areas for genocide as deportations began to the major killing centers established first at Chełmno in 1941 and then at Sobibór, Treblinka, and Belzec in 1942 in the wake of the German assault on the Soviet Union. In total, the Germans created over one thousand ghettos in eastern Europe as well as a more limited number in central and southeastern Europe, all sites of Jewish destruction [29–32].

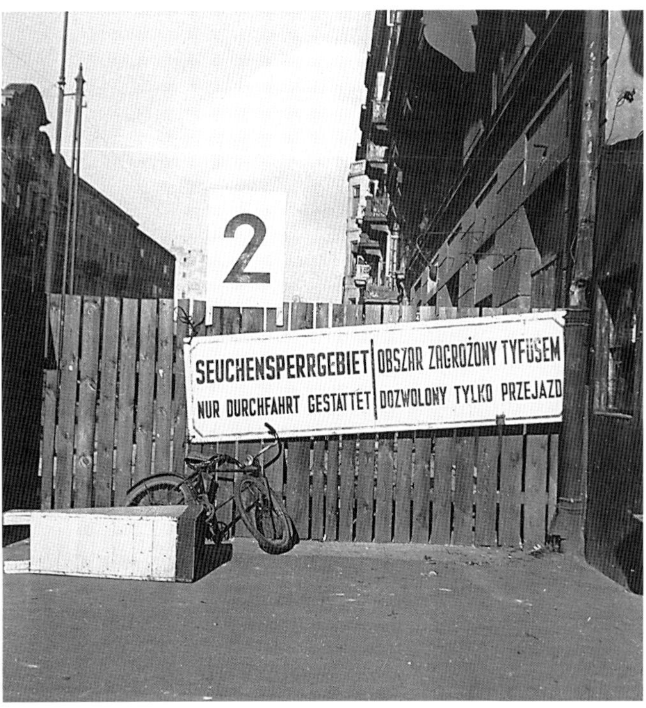

Fig. 3. Warsaw Ghetto: Sign reads: "Area closed because of epidemic. Only through traffic permitted. United States Holocaust Memorial Museum, courtesy of Guenther Schwarberg.

The large numbers of people moving into the ghettos, especially in Poland, led to overcrowding, starvation, and the outbreak of disease, a situation that the German-imposed Jewish Councils, known as *Judenräte*, established to oversee a variety of administrative and social welfare organizations including health services, never had the adequate resources to combat. One German rationale for the creation of ghettos was based on the racist belief that Jews were the carriers of disease, especially typhus, and TB. German propaganda conflated Jews with disease and identified them as "plague-boils" [29]. Many German doctors thus conceived ghettoization in part as a public health measure to protect the German and Polish populations from lethal epidemics that they argued the Jews spread. The Germans erected signs outside the ghetto walls stating: "Achtung! Seuchengefahr," or "Attention! Danger of Infection" or other similar warnings (Fig. 3). Conditions in the ghettos induced disease, a major ramification of the faulty German reasoning and one that ultimately led German authorities to seal the more populated ghettos [33].

The 2 largest ghettos were those at Warsaw, the Polish capital and center of Polish Jewry, and Lódz, 75 miles southwest of Warsaw. Other major Polish ghettos included

Kraków, Lvov, Lublin, Minsk, and Biaiłystok. The Lódz ghetto was sealed on May 1, 1940 enclosing over 220,000 Jews behind a wooden fence complete with barbed wire; the Warsaw ghetto sealed on November 16, 1940 trapped around 400,000 Jews behind a brick wall or 68,000 persons per square kilometer [34]. Refugees from other areas added to ghetto populations such as the 5,000 Roma sent to the Lódz ghetto in 1941. In the ghettos, multiple families were crammed into tiny rooms in dilapidated lodgings, most without heat, water, electricity, or plumbing. People with known cases of TB worked in the kitchens and factories actively spreading the disease. Food was severely rationed and there was never enough of it so that people without any way to make a living soon wasted away, especially in winter when many simply froze to death [32, 34]. The gaunt faces of TB victims became a common sight in the ghettos. Raul Hilberg estimated that 700,000 Jews died as a result of the harsh conditions of ghettoization or 13.7% of the 6 million killed in the Holocaust; the United States Holocaust Memorial Museum has raised the figure to 800,000 [35, 36].

Typhus is a central theme of ghetto histories even though TB was a serious problem. Squalid living conditions and lack of soap made a disease like typhus inevitable as it was spread by body lice and often epidemic in the ghettos. Authorities in the Warsaw ghetto registered 15,449 cases of typhus in 1941, for example, although historian and ghetto resident Emanual Ringelblum believed there were as many as an additional 4,000–5,000 unreported cases [36]. In terms of absolute numbers of victims, however, TB was likely far more widespread. TB was a common problem in eastern Europe before the war, with a death rate in Poland twice as high as that in Germany [39], (see Chapter 7). It is assumed that many persons carried latent TB in their bodies before the war, and poverty and starvation during the war caused immune systems to fail, which re-activated the disease. Crowded living conditions then stimulated epidemic TB turning it into a major killer [39]. Both chronic and acute forms of TB existed in the ghettos attacking children and adults alike. Isaiah Trunk indicates that in the 1930s, TB accounted for 8.3% of Jewish deaths, and this figure soared to 33.7% in the Warsaw ghetto by 1941 [37]. At least 50% of all those victims of infectious disease in the Lódz ghetto during 1940–1944 suffered from TB [40–42]. In 1943, Jewish doctors estimated that over 10,000 people had TB in the Lódz ghetto [43]. Dawid Sierakowiak, who kept a ghetto diary during this time and probably died of TB in 1943 wrote, "Lung disease (TB) is the latest hit in ghetto fashion; it sweeps people away as much as dysentery and typhus" [44].

Little reliable statistical data exist to track TB in the ghettos. There were never enough doctors and nurses to care for all the sick and those who did had little time to collect data; some of the material gathered by researchers in the Warsaw ghetto on hunger, disease, and TB did not survive the destruction of the ghetto in 1943. Medical professionals also often lacked the equipment such as X-ray machines with which to make accurate diagnoses or the time to conduct post-mortem autopsies to confirm causes of death. Many ill people never went to doctors, knowing they had few medicines for treatment. Others simply died in the streets with their deaths attributed to starvation when they very well might have had TB. Once the deportations began, sufferers of TB or those suspected of having it were often the first selected to be sent to the extermination camps [36]. In preparation for deportations to Chełmno in 1942 and speaking of the sick, including those with TB, Chaim Rumkowski, head of the *Judenrat* in Lódz, stated, "Give me these sick people, and perhaps it will be possible to save the healthy in their place" (cited in [45]).

Not all ghettos suffered from infectious disease to the extent of Warsaw and Lódz. The Vilna ghetto in Lithuania established in September of 1941 is noted for its resistance to Nazi oppression, and this resistance included vigorous attention to public health, which prevented typhus and TB from becoming an epidemic. Vilna was known as a center of advanced Jewish medicine before the war, and once the ghetto was established the *Judenrat* set up a Sanitation Commission and Epidemiological Section as part of the organization of public health. Through these entities, soup kitchens were opened, hot water was made available for washing and ghetto inhabitants needed proof of visiting a sanitation station to get daily food rations. Laundry facilities operated to sanitize clothing and quarantine was imposed when disease appeared. A TB station was also created to isolate known cases. Perhaps the Vilna ghetto was easier to manage because it only included 30,000 inhabitants. Nevertheless, creative public health helped to decrease the impact of TB and other diseases in Vilna before its liquidation in September of 1943 when the remaining inhabitants were sent to forced labor or death camps. Only a few hundred survived [46].

Defying all odds, inhabitants of other ghettos also addressed health problems with greater and lesser degrees of success. Jews in the Płońsk ghetto near Warsaw managed to set up a 2-story hospital with a forty-bed ward to treat patients with typhus and TB. Nevertheless, the Germans liquidated the Płońsk ghetto in the fall of 1942. The first transport that left on October 28 for Auschwitz consisted of the sick and elderly, including those with TB. Health care management in all of the ghettos was only a temporary solution to the epidemic outbreaks ghetto life stimulated. In the end, Nazi medicine eradicated the disease by eliminating human life [47, 48]. (For other comparisons, see [49]).

Concentration Camps

Disease Landscapes

There was no typical concentration camp (*Konzentrationslager* known as KZ or KL), during WWII although they all shared characteristics, and prisoners regularly faced death in all the camps. General readers often confuse the concentration camps with the death camps, although there were over 40,000 of the former and other incarceration sites inclusive of ghettos spread throughout Germany and the German occupied lands, and only 6 of the latter: Chełmno, opened in 1941 and the first mass gassing facility built; Belzec, Sobibór, and Treblinka, established in 1941–1942 under Operation Reinhard to exterminate Jews in the so-called *Generalgouvernement* of Poland; and, Majdanek and Auschwitz-Birkenau that operated as both labor and death camps. Auschwitz-Birkenau predated Operation Reinhard and was the largest of the camps comprising 3 enormous complexes and hundreds of slave labor subcamps. The Nazi state incarcerated over 2.3 million people in formal SS concentration camps between 1933 and 1945, where over 1.7 million died from a variety of causes including thirst, starvation, disease, exposure, arbitrary murder, experimentation, and extermination. Nearly one million were Jews killed at Auschwitz-Birkenau [50]. Approximately, 2 million more were killed by gas at the death camps, (Chełmno, Belzec, Sobibór, and Treblinka) most of them Jews. There were few survivors of the killing centers since most prisoners were murdered within hours of arrival, because Auschwitz-Birkenau was also a labor camp over 200,000 survived this camp. The camp system was never uniform and camps evolved over the course of the pre-war and wartime periods [36].

The concentration camps were first implemented as tools of political persecution to enforce political conformity after Adolph Hitler came to power; Dachau near Munich was the first to open its gates in 1933 and 5 other main camps were established in the 1930s. In Germany, these included Sachsenhausen, Buchenwald, Flossenbürg, and Ravensbrück, the latter for women prisoners, and Mauthausen in Austria. Beginning in 1936, the Nazi state sent persons identified as criminal or asocial to the camps and exploited prisoners for forced labor. Eventually the camp system was brought under the SS economic administration office known as the *Wirtschafts-Verwaltungshauptamt* or WVHA to manage the deployment of slave labor. This use of camp prisoners to boost the economy continued for the duration of the war just as territorial conquest brought a constant variety of people into the camps: Jews of various nationalities but also Roma and Sinti, German, Polish, and Soviet political prisoners, Communists and Socialists of various nationalities as well as homosexuals, Jehovah's Witnesses, and resistance fighters and POWs from all over Europe (Fig. 4) [24, 51–54].

After 1941, the war itself allowed the Germans to build their death camps in remote parts of Poland for the extermination of Jews and to dismantle most of them long before the war was over in an attempt to hide their crimes. Near the end of the war, the camp system collapsed as prisoner numbers grew in the Nazi state's desperate attempt to ramp up armament production through increased slave labor. But as the Allies advanced, camps were shut down and prisoners were sent on death marches back into Germany where camps like Bergen-Belsen in northern Germany were unequipped to handle the burgeoning prison population and massive death occurred. As such, the worst conditions in the camps came in 1944–1945 when overcrowding caused epidemic disease to soar and food became scarce in the final phase of Nazi genocide. The camp system was established in 1933 to create discipline and control in the Third Reich; it expanded throughout the war to institutionalize brutality, economic exploitation, and genocide ending in 1945 in complete chaos and exposing the Holocaust [51]. Overcrowding and starvation along with the filth of the camps made them breeding grounds for disease throughout the war. And disease threatened all the deportation camps in the occupied countries as well so that people often came into contact with TB before they were sent to the concentration camps. This early contact was especially true in occupied countries where no ghettos existed, but deportation camps were established to facilitate collection and transport to the East. Camps like Drancy (France), Westerbork (the Netherlands), and Mechelen (Belgium) were known for crowded conditions and TB [50, 52]. Due to elevated numbers of TB cases at the Drancy camp outside Paris in the fall of 1943, for example, a request was made for the installation of an X-ray machine to make more accurate diagnoses. In the end, the German authorities denied the request ensuring the spread of TB throughout the camp [54–56].

The T-4 euthanasia program is critical to understanding the escalation of murder in the camps during the war. Nazi doctors extended the T-4 euthanasia program into the con-

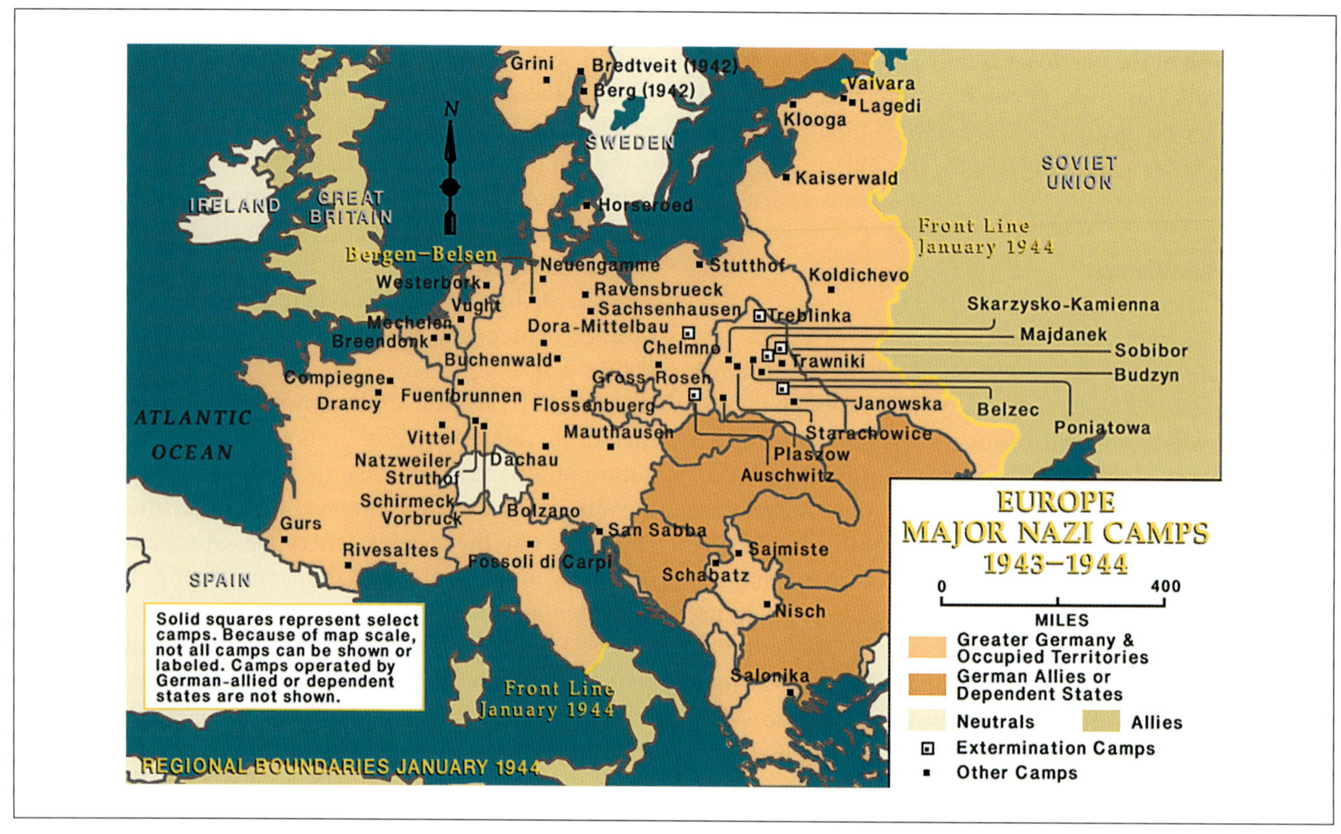

Fig. 4. Major Nazi camps in Europe, 1943–1944. Bergen-Belsen indicated, courtesy of United States Holocaust Memorial Museum.

centration camps in 1941, including the use of inmates in medical experimentation as part of the annihilation process thus establishing a direct relationship between euthanasia and genocide and revealing the key role medical personnel played in the "Final Solution." The T-4 killing project in the camps was given the code name 14f13 or officially "Operation Special Treatment," 14f being a prefix the Nazis created to indicate prisoner death, and "special treatment" gradually becoming the euphemism from this point forward for killing in general [50]. In the 14f13 program, Nazi doctors developed policies and processes that led to the death of millions, especially the 6 million Jews who died in the Holocaust [6].

The beginnings of 14f13 are tied to the history of the camp at Dachau in Germany [50]. In the summer of 1940, the Nazis used Dachau as a collection center for sick and invalid prisoners coming from other camps such as Sachsenhausen near Berlin and Buchenwald near Weimar. Due to the arrival of so many sick prisoners, Dachau quickly became overwhelmed by death and disease, and the other camps experienced only a temporary reprieve from high prisoner mortality. Nazi Police Chief Heinrich Himmler

toured Dachau in January of 1941 and soon after decided that the most logical solution to the epidemiological crisis was to send the experienced T-4 doctors into the camps. With Bouhler's approval, therefore, in the summer and fall of 1941 about a dozen T-4 psychiatrists made the rounds of the German and Austrian camps and began inspections, meeting with SS commandants and staff, studying prison files, evaluating prisoners, and inventing a process whereby prisoners determined too sick or weak to work, were dispatched to one of the euthanasia killing centers. To enhance the legitimacy of these medical killings, the T-4 doctors sent completed forms to Berlin on each prisoner selected for death, and SS guards accompanied the transports to the killing centers. Over 4,841 inmates from the Austrian camps Mauthausen and Gusen alone were euthanized during the war at Hartheim near Linz [57]. Originally intended for the sick and disabled only, many of the first transports from the camps to the killing centers included patients identified as having TB [58–61]. Before the end of 1941, however, the justification for killing was extended to those determined to be "social outsiders," a category most often reserved for the Jews. The Jews were especially vulnerable since German doctors also believed they were genetic carriers of TB. There was also interest in variances to susceptibility in different Jewish populations. By the autumn of 1941, therefore, Action 14f13 began to target more and more Jews and other racial minorities, and the T-4 doctors no longer bothered to make visual inspections but instead used racial profiling to determine selections. These measures preceded the Wannsee Conference held on January 10, 1942 in which the Nazi hierarchy met and formulated their plan to kill an estimated 11 million Jews in what they labeled the "Final Solution" [50].

The original 14f13 action lasted about twelve months and led to the murder of 6,500 prisoners in T-4 gas chambers, most killed with carbon monoxide. By the spring of 1942, however, the situation had changed as many of the T-4 doctors and administrators were transferred to the newly established killing centers in Poland at Belzec, Sobibór, and Treblinka to annihilate Jews after it had been determined at Wannsee that shooting them as was done in the Soviet Union was not cost effective. By then, the Camp SS men had also begun to initiate the murder process on their own without waiting for T-4 doctors to make decisions. In the summer of 1941, for example, the SS officials at Buchenwald felt overwhelmed by prison transports arriving with suspected cases of TB. In this environment, an SS doctor named Hans Eisele opted to kill the prisoners with lethal injections rather than wait for clearance from a T-4 doctor to send them to a killing center. During that summer, other SS doctors in numerous camps began using phenol injections in the heart to kill patients considered too sick or weak to work. TB patients were especially targeted for "special treatments." The so-called "invalid transports" to Dachau resumed, and the SS there used lethal injections and poison gas to exterminate the prisoners. Those in the medical blocks or TB patients in various camps were thus the most vulnerable in terms of selections for phenol injections, especially as camp infirmaries increasingly became murder sites [50, 51, 61]. Jay Lifton notes that the use of phenol on sick patients did not reduce the epidemic outbreaks in the camps, however, since prisoners realized quickly that going to an infirmary or doctor meant death and so avoided seeking medical assistance for any reason, thus exposing the general camp populations to infectious disease [6].

The completion of gas chambers at major camps like Auschwitz ended the use of phenol injections for mass murder, although it was continued as a procedure to conclude medical experiments on human subjects performed in the camps. By the end of the war, the 14f13 project resulted in the death of roughly 20,000 prisoners, a figure comprising killings that took place both inside and outside the camps. The T-4 operation overall accounted for more than 200,000 deaths, including the 14f13 victims and over 5,000 children. Moving the euthanasia program inside the camps, moreover, expanded methods of prisoner torture as SS doctors and SS staff experimented with killing methods and targeted diseased prisoners for murder. Eventually, the T-4 gas chambers were dismantled in the asylums in the West and reassembled in the death camps in the East, establishing another link between T-4 and the Final Solution. At that point, the camps became instruments of industrialized genocide when the killings reached proportions the euthanasia program could never have achieved. Six thousand people were murdered per day at Auschwitz-Birkenau at the height of the killing process [6, 51, 62].

Medical Ethics Unbound

Experiments in the Pathophysiology and Treatment of TB
During WWII, Nazi doctors discarded the fairly advanced medical ethical guidelines promulgated by the Weimar Republic in 1931 that protected the individual and replaced them with an ideology furthering the perverted primacy of societal good as defined by the Third Reich. Within a few years, Nazi medical ethics placing the state above the individual became part of the standard curriculum in all German medical schools [63]. In this context, Himmler realized that the concentration camps offered the perfect opportunity for medical research and he encouraged experimentation. Sound science, as the basis for experiments, was thus replaced by politics and anti-Semitism meaning that Jews from across all of Europe became experimental subjects. Other ethnic groups such as the Roma and Sinti were targeted for medical research as well as homosexuals, twins, dwarfs, and political prisoners of various nationalities, in particular the Poles. Much has been written about the variety of human experiments performed in the camps. Prisoners were injected with infectious diseases such as malaria, typhus, or yellow fever to study their effects in human blood or to search for a vaccine. Others were subjected to freezing temperatures in an attempt to better understand hypothermia. Prisoners were used as human test subjects in a variety of drug trials while more gruesome experiments involved castration and sterilization procedures. The best known medical experiments were those performed by Dr. Josef Mengele at Auschwitz on over 1,000 twins, who were in most instances only children. Death of the study subjects resulted in many experiments, and in the case of twins, if

one twin died during the experiment, the "control twin" was euthanized as well [22, 24, 28, 63]. Weindling estimates 4,364 prisoners died as a result of experimental science during WWII, while 23,395 survived horrific medical procedures tied to the medical depravity of the Third Reich [64].

Not surprisingly, TB was also a disease the Nazi doctors used prisoners to research. In 1941, a series of coordinated TB experiments began at Dachau, Sachsenhausen, and Buchenwald. In Sachsenhausen, 2 groups of camp prisoners followed different therapies in the medical research for a TB cure. Almost all of the study subjects died in the end. In Dachau, medical researchers performed a similar experiment using a homoeopathic therapy, although in this case orderlies injected research subjects with *M. tuberculosis.* The Buchenwald experiment tested the belief that breathing coal dust could cure TB. Some subjects received injections of coal dust extracts. At least 5 were killed and autopsied [11, 27]. During the same period, Friedrich Entress established a TB ward at Auschwitz to experiment with collapsing tubercular lungs. Once he mastered the technique, Entress murdered all the patients in the ward with phenol injections [6].

Josef Mengele also linked some of his twin research to TB. He arrived at Auschwitz in May of 1943 and soon began work on a TB project. Along with Otmar von Verschuer at the Kaiser Wilhelm Institute for Anthropology, Human Genetics and Eugenics, Mengele wanted to identify the genetic factors he believed caused resistance to certain diseases. This idea was a part of racial medicine predicated on the idea that some people were either more susceptible or less susceptible to disease. Mengele and von Verschuer researched elusive proteases called "defense enzymes" that they believed fought off TB. Mengele infected his study subjects with *M. tuberculosis* and sent the blood samples to von Verschuer in Berlin to test against dead TB bacteria. He and von Verschuer announced that they would isolate the sera of disease-resistant people and possibly cure TB, although the research was later proven to have been ill-conceived and fraudulently promoted. With some exceptions, the subjects of Mengele's experiments either succumbed to the infection that had been induced or were euthanized for the study of their organs [65].

Perhaps the most infamous experiment involving TB and the camps took place at Neuengamme, a subcamp of Sachsenhausen and at Hohenlychen, a sanatorium for TB patients outside Berlin [63]. During the Nazi era, part of Hohenlychen became a training center for athletes and a retreat for Nazi officials. The assistant-director of the institution and SS party member, Dr. Kurt Heissmeyer, proposed testing the already repudiated Kutschera-Aichbergen treatment of TB on patients from the Neuengamme concentration

camp [66]. In June of 1944, he began the experiments by driving the 104-kilometer journey to Neuengamme and bringing with him virulent tubercle bacilli he had obtained from Berlin. He began human testing on an unrecorded number of Polish and Soviet prisoners, several already quite ill with TB and tortured them by inserting a rubber tube down into their lungs. The therapy was based on a premise that advanced TB could be treated by artificially implanting TB in the skin to act as a vaccine. The experiment consisted of instilling *M. tuberculosis* into the trachea and injecting a suspension of tubercle bacilli under the skin of 4 groups of inmate-research subjects: inmates with known extensive bilateral pulmonary TB; inmates with unilateral pulmonary TB; inmates with extra-pulmonary TB; and inmates free of TB at the onset of the experiments. After 4 weeks of observing the spread of TB from the skin to the lungs, the inmate-subjects were anesthetized, then killed by hanging, and readied for autopsy. Heissmeyer repeated the process in November 1944 with 4 more inmates only to conclude that injecting tubercle bacilli into sick patients actually worsened their conditions [66].

Instead of accepting the negative results of these first trials and abandoning the experiment, Heissmeyer persisted and requisitioned twenty healthy Jewish children from Auschwitz to see if they were more likely to benefit from the Kutschera-Aichbergen treatment [27]. The children, aged 5–12, ten girls and ten boys originally from France, Italy, the Netherlands, Poland, and Yugoslavia, arrived in Neuengamme in November 1944. Heissmeyer made incisions in their arms and rubbed the incisions with tubercle bacilli. Within days the children developed local and constitutional symptoms. One week later, the doctor excised one lymph node from each child using only Novocain as a local anesthetic. He sent the nodes to Berlin where new cultures were grown from the lymph nodes. An emulsion of these cultures, specific for each child was then prepared, sent back to Neuengamme and injected bi-weekly in the same child where the lymph node had been. After 4–5 months, 80% of the children had pulmonary TB which turned cavitary by the 6th month. As the Allies approached in April 1945, Heissmeyer attempted to erase evidence of his terrible experiments and ordered the children to be taken to the Bullenhuser Damm school near Hamburg where they were injected with morphine and then hanged along with their 4 adult prisoner caregivers. The bodies were later taken back to Neuengamme for cremation [66].

The German pharmaceutical industry was also a driving force behind human experimentation during WWII, in particular the I.G Farben corporation (*Interessen-Gemeinschaft*

Farbenindustrie AG) that encouraged testing of a variety of drugs aimed at treating infectious diseases. I.G. Farben established a subsidiary called I.G Auschwitz Industries at the Auschwitz camp to try out new drug compounds. One of the SS doctors responsible for these experiments was also an I.G. Farben employee, Dr. Hellmuth Vetter. He experimented on inmates at Auschwitz to treat TB using a nitroacridine preparation called "3582" and "Rutenol," a mixture of 3582 with arsenic acid. Quite often the medication provoked vomiting in patients or bloody diarrhea when given as enemas. In July of 1943, working with the Bayer subsidiary of I.G. Farben, Vetter had twenty patients suffering from TB transferred to Block 20 in Auschwitz and treated with Rutenol. By the spring of 1944, 16 of the test subjects had died. Neither drug proved effective, although Vetter continued similar experiments at Mauthausen in Austria, and executives at Bayer encouraged him to stress the curative value of the drugs. I.G. Farben also manufactured the Zyklon B gas used at Auschwitz-Birkenau to exterminate nearly one million Jews [67].

Case Histories

Slave Labor and TB
The following case histories offer a glimpse into the personal experience of TB by camp victims. Simcha Minzer died of TB; Ruth Cohen was sent to a sanatorium after the war to recover. Both these cases reveal the connection between slave labor, the Nazi policy of "annihilation through work," and TB [68].

Simcha Minzer
Simcha (Siegfried) Minzer (Fig. 5) was the father of the co-author of this chapter, Alfred Munzer. Simcha's story derives from personal knowledge of the author and documents from the International Tracing Service. His case represents the likely reactivation of TB due to severe malnutrition.

Simcha was born on September 6, 1904 in Kanczuga, Poland. He immigrated to the Netherlands in 1926 and started a men's clothing business. He married Gisele Münzer in December 1932 and had 3 children, 2 girls born before the German invasion of The Netherlands and one son born after the invasion. The 2 daughters were hidden with a devout Catholic woman, but were denounced by the woman's husband and deported and killed at Auschwitz. Their son was rescued by a Dutch-Indonesian family and their Muslim nanny living in The Hague and survived the war. In January 1943, Simcha and his wife were deported to the transit camp

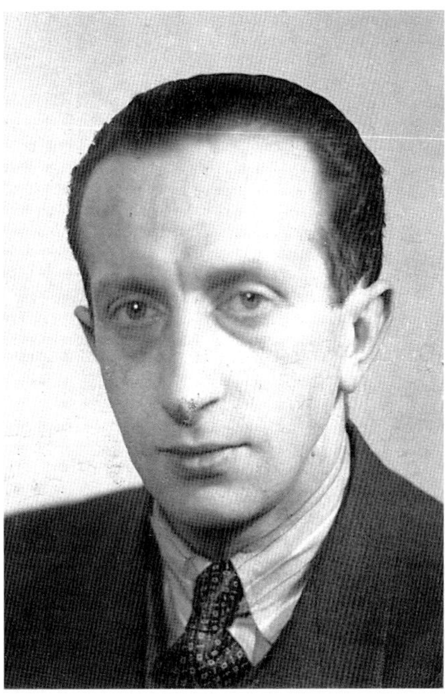

Fig. 5. Simcha (Siegfried) Minzer, before his deportation, courtesy of Alfred Munzer.

Westerbork, and shortly thereafter they were sent to do slave labor in Vught, the SS concentration camp in Holland that serviced northeastern Europe. From there Simcha and Gisele were deported to Auschwitz where they were separated. Gisele was assigned to do slave labor at the Telefunken factory in Reichenbach, eventually participated in the "death marches" as the German army retreated from Eastern Europe, and survived the war. Simcha remained in Auschwitz for 6 months where he performed slave labor at the IG Farben synthetic rubber factory. He was then sent to Mauthausen, Gusen, and Steyer concentration camps and finally to Ebensee in Austria continuing to do slave labor (see Fig. 6). In Ebensee, he worked on a project excavating underground tunnels created for the assembly of V2 rockets. He survived liberation by the US Army on May 6, 1945, but succumbed to pulmonary TB on July 25, 1945. His medical history prior to being imprisoned was entirely negative except for a hernia repair. Since Simcha was born in Poland, however, he probably had been infected with *M. tuberculosis* at a young age, like 80–90% of the Polish population (see chapter 7). Under the conditions of severe, debilitating malnutrition at Ebensee, his TB was reactivated and in the absence of treatment, it overwhelmed his immune system and led to his death.

The US Army Center for military history has documented the conditions of the Ebensee concentration camp on May 6, 1945 as witnessed by the 3rd Cavalry Reconnaissance Squadron [69]. Captain William O. Howk reported entering the town of Ebensee and hours later contacted his superiors with a key question. "There are 16,000 political prisoners in Ebensee…badly in need of food and med [sic] care. What shall we do about them…?" (cited in [69]). Ebensee was a subcamp of the Mauthausen concentration camp situated near Linz and established in late 1943. The camp's inmates had been put to work building underground tunnels. Food rations were poor and many inmates died of starvation, their bodies burned in a crematorium established in the camp. Conditions grew worse as transports arrived from other camps via trains and forced marches. The additional prisoners included Simcha Minzer. As the war effort collapsed, conditions deteriorated further and the camp's population tripled with inmates representing twenty different nationalities. There was virtually no food in the camp and according to US Army Records at liberation, "internees were dying of starvation at a rate of 300 daily" (cited in [69]).

On May 10, support arrived with the 80th U.S. Army, 30th Field Hospital (see Fig. 7), although it was already too late for Simcha Minzer whose TB was far too advanced and body too weak to recover. The Field hospital records state,

The unit rolled through the town of Ebensee on 10 May to discover the horror of the Concentration Camp. The place was a death camp for KZ-Mauthausen, the largest concentration Camp in Austria where prisoners came in to work excavating in the mountains. Most of the inmates were worked to death and resembled walking skeletons, and although the medical staff were more or less accustomed to illness, suffering, and even death, they were not only shocked but physically sick after their first view of the camp survivors. Most of the ex-inmates, emaciated survivors of the camp's inhuman regime, were still crammed in disease-ridden overcrowded barracks. [70]

Army doctors set up 3 hospitalization units and worked to try and save the Ebensee victims for 6 weeks in 1945 before transferring the remaining patients to a civilian hospital in Austria.

Ruth Cohen
Ruth Cohen (née Friedman; Fig. 8) is an example of the likely hematogenous spread of newly acquired TB due to crowded living conditions and malnutrition [71]. Ruth was born on April 26, 1930 in Mukachevo, then part of Sub-Carpathian Ruthenia, Czechoslovakia, now part of Ukraine. In 1939 Hungary, then an ally of Nazi Germany, annexed Sub-Carpathian Ruthenia as part of the dismemberment of Czechoslovakia. In spite of anti-Semitic legislation by the Hungarian government, Jews remained fairly safe until 1944 when

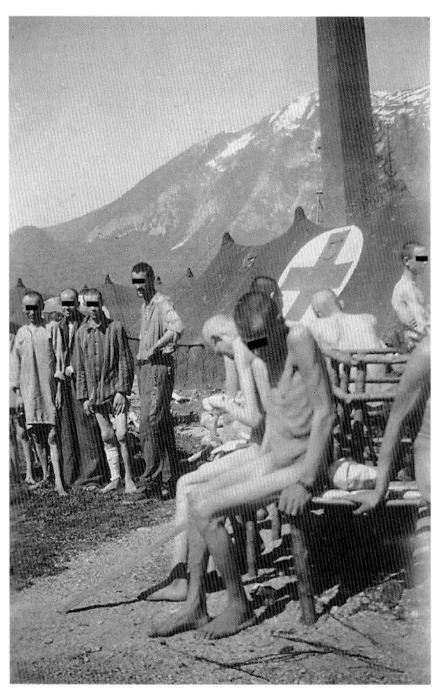

Fig. 6. Simcha Minzer's camp registration card at Mauthausen, courtesy of Alfred Munzer.

Fig. 7. Ebensee: A group of survivors outside tent set up by 30th Field Hospital. United States Holocaust Museum, courtesy of Lillian Pressman.

Germany invaded Hungary. Just before Passover in April 1944, Ruth and her family were ordered to move to the Munkács Ghetto. On May 15, all Jews were rounded up in the local brick factory and from there deported to Auschwitz. During the selection process on arrival in Auschwitz, Ruth's father and sister were sent right to the labor

Finley-Croswhite · Munzer

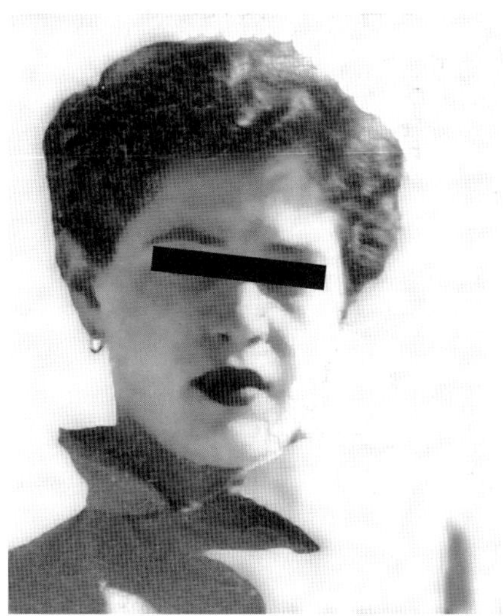

Fig. 8. Ruth Cohen (née Friedman), about 20 years old. United States Holocaust Memorial Museum, courtesy of Ruth Cohen.

camp while her mother, brother, and cousins were sent left to the gas chamber. Fortunately, a barrack's supervisor recognized Ruth and made her a messenger. At the end of November, Ruth and her sister were transferred to Nuremberg to work in a spool factory. While there Ruth developed excruciating back pain without any other symptoms. Because Nuremberg was under constant bombardment by the Allies, Ruth and her sister were moved to Holleischen concentration camp in Bohemia near Pilsen (Czechoslovakia) to work in a similar metallurgical factory. By February 1945, the pain was so excruciating that Ruth could no longer work.

Holleischen was liberated in May 1945 initially by Polish partisans, then the US Army, and one month later Ruth and her sister returned to Mukachevo where they were reunited with their father. Ruth's back pain persisted and she was admitted to the Budapest Children's Hospital where doctors diagnosed her with a "congenital anomaly" of her spine. She was prescribed bedrest without any improvement. She then went to the Jewish Hospital in Bratislava where "an abscess" was drained from her back and the diagnosis of TB of the spine was established. She was placed in a long cast for 6 months and remained in the hospital for one year before she was transferred to a TB sanatorium. Ruth had been in excellent health prior to her deportation and had no known contact with TB. Chances are she came into contact with the disease in Auschwitz or Holleischen or in her role as a slave laborer in Nuremberg. Ruth recovered from TB and immigrated to the United States in 1948 where she lived first in New York City and later in Washington, D.C. [72].

Horror Camps

TB and Liberation

Although freedom was the dream of all camp inmates, liberation itself created a unique set of challenges for camp populations, and what preceded liberation often put prisoners in the most disease-ridden environments of the whole war [73]. In late 1944, when it was clear that Germany was losing, Himmler ordered camp officials to empty the camps in the East by moving hundreds of thousands of prisoners, POWs, and forced laborers back towards Germany inclusive of Jews and people of all nationalities. In this situation, often the sick in the camp hospital blocks were merely shot or abandoned to fend for themselves. By that point, most of the killing centers had been shut down; Belzec and Sobibór were dismantled in 1943 and Chełmno and Treblinka in 1944 once the murder of Jews in the surrounding areas was complete. The camp grounds were plowed over to cover the crime scenes; in the case of Belzec, the Nazis erected a manor house on the site of the notorious camp to camouflage it as a farm. The Red Army liberated Majdanek in July of 1944 and took Auschwitz-Birkenau in January of 1945, but by that time the camps had largely been abandoned by their SS guards and prison populations. In mid-January of 1945, for example, before the Soviets arrived, SS guards evacuated around 65,000 prisoners from Auschwitz-Birkenau, about one half of them Jews, to camps like Buchenwald, Dachau, Bergen-Belsen, and Mauthausen in the West [50].

As the concentration camp system collapsed, these death marches presented prisoners with some of the most difficult situations of the war as they walked and sometimes rode in open trains or trucks enduring horrible cold or heat with little or no food to sustain them and few clothes or shoes to protect them from the elements. The death marches turned prison populations into mobile camps. Guards used extreme brutality to keep a murderous pace and shot prisoners who fell behind. Others died along the way of hunger, disease, and exhaustion. The arrival of these prisoners flooded the camps in Germany and Austria with greater numbers of sick and starved persons adding to the chaos and deprivation of war's end. As the Germans retreated further into Germany itself, prisoners on the death marches were moved from one camp to another, their unwell numbers dwindling with each transfer as so many succumbed to death. In the spring of 1945, thousands and thousands of bodies lined retreat routes, visual testimony to the end of the camp system. When the Americans liberated Dachau on April 29, 1945, one of the most appalling sights they encountered was a train load of 2,000 corpses, the bodies of prisoners transferred 3 weeks earlier from Buchenwald who did not survive the journey and were left to rot in the boxcars. It is estimated that 250,000 to 275,000 people died in the death marches. Tens of thousands more perished in the weeks after liberation due to their pitiful physical conditions that the liberators could not restore. The survivors of Bergen-Belsen, for example, had been living on less than 800 calories a day since January of 1945 consisting of 200 g of rye bread and a bit of soup made from a beet root generally reserved for cattle-fodder. Even these stores had been depleted by the time the Allies arrived on April 15 [50, 61, 73–75].

The camps liberated by the Western Allies exposed scenes of utter horror in which the camp populations were either dead or dying. Belsen (see Fig. 4) was the largest of the concentration camps liberated in the West with about 57,500 prisoners in 2 camps when the Allies marched in and up to 10,000 corpses that needed immediate burial (see chapter 5). Descriptions of the British first encounter with Belsen in April 1945 are well known. British military photographers captured images of severely emaciated bodies being bulldozed into mass graves that were then broadcast around the world. In time, these pictures of Belsen's liberation became iconic emblems of the crimes against humanity [76]. Weindling calls Belsen a "medical calamity" presenting a "lethal cocktail of diseases" including a minimum of 3,500 cases of typhus, 10,000 cases of severe malnutrition, 20,000 cases of dysentery, and 10,000 cases of TB [77]. One nurse sent to Block 61 of the immense Belsen complex reported that 90% of her patients suffered from TB (cited in [78]).

The horror the Allies experienced at Belsen was repeated in camp after camp, large and small, each riven with filth and disease, some covered in layers of excrement that reached the tops of the soldiers' boots [76]. Liberators consistently remarked on the nauseating smell of the camps that reached their noses long before they saw the sources with their eyes, barren landscapes mired in mud and rotting bodies, the emaciated victims still alive often naked and covered in vermin. Gunskirchen Lager, for example, was a subcamp of Mauthausen. Major Cameron Coffman and the U.S. 71st Infantry Division liberated it on May 4, 1945. The camp held around 15,000 prisoners, mostly Hungarian Jews and German Austrian, Czech, and Yugoslavian political prisoners. By the time the Americans arrived, none of the prisoners had had any water for 4 days and several hundred bodies were stacked in piles around the camp. Coffman observed: "The living and the dead, evidence of horror and brutality beyond one's imagination [were] there, lying and crawling and shuffling in stinking, ankle-deep mud and human excrement" [79]. Decades later, Bill Jucksch, another American

solider at Gunskirchen Lager that day remembered, "When I went into one building there was a stack of bodies over at the end one on top of another, stinking…all their waste, all their bowel movements, everything was right there" [80].

While the camps were cleaned and disinfected, the Allies established evacuation hospitals to care for the sick. Doctors and nurses confronted enormous problems, especially trying to re-feed persons who had been starving for so long [75]. Even so, infectious disease was their greatest fear. The TB cough was a constant sound that echoed throughout the hospital wards. The 131st Evacuation Hospital attached to the 11th Armored Division of Patton's Third Army brought medical care to Mauthausen and the subcamps of Gusen 1 and 2. The unit history of the 131st confirms the crisis tied to infectious disease. "We found this to be a typical German concentration camp with victims dying rapidly from the lack of food, TB and typhus. The TB cases were the biggest problems" [81]. Mauthausen was anything but typical, however. A slave-labor camp tied to the surrounding stone quarries, by March of 1945 the main camp and its subcamps held 84,000 prisoners. At that point, Mauthausen had become a depot for prisoners in transit at the end of the war, those coming from Auschwitz, Sachsenhausen, and Gross-Rosen on death marches [58]. Franklin Clark who liberated Mauthausen observed, "The people were more dead than alive. I remember seeing one, it looked like a pile of rags on the floor, but it was actually a man" [82].

Once the Americans took over the camp on May 5, 1945, Mauthausen and its subcamps held around 28,000 prisoners, 5,000–6,000 in serious need of medical attention [81]. The doctors of the 131st Evacuation Hospital went to work immediately setting up hospital wards, although they kept their nurses away for days because they believed the situation was too unsanitary and dangerous. They erected a 1,500-bed hospital, but it was hardly enough, and this main hospital was supplemented by a 600-bed female hospital and a number of tent hospitals. Eventually a large warehouse and former SS barrack were converted into hospital wards. While the medical records speak of TB, the most common diagnosis made at Mauthausen was severe malnutrition [81]. On May 18, 1945, for example, the doctors of the 131st recorded the medical situation of 1,095 admitted patients. They identified 1,048 as having "severe malnutrition," while 47 others were diagnosed with a variety of other specific illnesses, enterocolitis being the chief problem along with eleven cases of typhus and 6 cases of TB.

The doctors knew, however, that when they had time to X-ray many of the malnourished patients that they would find TB [81] (see Fig. 7). At Buchenwald, for example, where

1 in 10 of the 21,500 prisoners suffered from TB, Army medical officer Abner Zehm wrote, "The conditions under which the prisoners lived were conducive in every way to the development and spread of TB " (cited in [74]) [60, 61] (Fig. 9).

Lack of food and harsh working conditions activated TB in prison populations, while poor ventilation in crowded barracks and factories ensured its spread. X-rays of 2,267 patients at Dachau revealed that 30% showed signs of TB while 6% of those admitted to Belsen's evacuation hospitals were diagnosed with the disease, although medics speculated that many others had already died of it [74, 83]. In fact, it was quite routine for newly liberated prisoners and displaced persons to suffer simultaneously from a variety of diseases and health problems, malnutrition and TB being the 2 most common to present in tandem [74]. Such misery meant that many victims who survived the liberation, like Simcha Minzer, did not live long thereafter. Of the 21,500 prisoners liberated at Buchenwald, for example, 4,700 died within the first month even with doctors and nurses doing everything they could to try and save them [60]. And for those victims of TB who did survive, like Ruth Cohen, many faced long periods of convalescence and compromised health for years to come. The end of the war did not, after all, put an immediate end to TB. In many instances, TB followed survivors for the rest of their lives, the most profound reminder inside their bodies of the Nazi deployment of medical genocide during WWII [77, 84].

Crimes against Humanity

Post-War Trials

At the end of the war, a number of post-war trials defined and prosecuted what came to be known as "crimes against humanity," tackling difficult questions about individual responsibility during wartime. The Americans, for example, took the town of Hadamar in April of 1945 and stumbled on the euthanasia center where Nazi doctors used false diagnoses of TB to legitimize the murder of patients at the institution (Fig. 10).

The Hadamar trial opened in October 1945 and was the first of many mass atrocity trials. American judges prosecuted 7 members of the medical staff at Hadamar including the head nurse, Irmgard Huber. Three of the 7 including the head doctor were sentenced to death by hanging and 4 others received significant jail time. Huber was sentenced to 25 years, one of the few women convicted of war crimes, although she was released in 1953. The International Tribunal at Nuremberg also conducted a Doctors' Trial in 1946–7 that

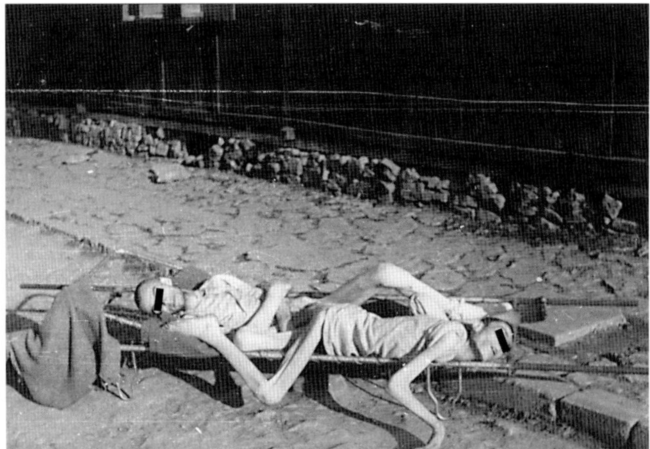

Fig. 9. Buchenwald, April 1945. Photo belonging to U.S. Army medic John E. Chapman of the 120th Evacuation Hospital. Given to Annette Finley-Croswhite by Chapman's son, Dr. Thomas Chapman.

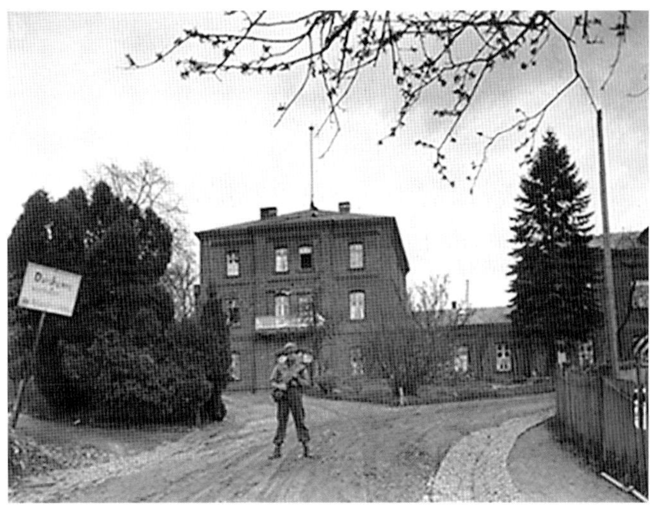

Fig. 10. An American soldier stands guard in front of the Hadamar Institute, April 5, 1945. United States Holocaust Memorial Museum, courtesy of Rosanne Bass Fulton.

led to the conviction of 23 German doctors and T-4 administrators [22]. Sixteen received sentences and 7 were hanged including T-4 chief administrator, Karl Brandt (Fig. 11).

That same year, 24 executives from I.G. Farben were also prosecuted at Nuremberg for crimes against humanity inclusive of experiments on prisoners, although the sentences were lighter and thirteen were acquitted of wrongdoing. The Allied powers held other trials and many other nations that Germany occupied, like Poland, also conducted trials in the post-war years; however, the Cold War ended the most vig-

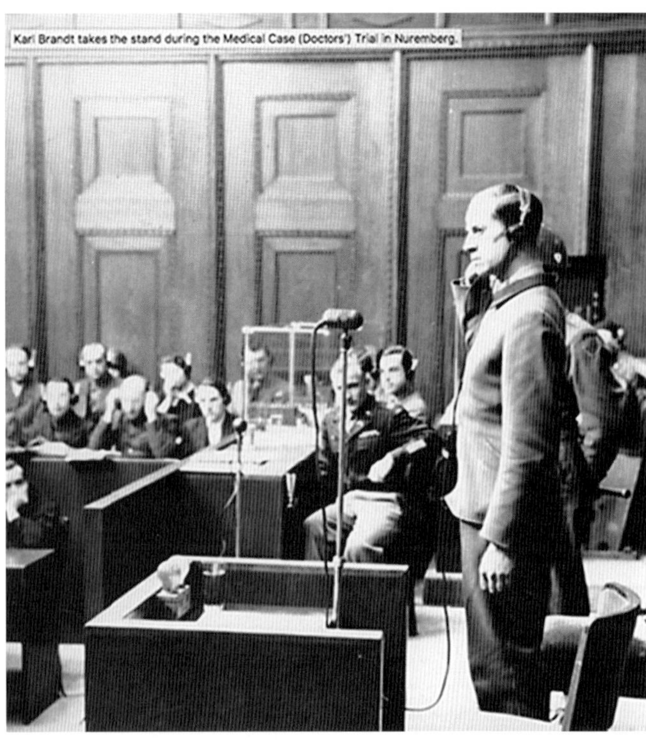

Fig. 11. Karl Brandt takes the stand at the Nuremberg Doctors' Trial. United States Holocaust Memorial Museum, courtesy of Hedwig Wachenheimer Epstein.

orous prosecution, and many Nazi doctors, nurses, and other health care professionals thus escaped prosecution and went back to practice medicine in the post-war world [67, 85, 86].

The scarcity of medical resistance to the Nazi regime has been explored, but remains a troubling mystery [87]. The only medical publication that has been identified as opposing the Nazi regime was the International Medical Bulletin published in Prague by the International Medical Union, a successor to an earlier organization, the Socialist Medical Association. Karl Friedrich Rittmeister was a psychiatrist who was the co-author of leaflets that were distributed by him and a handful of other physicians that described the torture and atrocities of the Third Reich. He was caught, imprisoned, and then executed on May 13, 1943.

As part of the judgment in the case of the Doctors' Trial, the International Tribunal issued a ten-point set of rules that became known as the Nuremberg Code [88]. These rules for the conduct of medical research drew on the guidelines that had been promulgated by the pre-Nazi, Weimar Republic but had been discarded during the Nazi era. The Nuremberg Code, like the subsequent United Nations Universal Declaration of Human Rights, was a foundation stone of the mod-

ern democratic state and a milestone in the advancement of medical ethics focused on human rights. In 2017, the "Galilee Declaration" was published [89]. Produced by 140 scholars from 17 countries during the Second International Scholars Workshop on "Medicine in the Holocaust and Beyond" held in Israel in May 2017, it is the most recent attempt to bring the lessons of the Holocaust to the medical and scientific professions. "The Galilee Declaration" calls on all institutions of higher learning in the medical sciences and allied fields to develop curricular programs on medicine and the Holocaust to undergird critical discussions of ethics and medical practice.

Conclusion

TB and the Final Solution

Figuring out an accurate number for how many people lost their lives to or suffered from TB because of the unethical medical practices of the Third Reich is probably an impossible task. So many deaths from TB went unrecorded, and there is no way to know how many TB victims acquired the disease in the ghettos and work camps but were exterminated in the gas chambers, their numbers later tallied as victims of genocide but not necessarily as sufferers of TB. Statistics taken from the camp hospitals are useless in this regard because so often TB was employed as a convenient diagnosis to murder whether the victims had the disease or not just as deformed and mentally ill patients were often euthanized under false diagnoses of TB. In addition, so many victims died in the final days before liberation, creating such chaos and epidemiological crises at the end of WWII that countless sufferers of TB were buried in mass graves in which the specific causes of their deaths went undocumented.

What the history of Nazi medicine and TB so clearly reveal, however, is the way in which Nazi doctors and health professionals used the disease to promote a racial agenda that led to genocide. As the war expanded, more and more opportunities existed for the Third Reich to stimulate TB epidemics. Ethnic cleansing via genocide was conceived as science, and TB became a powerful weapon in the Nazi biological wartime arsenal. Predatory medical staff also engaged in torturous experimentation on human beings suffering from TB; many victims contracted the disease through exposure as human test subjects. The war increased the risk of infection from TB, especially in 1944–1945 when many of the camps in Germany and Austria were overcrowded following the death marches as the KZ system collapsed. TB was a disease that Nazi science did not try to eradicate for public good but rather one they used to justify murder.

The Nazi medical profession's ready acceptance of ethical guidelines that substituted the interests of the state and racist ideologies for those that primarily protected the individual led to the practice of targeting disease by killing people. Medicalized brutality and torture are legacies of the Nazi era and part of the history of the Holocaust. The ghetto and concentration systems developed by the Nazi state spread many diseases; TB was especially deadly. TB was incorporated into the implementation of "Final Solution" and became intricate to the Third Reich's exploitation and extermination of victims on a manufactured disease landscape, one that linked health, race, destruction, and ultimately, genocide.

References

1 Jäckel E, Kuhn A (eds): Hitler. Sämtliche Aufzeichnungen 1905–1924, Stuttgart, Deutsche Verlags-Anstalt, 1980.

2 Hitler A: Mein Kampf, Manheim R (Trans), Boston, Houghton and Mifflin Company, 1971.

3 Bergen DL: War and Genocide: A Concise History of the Holocaust, ed 3. New York, Rowan & Littlefield, 2016.

4 Friedlander H: The Origins of Nazi Genocide: From Euthanasia to the Final Solution, Chapel Hill, University of North Carolina Press, 1995.

5 Proctor R: Racial Hygiene: Medicine Under the Nazis. Cambridge, Massachusetts, Harvard University Press, 1988.

6 Lifton R: The Nazi Doctors: Medical Killing and the Psychology of Genocide. New York, Basic Book, 1986.

7 Wilson PK: Confronting "Hereditary" Disease: Eugenic Attempts to Eliminate Tuberculosis in progressive era America. J Med Humanit 2006;27: 19–37.

8 Lerner BH: Constructing medical indications: the sterilization of women with heart disease or tuberculosis, 1905–1935. J Hist Med Allied Sci 1994; 49:362–379.

9 Bruinius H: Better for All the World: The Secret History of Forced Sterilization and America's Quest for Racial Purity. New York, Vintage Books, 2007.

10 Moser G: Tuberkulosebekämpfung zwischen "Volksröntgenkataster" und SS-Röntgensturmbann. Fortschr Röntgenstr 2014;186:329–333.

11 Wolters C: Tuberkulose und Menschenversuche im Nationalsozialismus. Stuttgart, Franz Steiner Verlag, 2011.

12 Schmidt M, Winzen T, Gross D: The SS x-ray unit as an instrument for "total registration" and "race selection." Strahlenther Onkol 2015;191:437–441.

13 Haque O, De Freitas J, Viani I, Niederschulte, B, Bursztajn, H: Why did so many German doctors join the Nazi party early? Int J Law Psychiatry 2012;35:473–479.

14 Post S: The legacy of racial hygiene: hearing the voice of the victims. Soundings An Int J 1991;74: 541–558.

15 Hanauske-Abel HM: Not a slippery slope or sudden subversion: German medicine and national socialism in 1933. BMJ 1996;313:1453–1463.

16 Freidl W, Poier B, Oelschläger T, Danzinger R: The fate of psychiatric patients during the Nazi period in Styria/Austria: part I: German speaking Styria. Int J Ment Health 2006;35:30–40.

17 Kessler K: Physicians and the Nazi Euthanasia Program. Int J Ment Health 2007;36(1) The Holocaust and the Mentally Ill: Part III Euthanasia, 4–16.

18 Slavko Z, Zdenky CT, Zvonka Z: The extermination of psychiatric patients in patients in occupied Slovenia in 1941. Int J Ment Health 2007;36(1) the holocaust and the mentally Ill: part III Euthanasia: 99–104.

19 Benedict S, Chelouche T: Meseritz-Obrawalde: a "wild euthanasia" hospital of Nazi Germany. Hist Psychiatr 2008;19:68–76.

20 Kaelber L: The Hadamar "Mixed-Race Ward" Mischlingsabteilung in Nazi Germany: Persecution, Fate, and Memory of Jewish Mischlinge and Their Parents. Bulletin of the Carolyn and Leonard Miller Center for Holocaust Studies. 2014 (Spring); 9. https://www.uvm.edu/~lkaelber/CHS-BULLETIN.2014-Kaelber.pdf (cited August 11, 2017).

21 Kintner EW: The Hadamar Trial, London, William Hodge and Company, 1948.

22 Mitscherlich A, Mielke F: Doctors of Infamy: The Story of the Nazi Medical Crimes. Norden H (trans): New York, Henry Schuman, 1949.

23 Noakes J, Pridham G (eds): Nazism 1919–1945, vol 3, Foreign Policy, War and Racial Extremism, Exeter, Exeter University Press, 1984.

24 Dahl M: Behinderte Kinder als Versuchsobjekte und die Entwicklung der Tuberkulose. Medizinhist J 2002:37:57–90.

25 Rieder HL: Die Abklärung der Lübecker Säuglingstuberkulose. Pneumologie 2003;57:402–405.

26 Moegling A: Die "Epidemiologie" der Lübecker Säuglingstuberkulose. Arbeiten aus dem Reichsgesundheitsamt 1935;69:1–24.

27 Weindling P: Victims and Survivors of Nazi Human Experiments: Science and Suffering in the Holocaust. New York, Bloomsbury, 2015.

28 Czech H: Abusive Medical Practices on "Euthanasia" Victims in Austria during and after World War II; in Ruberfeld S, Benedict S (eds): Human Subjects Research after the Holocaust. Heidelburg, Springer International Publishing Switzerland, 2014, pp 109–125.

29 Browning CR: Before the "Final Solution" Nazi Ghettoization Policy in Poland (1940–41) in Ghetto 1939–1945: New Research and Perspectives on Definition, Daily Life, and Survival, Symposium Presentations, Washington, DC, United States Holocaust Memorial Museum, 2005, pp 1–14.

30 Browning CR: Introduction; in Dean M, Hecke M (eds): Encyclopedia of the Camps and Ghettos, 1933–1945, Volume II, Ghettos in German-Occupied Eastern Europe, Bloomington and Indianapolis, Indiana University Press, 2012, pp xxvii–xxxix.

31 Desbois P: The Holocaust by Bullets: A Priest's Journey to Uncover the Truth Behind the Murder of 1.5 Million Jews. New York, St. Martin's Griffin, 2008.

32 McDonough F, Cochrane J: The Holocaust, New York, Palgrave Macmillan, 2008.

33 Browning CR: Genocide and public health: German doctors and the polish jews, 1939–41. Holocaust Genocide Stud 1988;3:21–36.

34 Fein H: Genocide by attrition 1939–1993: the Warsaw ghetto, Cambodia and Sudan: links between human rights, health, and mass death. Health Hum Rights 1997;2:10–45.

35 Hilberg R: The Destruction of European Jewry. Chicago, Quadrangle, 1961. Appendix 3.

36 United States Holocaust Memorial Museum: Documenting the Numbers of Victims of the Holocaust and Nazi Persecution. https://www.ushmm.org/wlc/en/article.php?ModuleId=10008193 (cited June 25, 2017).

37 Trunk I: Epidemics and mortality in the Warsaw ghetto. Yivo Annu Jew Soc Sc 1953;8:82–122.

38 Roland C: Courage under Siege: Starvation, Disease, and Death in the Warsaw Ghetto. New York, Oxford University Press, 1992.

39 Flynn JL, Chan J: Tuberculosis: latency and reactivation. Infect Immun 2001;69:4195–4201.

40 Dwork D, Van Pelt JR: Holocaust: A History. New York, W.W. Norton & Company, 2002.

41 Lenski M: Problems of disease in the Warsaw ghetto. Yad Vashem Stud 1959;3:283–294.

42 Trunk I: Judenrat: The Jewish Councils in Eastern Europe Under Nazi Occupation. New York, Macmillan, 1972.

43 Truck I: Lódź Ghetto, A History Shapiro RM (Trans), Bloomington, Indiana University Press, 2006.

44 Sierakowiak D: The Diary of Dawid Sierakowiak. Adelson A (ed), New York, Oxford University Press, 1996.

45 Arad Y, Gutman Y, Margaliot A (eds): Documents on the Holocaust: Selected Sources on the Destruction of Jews of Germany and Austria, Poland and the Soviet Union. Jerusalem, Yad Vashem, 1981, Doc. 129.

46 Longacre M, Beinfeld S, Hildebrandt S, Glantz L, Grodin M: Public health in the Vilna ghetto as a form of jewish resistance. Am J Public Health 2015;105:293–301.

47 Schalkowsky S, Kraemer J: Płońsk; in Dean M, Hecker M (eds): Encyclopedia of the Camps and Ghettos, 1933–1945, vol II, Ghettos in German-Occupied Eastern Europe, Bloomington, Indiana, Indiana University Press, 2012, pp 24–26.

48 Yad Vashem: The Community of Płońsk during the Holocaust: Health Institutions in the Płońsk Ghetto. http://www.yadvashem.org/yv/en/exhibitions/communities/plonsk/health.asp (cited August 8, 2017).

49 Bender S: Similarity and Differences: A Comparative Study between the Ghettos in Białystok and Kielce; in Goda N (ed): Jewish Histories of the Holocaust: New Transnational Approaches. New York, Berghahn, 2014, pp 73–90.

50 Wachsmann N: KL: A History of the Nazi Concentration Camps. New York, Farrar, Straus and Giroux, 2015.

51 Pingel F: The Concentration Camps as Part of the National-Socialist System; in Marrus M (ed): The Nazi Holocaust: Historical Articles on the Destruction of European Jews, Part 6: the Victims of the Holocaust. Westport, Connecticut, Meckler, 1989, vol 2, pp 909–923.

52 Mass Z: Passeport pour Auschwitz. Correspondance d'un médecin du camp de Drancy; in Laffitte M (ed): Paris, Le Manuscrit – Fondation pour la Mémoire de la Shoah, 2012, p 410.

53 Hájková A: "Das Polizeiliche Durchgangslager Westerbork"; in Benz W, Distel B (eds): Terror im Westen. Nationalsozialistische Lager in den Niederlanden, Belgien und Luxemburg, 1940–1945, Berlin, Metropol, 2004.

54 Caplan J, Wachsmann N: Introduction; in Caplan J, Wachsmann N (eds): Concentration Camps in Nazi German: The New Histories. New York, Routledge, 2010, pp 1–16.

55 Blatman D: The Death Marches and the Final Phase of Nazi Genocide; in Caplan J, Wachsmann N (eds): Concentration Camps in Nazi German: The New Histories. New York, Routledge, 2010, pp 167–185.

56 Yad Vashem: Union Généale des Israèlites de France (UGIF-General Union of Jews in France), Zone Nord correspondence with the Red Cross regarding supply an X-ray machine to the Drancy Camp. 3689115, Record Group O.9 France Collection. Available from: http://collections1.yadvashem.org/list.asp (cited Auguest 11, 2017).

57 United States Holocaust Memorial Museum: Mauthausen Killing Operations. Available from: https://www.ushmm.org/wlc/en/article.php?ModuleId=10007729 (cited August 4, 2017).

58 Bouard M: Mauthausen. Revue d'Histoire de la Deuxième Guerre Mondiale. 1954;4e Année 15/16:39–80.

59 Kulish N, Mekhennet S: The Eternal Nazi: From Mauthausen to Cairo, The Relentless Pursuit of SS Doctor Aribert Heim, New York, Doubleday, 2014.

60 Stein H (ed): Rosenthal J (Trans): Buchenwald Concentration Camp, 1937–45: A Guide to the Permanent Historical Exhibition. Göttingen, Wallstein, 2004.

61 Hackett D (ed and trans): The Buchenwald Report. Boulder, Colorado, Westview Press, 1995.

62 Müller-Hill B: Murderous Science: Elimination by Scientific Selection of Jews, Gypsies, and Others in Germany, 1933–45, Fraser R (Trans), Oxford, Oxford University Press, 1988.

63 Pasternak A: Inhuman Research: Medical Experiments in German Concentration Camps, Budapest, Hungary, Akademia Kiadó, 2006.

64 Weindling P: Surviving Nazi Medical Atrocities: Compensation and Care in the German Federal Republic after 1945. Conference Paper given at the Second International Conference on Medicine in the Holocaust. Akko, Israel, 2017.

65 Müller-Hill B: Genetics of susceptibility to tuberculosis: Mengele's experiments in Auschwitz. Nat Rev 1981;2:631–634.

66 Schwarberg G: The Murders at Bullenhuser Damm: The SS Doctor and the Children, Rosenfeld E, Rosenfeld A, (trans). Bloomington, Indiana University Press, 1984.

67 López-Muñoz F, García-García P, Alamo C: The pharmaceutical industry and the German National Socialist Regime: I.G. Farben and pharmacological research. J Clin Pharm Ther 2009;34;67–77.

68 Munzer A: Personal Communication, International Tracing Service. United States Holocaust Memorial Museum, June 16, 2017.

69 Nawyn KJ CMH: The Liberation of Ebensee Concentration Camp May 6, 1945, CMS News and Features, U.S. Army Center of Military History, May 1945.

70 Second Hospitalization Unit, 30th Field Hospital Unit History, World War II Medical Research Centre. https://www.med-dept.com/unit-histories/30th-field-hospital-second-hospitalization-unit-platoon/ (cited August 8, 2017).

71 Cohen R: Personal Conversation with Alfred Munzer, June 16, 2017.

72 Cohen R: Oral History with Ruth Cohen, United States Holocaust Memorial Museum. https://collections.ushmm.org/search/catalog/irn44295 (cited July 8, 2017).

73 Stone D: The Liberation of the Camps. The End of the Holocaust and its Aftermath, New Haven, Yale University Press, 2015.

74 Byerly CR: Camp Follower: Tuberculosis in World War II, Chapter Eight in "Good Tuberculosis Men": The Army Medical Department's Struggle with Tuberculosis, Fort Sam Houston, Texas: U.S. Army Medical Center Department and School, 2013, pp 205–232.

75 Brooks J: "Uninterested in anything except food:" the work of nurses feeding the liberated inmates of Bergen-Belsen. J Clin Nurs 2012;21:2958–2965.

76 Kemp P: The British Army and the Liberation of Bergen-Belsen in April 1945; in Reilly J, Cesarani D, Kushner T, Richmond C (eds): Belsen in History and Memory. Lincoln, Frank Cass, 1997, pp 134–148.

77 Weindling P: Epidemics and Genocide in Eastern Europe, 1890–1945. New York, Oxford University Press, 2000.

78 Hay I: One Hundred Years of Army Nursing: The Story of the British Army Nursing Services from the time of Florence Nightingale to the Present Day. London, Cassell, 1953.

79 United States Holocaust Memorial Museum Archives, RG-09.24, Liberation: 71st Infantry Division records relating to the liberation of Gunskirchen.

80 Jucksch W: Interview (1979, 9 April), Witness to the Holocaust Project Files (1939–2005) (bulk 1978–1983), Emory University. http://witness.digitalscholarship.emory.edu/items/show/63 (cited August 15, 2017).

81 National Archives and Records Administration, [NARA], College Park, Maryland: RG112 Records of the Office of the Surgeon General (Army); Records Used for Preparing WWII-Era Medical Unit Histories, UD1012 (HUMEDS), Boxes 86 and 87, Evacuation Hospitals, 121–131, Unit History of the 131st Evacuation Hospital.

82 Clark F: Interview (1981, 21 May), Witness to the Holocaust Project Files (1939–2005) (bulk 1978–1983), Emory University, http://witness.digitalscholarship.emory.edu/items/show/40 (cited August 15, 2017).

83 Harrison M: Medicine and Victory: British Military Medicine in the Second World War. New York, Oxford University Press, 2004.

84 Keinan-Boker L, Shasha-Larsky H, Eilat-Zanani S, Edri-Shur A, Shasha SM: Chronic health conditions in Jewish Holocaust survivors born during World War II. Isr Med Assoc J 2015;17:206–212.

85 Koessler M: Euthanasia in the Hadamar Sanatorium and International Law. J Crim Law Crim 1953;46:735–755.

86 Weindling P: Nazi Medicine and the Nuremberg Trials: From Medical War Crimes to Informed Consent. New York, Palgrave Macmillan, 2004.

87 Ernst E: Commentary: The Third Reich – German physicians between resistance and participation. Int J Epidemiol 2001;30:37–42.

88 Moreno, JD, Schmidt U, Joffe S: The Nuremberg Code 70 Years Later. JAMA 2017;17 Aug. DOI: 10.1001/jama.2017.10265.

89 Second International Workshop on Medicine in the Holocaust and Beyond: "The Galilee Declaration." http://english.wgalil.ac.il/?catid=%7b689D6CB5-A7BD-466A-9297-AFEABA2C0257%7d

Annette Finley-Croswhite, PhD, Professor of History
Department of History, BAL 8000
Old Dominion University
Norfolk, VA 23529-0091 (USA)
E-Mail acroswhi@odu.edu

Reflections about Belligerent Countries in Order of Appearance

Murray JF, Loddenkemper R (eds): Tuberculosis and War. Lessons Learned from World War II.
Prog Respir Res. Basel, Karger, 2018, vol 43, pp 64–85 (DOI: 10.1159/000481475)

Tuberculosis in Germany before, during and after World War II

Robert Loddenkemper[a] · Nikolaus Konietzko[b]

[a]German Central Committee against Tuberculosis, Berlin, and [b]Essen, Germany

Abstract

In 1939, the year Germany started World War II, tuberculosis (TB) mortality was at its lowest, only a few countries had lower TB mortality rates. When the Nazis came into power in 1933, they took over under the main health-related motto "Public interest ahead of self-interest" ("Gemeinnutz vor Eigennutz"). In the first years, there was an intense discussion as to whether TB was caused more by hereditary disposition or by infection. Finally, the arguments by leading TB specialists were accepted that TB is predominantly an infectious disease. As TB mortality was increasing during the war in all sectors – in the civilian and military populations as well as among prisoners of war, foreign forced (slave) laborers and those in the concentration camps – multiple, partly inhuman measures for TB control were introduced, for example, compulsory isolation of so-called "anti-social" TB patients or even patients with infectious TB were forced to work. TB was one of the prevailing diseases in the concentration camps due to the crowded, filthy living conditions, and severe malnutrition. Overall, TB mortality increased by 160–240% compared with pre-war figures. With the help of the victorious Allied powers, the TB control system was restructured and the situation improved slowly over the following years.　　　　　　　　　　　© 2018 S. Karger AG, Basel

Germany started the Second World War (WWII) on September 1, 1939, with the invasion of Poland. As a result, the XIth Conference of the International Union against Tuberculosis (IUAT), which was due to be held in Berlin in the second half of September, had to be cancelled. In preparation for the conference, the Tuberculosis Committee of the German Reich (Reichs-Tuberkulose-Ausschuss [RTA]) had already had a booklet printed, entitled "The fight against tuberculosis (TB) in Germany" [Der Kampf gegen die Tuberkulose in Deutschland], which described the TB situation in some detail [1]. The "German Central Committee for the fight against Tuberculosis" (Deutsches Zentralkomitee für den Kampf gegen die Tuberkulose [DZK]), founded in 1895, had already been replaced by the RTA in 1933, shortly after the Nazi regime came into power in January 1933.

All non-governmental health organizations and scientific societies lost their legitimacy, and the government took over full responsibility under the main health-related motto "Public interest ahead of self-interest" ("Gemeinnutz vor Eigennutz"). This edict also changed the existing concepts of TB control in many ways as new control measures were decreed by new laws, as outlined below.

Tuberculosis before the War

Epidemiology

As described in chapter 1, death rates from TB peaked in Western Europe at the beginning of the 19th century, and

Nikolaus Konietzko is a Professor Emeritus of Universität Duisburg-Essen and a former Medical Director of Ruhrlandklinik, Essen.

then declined at a nearly constant rate for more than 100 years. A schematic model showing this trend of mortality from 1740 to 1985 is illustrated in Figure 2 in chapter 1 [2]. The challenges in the assessment of appropriate epidemiological data are described in detail in chapter 2.

The development of the TB situation in Germany was quite similar. Figure 1 illustrates the development in Prussia after the discovery of the TB bacillus by Robert Koch in 1882. This figure is taken from his last presentation a few weeks before his death [3]. It shows an almost constant decrease in mortality between 1882 and 1907.

This decline continued over the following decades, and was only interrupted in the years of World War I (WWI; 1914–1918) and during the hyperinflation crisis (the Great Depression) in 1923–1924 (Fig. 4 in chapter 1 and 10 in chapter 2).

In 1939, the year WWII began, TB mortality was at its lowest level to date, at 60 per 100,000 population; by 1940, it had increased to 68/100,000. TB mortality in the Greater German Reich (Grossdeutschland), which included Austria and Sudetenland (part of Czechoslovakia) from 1938 after the annexation, was estimated in 1939 at 64/100,000 (and in 1943 and 1945 at, respectively, 80 and 100/100,000 [4].

In 1948, US TB specialist Esmond R. Long, who was appointed Head of a TB commission by the Secretary of the Department of the US Army, was asked to investigate the incidence of TB and recommend control measures in the German civilian population. He cites in his report:

Currency stabilization and resumption of a normal economic state in 1923, with ordinary employment and disappearance of some of the factors supposedly responsible for the 1922 rise in mortality, were accompanied by the development of one of the strongest TB control programs in the world. A nationwide system of TB dispensaries (Fürsorgestellen), a generous provision of sanatorium beds, an insurance system financing treatment of all social levels, and a centralized authority for maintenance of a control program (RTA) all had contributed to this success. Within Germany, excessive rates prevailed in a few places, like Berlin, but the national average compared with most other countries was low. [5]

The 1949 report of the US Commission came to the conclusion that "in 1939 only 4 countries – Denmark, Australia, The Netherlands and the United States – had lower TB mortality rates than Germany" [6].

However, in 1933, the speed of the annual decline in TB mortality had begun to slow down, from 73 to 60/100,000 in 1939. Between 1935 and 1937, an increase had been seen in 15–20 year olds: in males from 31.7 to 36.4/100,000 and in

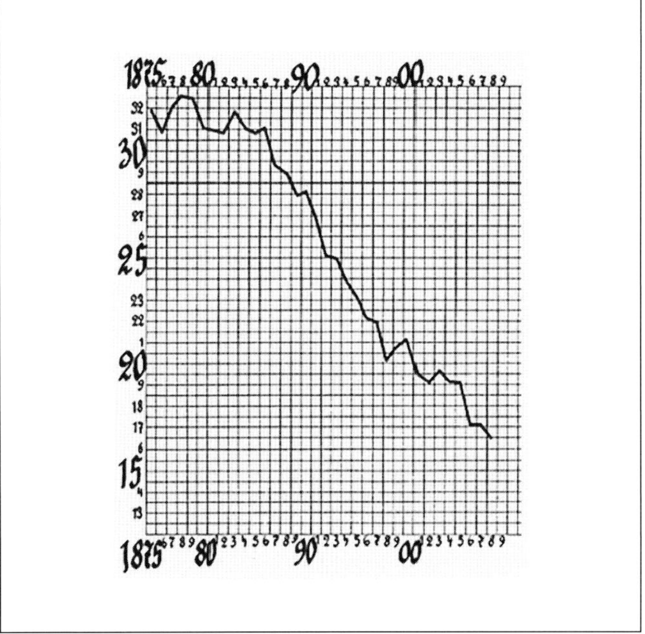

Fig. 1. TB mortality in Prussia, 1875–1907 (*n*/10,000) [3], with permission of Springer.

females from 43.6 to 55.5/100,000. Increased physical stress was assumed as the most likely explanation for the increase in this age group – in the newly founded youth organizations of the Nazi regime (Hitlerjugend [Hitler Youth] for boys and the Bund deutscher Mädchen [League of German Girls] for girls, and in the labor service (Arbeitsdienst), which was compulsory by law from 1935 for adolescents between 18 and 25 years of age [7]. Therefore, special regulations were decreed in 1938 to protect young workers (Erlasse zum Schutz jugendlicher Arbeitnehmer).

In 1938, the "Regulation on the control of communicable diseases" (Verordnung zur Bekämpfung übertragbarer Krankheiten) was decreed, sharpening the obligation to notify all new cases (and even suspected cases) of infectious pulmonary and laryngeal TB, TB of the skin, and of other organs. The registration of notified new TB cases (TB incidence or morbidity) was started throughout Germany already in 1934, and was discontinued only in 1943. In 1938, 65,866 cases of all forms of TB were registered (pulmonary 60,782, extrapulmonary 5,084). In 1939, these figures had increased to 80,798 (72,700 and 8,098) due to the annexing of Austria and the Sudetenland. Table 1 shows that in 1942–1943, the number of new notified cases had almost doubled compared to 1939, with a corresponding increase in incidence (Table 1). These numbers apply only to the ci-

Table 1. Annual new TB cases and incidence, Germany, 1938–1943 (from 1939 including Austria and Sudetenland)

Year	New TB cases, n	Incidence (n/100,000)
1938	65,866	963
1939	80,798	1,166
1940	109,508	1,568
1941	134,979	1,922
1942	146,121	2,063
1943	143,171	2,033

Modified from Pöhn and Rasch [9].

vilian population; the military services had their own statistics [8].

Otto Walter, President of the RTA, estimated that in 1935 there were 300,000–400,000 open (infectious) TB cases (probably, largely sputum smear-positive cases, as culture was not yet routinely available), and more than one million persons at risk of becoming infectious. Approximately, 50,000 were entirely and 500,000 partly unable to work [10]. This caused a severe penury of workers, and measures were later taken to integrate most of these into the labor market (see below).

Pre-War Political Measures and TB Control Measures
Political Measures
After coming into power in 1933, the Nazi government issued a series of laws, decrees, and directives that affected the control of TB both directly and indirectly. As early as April 1933, the "Law for the Restoration of the Civil Service" (Gesetz zur Wiederherstellung des Berufsbeamtentums) was passed, "a law that excluded anyone either of non-German heritage (Jews) or of questionable political sympathies (communists) from employment in the civil service" [11]. The most intrusive edict was the law for the "Unification of Health Affairs," decreed in July 1934 (Gesetz über die Vereinheitlichung des Gesundheitswesens), which ensured that the health system came under almost complete control of the central government (Ministry of the Interior). By an executive order, most of the communal TB dispensaries (Fürsorgestellen) were incorporated into the local public health offices (Gesundheitsämter), thus transferring decision-making power to the central government, with potentially significant consequences for the individual TB patient.

The most intrusive laws for the individual were the "Law on the prevention of genetically diseased offspring" (Gesetz zur Verhütung erbkranken Nachwuchses), issued in July 1933, allowing the sterilization of persons with mainly psychiatric diseases, which was followed in 1935 by the "Law for the protection of the genetic health of the German Volk" (Marriage Health Law) (Gesetz zum Schutze der Erbgesundheit des deutschen Volkes [Ehegesundheitsgesetz]) [12], on the basis of which a marriage could be forbidden (or divorce allowed) when one of the partners suffered from an infectious (or mental) disease that could substantially threaten the health of the (future) spouse and/or potential descendants. Thus, before being married, both partners had to produce a certificate from the health office to the effect that there were no impediments to the marriage. In 1937, Julius Kayser-Petersen, Secretary General of the DTG, postulated that in almost all cases – except in the case of obviously infectious patients – an examination should be performed by a specialist and that in case of unclear results, the decision to allow the marriage should be postponed followed by careful observation [13]. It is not exactly known how many TB cases were affected by these and the corresponding decrees. In any case, there were many fewer than among psychiatric patients, many of whom were sterilized or even killed as terrible consequence of the Marriage Health Law and other, similar decrees. As cited by Susanne Hahn [14], the suggestion was made that women diagnosed with TB during pregnancy should have their babies taken away immediately at birth to allow them to grow up in a healthy environment [15]). In theory, therefore, termination of pregnancy was strictly prohibited. However, in practice, TB was in fact the most frequent medical indication for abortion [16].

The whole topic was connected to the debate as to whether certain diseases are of hereditary origin, an international debate which had already started at the turn of the century, stimulated by Darwin's Law of Evolution by Natural Selection [11, 17]. On the basis of the results of research in animals and twins [18, 19], there had also been intense discussion, particularly in Germany during the 1930s, as to whether TB was caused more by hereditary disposition or by infection. Finally – and fortunately – the arguments by leading TB specialists were accepted by the Nazi regime that TB is predominantly an infectious disease [10, 20–22]. This prevented far-reaching measures such as sterilization of TB patients or – as was the case for the thousands of people with mental disease – euthanasia for genetic reasons. This approach was endorsed in 1920 in a book entitled "Die Freigabe der Vernichtung lebensunwerten Lebens" – "Allowing the Destruction of Lives Unworthy of Life" [23] – in which, in addition to mentally ill, psychotic patients, those with incurable cancer and fatally wounded patients, even incurable TB patients ("unrettbare Phthisiker") were listed as potential candidates for destruction (cited in Ref. [24]). This later provided the intellectual foundation for the Nazi T4 "euthanasia" program [25, 26], and through this, the Holocaust [11] (for more details, see chapter 4).

Tuberculosis Control Measures

The above-mentioned "Regulation on the control of communicable diseases" enabled the compulsory isolation of so-called "anti-social" ("asozial") TB patients in closed TB institutions, often together with psychiatric patients [27]. Possible consequences for these patients were that they were purposefully undernourished, and ran the very real risk of dying of starvation.

How seriously the problem of incapacity to work in TB patients was discussed before the war is illustrated in 2 of the 5 articles in the booklet of the RTA, which had been prepared for the cancelled XIth Conference of the IUAT, which ended with the statement that the aim of most measures was the reintegration of cured TB patients and – perhaps – those who had shown improvement in the work force. Later, in 1941, when the shortage of workers during the war was accelerating, a decree on the employment of labor was issued which allowed even patients with open pulmonary TB to be forced to work (Erlass zum Arbeitseinsatz von Tuberkulösen). On the contrary, in 1942, the care of TB patients was secured by a decree on the financial assistance by the state (Verordnung über Tuberkulosehilfe) in cases with low income and without appropriate insurance to cover the costs of treatment (except in the case of Jews).

In 1938, all supreme authorities of the Reich involved in the fight against TB – the Ministries of the Interior, of Labor and of Education and Propaganda, the Office of the Nazi Party as well as the Supreme Command of the Armed Forces, the Wehrmacht – were coordinated in one working group, the Reichs-Tuberkulose-Rat (Reichs Tuberculosis Advisory Board), which set out the guidelines for Germany's fight against TB (and better control) with support of the RTA and under the presidency of the Reichs Health Leader (Reichsgesundheitsführer), Leonardo Conti.

Further Control Measures

To eradicate bovine TB, a law (Tuberkulosetilgungsverfahren) was issued in Prussia in 1912, which recommended the culling of tuberculin-positive cattle on a voluntary basis. This law was applied only after WWI, but was abandoned in 1939 due to a lack of success, although it is estimated that about two thirds of the country's cattle were infected (Ferlinz [28]). The pasteurization of milk was introduced in 1930, but was not applied systematically before 1947. An investigation that started in 1943 in cooperation with the Statens Serum Institut in Denmark showed that of 1,000 adolescent patients with open pulmonary TB, about 4% were infected by *Mycobacterium bovis* (*M. bovis*)[29]. It is estimated that 10% of TB disease was caused by the bovine bacillus [28]; it can be assumed that the proportion in children was much higher.

Serial X-ray examinations with mass screening to detect TB diseased persons were postulated in 1926 by Franz Redeker [30, 31]. Photofluorography (mass miniature radiography) was used first on a broad basis in the military services in fitness tests for the army and the navy [32], then, from 1933, in the police, and in the Reichs workforce (Reichsarbeitsdienst) due to the high risk of TB infection in the crowded housing situation, in the SA (Sturmabteilung, the "Storm Detachment," which functioned as the original paramilitary wing of the Nazi Party), SS (Schutzstaffel, the "Defense Squadron" of the Nazi Party), students, candidates for teaching posts, students in vocational schools, marriage candidates, and children aged over 6 years [33]. During the Nazi party convention in Nuremberg in 1938, mass screening by X-ray was performed in 10,736 members of the SS and changes suggestive of active TB were observed in 92 men (0.9%) [34]. In 1939, Holfelder published a report on the experiment, along with more than 900,000 photofluorographies [35]. According to Blome, 3 million individuals were examined from the mid-1930s until 1941 [36].

The TB department of the Robert Koch Institute recommended regular application of the tuberculin test for screening of the general population in 1939 to identify tuberculin converters in whom further examination by X-ray was indicated [37]. This type of screening was not introduced into routine practice. However, in recommendations on performing of tuberculin testing in staff working in TB wards, a chest X-ray was requested first, and only if this did not show tuberculous changes was the tuberculin test regarded as being indicated (Anweisung für die Durchführung der Tuberkulinprüfung (Ausgabe 1941 BG Gesundheitsdienst und Wohlfahrtspflege [Instruction for the performance of tuberculin testing. Edition 1941 Employers Mutual Insurance Association Health and Welfare Services]).

In December 1930, the introduction of the BCG vaccination was officially rejected by the Ministry of the Interior because no permanent immunity had been shown and, in particular, because of the Lübeck vaccination disaster, when virulent human mycobacteria were accidentally given orally to 251 neonates, causing the death of 72 [38–40]. Vaccination was discussed in view of the worsening TB situation during the war. Just before the end of the war, the decision was taken by the RTA to introduce BCG, but it was never undertaken. Karl Auersbach, who had been a member of the RTA as second secretary, expressed his skepticism about the efficacy in an article published in 1946, in which he mentioned the negative approach of the Americans to BCG [41].

Tuberculosis during the War

Epidemiology
There are considerable difficulties in obtaining accurate TB statistics for Germany during the war and post-war periods (see also chapter 2). Population movements, and the exclusion of non-civilians and of TB cases in refugee camps, prison camps, and concentration camps were an impediment to collecting precise data during the war [6]. It can also be assumed that the Nazi regime was not particularly interested in reporting the substantial rise in TB cases and deaths.

The members of the US American Commission identified several reasons for the rise in TB cases and deaths:

With the outbreak of war in 1939, deterioration in the (TB control) program began. Military mobilization led to a decrease in professional personnel for TB control, and with the continuation of hostilities, hospital beds once used for TB were employed for the accumulating casualties. The continuous bombing of German cities was a factor of as yet unmeasured importance. After large raids thousands of injured civilians crowded the hospitals, already undermanned through military necessity.

And they continue:

As time went by, other factors came into play which are believed to have had a seriously adverse effect on the incidence of TB. Prior to the war Germans with active TB were not allowed to participate in many forms of domestic and industrial employment. During the war, as manpower needs grew, documents were published in which the element of contagion was minimized. Germans with active TB were again permitted employment. Manpower needs could not be met from the German civilian population and importation of labor from adjacent allied or occupied countries followed. Little if any screening for TB was carried out and subsequent critical study has indicated that much TB was imported in this way.

During the war, TB mortality was recorded continuously in only a few regions (Berlin, Hamburg, Bavaria, Württemberg) and for only the civilian population. Although the absolute rise in TB mortality recorded during WWI was not reached in WWII, the increase over the pre-war rate was proportionately even greater [6]. In general, the increase in cities was much larger than in rural regions, presumably due to the less crowded living conditions and the better food situation in rural areas.

Berlin, the largest German city, with 4.3 million inhabitants, already had the highest TB mortality rates in the country before the war (82/100,000 in 1938). During the war, this increased to 127 in 1943 and to 162 in 1944, reaching its peak in 1945, with a rate of 291/100,000 [42]. TB, which had shown a more chronic course before the war, became a more acute disease during the war. TB killed about 70,000 men and women between 1939 and 1950. In 1945, TB morbidity in males was about 3 times (3.06) higher than in females (in 1938–1940, it was only 1.75 times higher). One possible reason for this considerably greater proportion in males during the war was the assumption that only healthy men were drafted to the army. Some were killed in the war, and some returned sick, thus augmenting the number of TB cases in the non-drafted male population. Typically, males in their third decade predominated. The corresponding fatality rate increased stepwise during the war from 19.0% in 1939 to 49.5% in 1945, when almost half of TB patients died from the disease, most probably due to the lowered resistance caused by undernourishment, and in particular protein deficiency [42].

A further reason for the deterioration of the TB situation in Berlin was the considerable loss of about 43% of total available housing due to the massive bombing raids of the allies as of 1943. In the different districts, 25–50% of houses were destroyed. The air raids – with the bombing of most big German cities – were followed by mass evacuation to the countryside; in Berlin, about one million inhabitants left the city. As a consequence, the basis for comparative mortality statistics became very fragile (in 1942, Berlin had 4.5 million inhabitants, but by August 1945 this figure had decreased to only 2.8 million). The population lived in overcrowded housing conditions – and in overcrowded bunkers during the raids – facilitating the spread of TB. However, the loss of housing space was partly counterbalanced by the 26.5% decrease in population between 1943 and 1946.

In Bavaria, as in most other largely agricultural regions of Germany, TB mortality rose less dramatically, from 59/100,000 in 1939 to 90/100,000 in 1945. The increase in TB mortality in the cities was almost twice as high as in the rural regions [43]. Here, the TB increase in males was also much more pronounced than in females, particularly among those aged between 15 and 25 years. The estimated number of extra-pulmonary cases remained almost stable, probably in part due to a lack of diagnostic investigations.

As already shown in Table 1, the number of new TB cases in Germany was 65,866 in 1938, with a corresponding TB incidence of 963/100,000. With the annexing of Austria and the Sudetenland in 1938, this rose to 80,798 and 1,166/100,000, respectively, and finally to 143,171 and 2,033/100,000, respectively in 1943, the last year notification data were collected. Thus, the figures in the civilian population had already almost doubled from the beginning of the war until 1943. The fact that TB became – as mentioned – a more acute disease is underlined by an interesting observation from the Moselle region, where the survival time from diagnosis to death became much shorter during the war period (1940–1945) than in comparable periods before and after [44]. This was also observed by Froelich in Chemnitz/Saxony (cited in Ref. [45]; Fig. 5 in chapter 3).

TB Control Measures during the War

As TB mortality was increasing in all sectors – in the civilian and military populations as well as among prisoners of war (POW), foreign forced (slave) laborers and those in the concentration camps – multiple measures for TB control were introduced.

Several decrees were issued for the civilian population: in 1940, the

Decree on nutrition of hospitalized tuberculous patients (and those in care of) ("Erlass zur Krankenernährung") was enacted, with the purpose of improving the quantity and quality of food for patients as well as for the doctors and nurses who took care of them. However, due to food shortages during the war, this could often not be achieved, and the decree was modified in 1943 to reduce the amount of food made available for the nutrition of TB patients (General and medical indications for the permission of supplementary food for sick persons). [46]

The most meager food rations were provided to those unable to work, those with steadily deteriorating status and possibly those of an age when the ability to work was no longer expected (and to those who had recovered completely from TB, as they were now back in the workforce).

One particularly inhuman act, typical of the Nazi regime, must be mentioned: as was already done during the pre-war period, but was now taken to another level; in some TB hospitals, nutrition was purposely restricted among severely ill patients with a poor prognosis and among the so-called un-

social ("asozial") cases, with a view to accelerating an early death [27, 47].

In 1940, the decree "Notification of admission and discharge of TB patients by hospitals" (Anzeige der Aufnahme bzw. Entlassung von Tuberkulosekranken durch die Krankenhäuser) was issued to improve the overall TB notification rate; the registration system had become inefficient and did not allow an overview of all TB cases.

Due to the increasing need for labor, TB patients were assessed in 1941 as being capable of working on the basis of the new "Decree on labor of tuberculous persons" (Erlass zum Arbeitseinsatz von Tuberkulösen). With very few limitations even patients with open (infectious) TB were considered capable of working. One prerequisite was that these patients should work in areas where they could not infect others. It was estimated that only about 20% of all notified TB cases were actually capable of returning to work [48].

To protect frail, underweight adolescents, a decree was issued in December 1941 to provide supplementary food for those in close contact with tuberculous persons (Zusätzliche Lebensmittel für tuberkulosegefährdete Jugendliche). However, this benefit was modified less than a year later, in November 1942, to include isolated cases only.

In addition, in 1942 the care of TB patients was improved by a decree on financial assistance by the state (Verordnung über Tuberkulosehilfe) for cases with low income and without appropriate insurance coverage of treatment costs. However, in 1943, this support was classified in different levels in relation to disease status and prognosis. Those patients who were not able to work had almost no chance of surviving. And Jewish TB cases were completely excluded [49].

Educational information about TB distributed to doctors and laypersons was intensified by the RTA, for example, by a fact sheet for doctors on the early diagnosis of pulmonary TB (Merkblatt für Ärzte zur Früherkennung der Lungentuberkulose), which ended with the threatening sentence that neglecting to order a chest X-ray for cases with even minimal suspicion of TB would be seen as malpractice and as a severe offense against the health of the whole nation (Volksgesundheit). An information sheet was published for the general population entitled "What everybody must know about TB" ("Was jedermann von der Tuberkulose wissen muss"), which was available through the RTA at the very low price of 1 Pfennig (1,000 leaflets for 10 Reichsmark).

In 1942, a detailed directive against the spread of communicable diseases in schools, orphanages, holiday camps for children and similar institutions was decreed, with particular emphasis on TB (Vorschriften gegen die Verbreitung übertragbarer Krankheiten durch Schulen, Kinderheime und ähnliche Einrichtungen [Schulseuchenerlass]), indicating once again that TB had become a growing problem during the war.

According to Johannes Holm, of the Tuberculosis Division of the Statens Serum Institut in Copenhagen, Denmark, tuberculin tests performed in the normal population before and during the war showed that the percentage of reactors was relatively low in many areas of Germany [50]. Tuberculin tests performed among recruits of the German army in 1942 showed only 60% reactors in the 20-year age-group. In Schleswig-Holstein in 1942–1943, 38% of the schoolchildren examined were reactors at the age of 14. This figure had increased among the same groups to more than 50% in 1946.

Schrag reports in 1953 that Holfelder performed more than 20 million examinations during mass screening by photofluorography before and during the Second World War in different regions of Germany. A very high number, about 200,000 of the first 10.6 million cases, showed findings suspicious of active TB. In 1940–1941, Schrag himself found about 1% of cases with suspicion of open, active or inactive TB in Stuttgart [51].

After the occupation of Paris in 1940, the Paris Office of the IUAT was closed by the Germans. In November 1941, a new Union (Vereinigung) was founded with its headquarters in Berlin. Fifteen states, all belonging to the Axis Alliance, became members. Raffaele Paolucci from Italy was elected as President. The IUAT's official journal was named "Tuberculosis," edited by Walter, Kayser-Petersen, and Redeker [52]. After the war, the IUAT resumed its activities as of 1946 and became – after the founding of the World Health Organization in 1946 – the first NGO to be officially recognized by the World Health Organization [53].

TB in the German Armed Forces (Wehrmacht)
TB in the armed forces was a special problem because predominantly young men, one of the most vulnerable groups for TB, were drafted to military service where they usually lived in crowded accommodation (barracks or tents), which facilitated the spreading of TB bacilli. The principal aim was, therefore, to exclude those with active TB from military service, after a medical examination. The newly introduced method of photofluorography was ideally suited to this purpose, and in Germany it was first used on a broad basis in the military service of the army and the navy at the beginning of the 1930s [32]. Several reports were published

on the results: on average about 1 in 1,000 candidates had findings suspicious of active pulmonary TB and, if confirmed, were not accepted for military service. The efficacy of the examination depended upon the experience of the radiologists, and it emerged later that in about 7% of TB cases, X-ray changes suggestive of TB, had been overlooked [54].

Exact numbers on the TB cases that occurred during military service have not been published; one reason may have been to avoid causing too much anxiety in the army. However, TB was an important subject in several meetings of military doctors (e.g., in Ref. [55]) and of multiple publications [56]). In the former, the report by Steinmeyer [54] reported that 1282 cases were diagnosed between June 1941 and September 1942 at the Russian front, mentioning that the situation there was of particular concern. Szerreiki [57] highlighted the lack of X-ray equipment and of medical specialists at the front, but reported that among 30,000 soldiers, 1.5/1,000 had active TB. To avoid fear among the soldiers, he recommended performing photofluorography during the routine delousing that soldiers underwent before going on leave. Kreuser [58] reported that since spring 1942, the number of new active TB cases was increasing and highlighted the diagnostic difficulties. He recommended sputum microscopy to identify TB bacilli and careful transportation back from the front for treatment.

Active cases, particularly those with open pulmonary TB (50–57% of all cases), were either discharged [59] or admitted to military TB hospitals/sanatoria, in which all conservative and surgical treatment methods were used [60]. However, one precondition for admission was a high probability that the patient would quickly return to working capacity or sputum negativity. Apparently, quite a number of soldiers became apathetic after being in action and neglected the seriousness of their disease, as a result of which some had to be admitted to closed TB wards (compulsory isolation) [61].

TB in Prisoners of War
There are a few reports on TB among prisoners of war (POWs) in German camps. Between 1941 and 1945, more than 5 million Soviet soldiers were incarcerated in German camps; 3.3 million died in the camps from starvation and infectious diseases, weakened by heavy forced labor [62]. Approximately, 80,000 Jewish POWs from the Red Army were murdered (http://www.yadvashem.org/yv/de/holocaust/about/07/jewish_soldiers.asp).

Nicol reported [63] that more than 75,000 X-ray examinations were performed among Soviet POWs who worked as forced laborers and that more than 3,860 deaths were caused by acute TB, accelerated by malnourishment. He warned that TB among the Soviet prisoners working under forced labor represented a real risk of infection among the general population. In addition, there were camps for 7–11 million slave laborers in whom TB was also frequently seen. In a report from 1944 a continuous rise of TB in foreign workers is described, particularly among workers from the East and Poland; the total number was estimated at 8–10,000 (cited in Ref. [49]).

In contrast to the conditions for Soviet POWs, the treatment of prisoners from the countries of the Western Allies was usually in accordance with the Geneva convention. Of the 232,000 US, British, Canadian, and other POWs, 8,348 (3.5%) did not survive the war [64]. In 1944 and 1945, TB mortality in the US Army showed a sharp increase among those who had served in foreign countries; it was assumed that this was the result of high TB incidence among released POWs, in particular among the whites [65].

Of 400,000 Polish POWs, about 10,000 died, and of 600,000 Italian prisoners about 45,000 lost their lives.

Roloff [66] estimated that about 3% of captive colored soldiers from different parts of the world had active TB, which, at 1–3%, was the leading disease in the camps. He recommended separating the races in the camps. Leyton reported in 1946 that Russian POWs had more frequent and more severe TB than British POWs, and that there were large differences in the prevalence of TB among British and Russian POWs; he assumed that the only causative factor was malnutrition among the Russian POWs [67].

Archie Cochrane, a Scottish doctor who was captured during the Battle of Crete in 1941 and subsequently worked as a Medical Officer in different German prisoner of war camps and hospitals, wrote a highly interesting report on his 4-year experience [68]. In all of the sites, he looked after TB patients from different nations. Their living conditions varied depending on the area of Germany, the type of work, the nationality of the prisoner, and the character of the supervisor. The Russians' housing conditions were the worst: overcrowded, badly ventilated, and dark. Cochrane gave no figures, but mentioned that mortality was high.

It is worth mentioning here that Cochrane's experience in the camps led him to believe that much of medicine did not have sufficient evidence to justify its use [69]. His advocacy of randomized controlled trials eventually led to the development of the Cochrane Library database of systematic reviews.

In the chapter "Camp Follower: Tuberculosis in World War II (WWII)" in her comprehensive book entitled "Good Tuberculosis Men: The Army Medical Department's Struggle with Tuberculosis," Carol R. Byerly describe how that American POWs in Japan suffered even more from TB [70]:

Exact TB rates among American POWs are not known because the rush of events surrounding the liberation of prisoners from German and Japanese control prevented a systematic X-ray survey. Rates did appear to be higher, though, for prisoners of the Japanese than for prisoners of the Germans. Long reported that about 0.6 percent of recovered troops from European POW camps had TB, whereas data from the Pacific theater suggested that 1% of recovered prisoners had TB.

She concludes:

Tuberculosis continued to take its toll on [US American] POWs for years after the war. The VA (Veterans Association) followed POWs as a special group because, explained Long, of "the hardships that many of these men endured, and the notorious tendency for TB to make its appearance years after the acquisition of infection." A follow-up study published in 1954 reported that, for American POWs during the 6 years after liberation, TB was the second highest cause of death, after accidents.

TB in Concentration Camps

About 6 million Jews and 500,000 Sinti and Roma were imprisoned in concentration camps, and most were murdered (for more details, see chapter 4). TB was one of the prevailing diseases in the concentration camps due to the crowded, filthy living conditions, and the severe malnutrition; it is estimated that about one in ten inmates was affected by TB (Fig. 2 and 3 of malnourished TB patients in the concentration camp in Sachsenhausen).

The alarming situation is described in detail by Carol R. Byerly in the subchapter "From Concentration Camp Prisoners to Sanatorium Patients:"

If the challenges Army medical personnel faced in caring for sick and starving POWs and refugees were unprecedented, the scale of disease and suffering they encountered in the Nazi concentration camps was almost unimaginable. Allied troops had heard about secret and deadly camps but were not prepared for what they found. As the Allies converged on Berlin from the East and the West, the Nazis evacuated thousands of prisoners – most of them Jews seized from across Europe, as well as POWs – to interior camps to hide their crimes and prevent the inmates from falling into Allied hands. These evacuations became death marches as SS (abbreviation of *Schutzstaffel,* which stood for "defense squadron") guards beat and murdered people, and failed to feed them for days on end. Survivors were crowded into camps such as Buchenwald and Dachau, making them even more chaotic and deadly. Americans, therefore, liberated camps that were riven with disease, especially typhus,

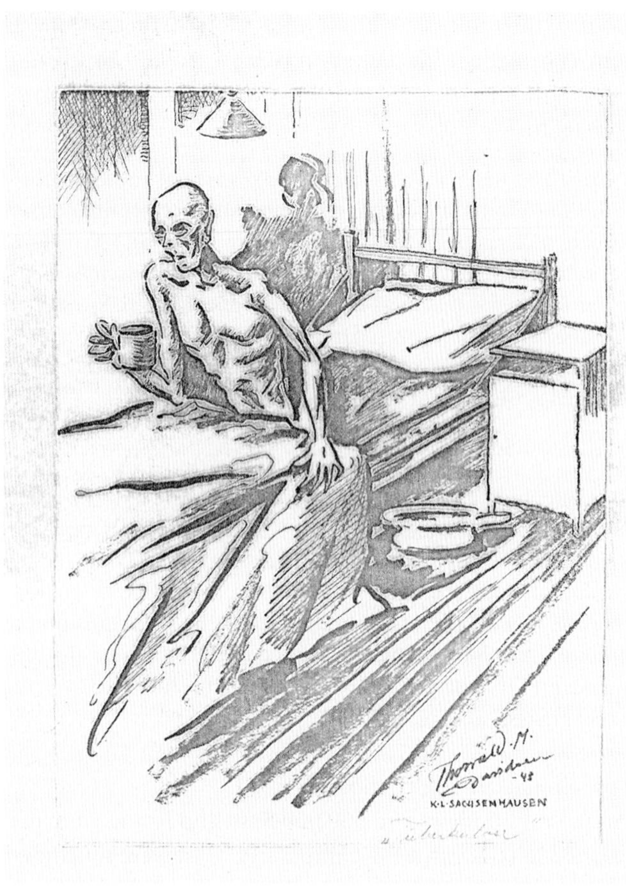

Fig. 2. "Tuberculosis." Drawing by Thorwald Davidsen, prisoner in the concentration camp at Sachsenhausen, 1943. Memorial and Museum Sachsenhausen [71], with permission.

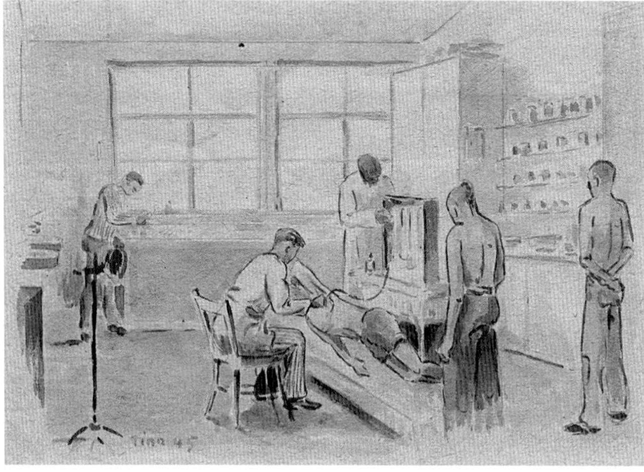

Fig. 3. Gas filling of therapeutic pneumothorax. Watercolor by Walter Timm, prisoner in the concentration camp at Sachsenhausen, 1943. Memorial and Museum Sachsenhausen [71], With permission.

TB, and malnutrition. An examination of Army Medical Department activities in one of these camps, Dachau, where evacuation hospitals spent the most time and confronted large numbers of people with TB and typhus, brings the American experience to light.

This even had an impact on the later TB situation in Europe, USA, and in particular Israel:

As with the American POWs, TB continued to follow Dachau survivors into their new lives. Thousands of Jewish survivors emigrated to what would become the state of Israel. Fifteen years after liberation, the Israeli Minister of Health reported that although concentration camp survivors comprised only 25% of the population, they accounted for 65% of the TB cases in the country. Tuberculosis continued to thrive in Europe as well. [70]

Daniels [72] quoted in his 1947 report on TB in post-war Europe, in the subchapter "Concentration Camps:"

We have all read of the horrors in the concentration camps – the mass extermination, the brutalities, the starvation, the herding together in filthy hutments, the reduction to the lowest bestial level. What was the extent of TB there we shall never know. We know only that, after the liberation, a number of autopsies at Belsen showed widespread tuberculous disease in the lungs of a very high proportion of cases of starvation.

The British Medical Officer, F.M. Lipscomb described the most horrible situation at the Belsen concentration camp which "comprised 2 portions – Camp I, which came to be known as "The Horror· Camp," housing about 22,000 females, 500 children, and 18,000 males in huts; and Camp II, containing about 17,000 males in brick buildings. Russians and Poles predominated. Czechs, Belgians, French, Italians, and Yugoslavs were also present. The great majority were Jews. The state of the inmates of Camp I was described by the Senior Medical Officer after his first survey as

a dense mass of emaciated, apathetic scarecrows huddled together in wooden huts, in many cases without beds or blankets, in some cases without any clothing whatsoever. The females in worse condition than the men, their clothing, if they have any, only filthy rags. The dead lie all over the camp…. On further investigation many more corpses were found inside the huts among the living who had not the strength even to drag them outside. Some 10,000 dead were lying in the camp when we took over and thousands more died before it could be cleared…. Some 70% of the internees in Camp I and 20% in Camp II would ordinarily have been regarded as "hospital cases" but it was impracticable to admit such a vast number to hospital at one time.

Among those who could be admitted, "the prevailing morbid conditions were deficiency diseases, typhus, and pulmonary TB." Lipscomb reported that "about 6% of admissions to the (improvised) hospital at Belsen had clinically obvious pulmonary TB in an advanced stage." And he continued,

Subsequent radiological examination of a cross-section consisting of 331 miscellaneous patients taken in groups at random from various parts of the hospital and unselected except that they were not too ill to be screened showed 6.6% positive, 5.3% probably positive, and 7.7% possibly positive. Assuming that all the probables and half the possibles would eventually prove positive, and adding 4% for the clinical cases too ill to be screened, means an over-all rate of some 20%. [73]

As cited by Daniels, shortly after the liberation of the Belsen concentration camp,

the Swedish Government permitted the entry of 10,000 displaced persons from the concentration camps, some 5,000 of these being hospital cases; of these some 40–50% had TB. It is not surprising then that among the displaced persons who remained to stay on for long periods in United Nations Relief and Rehabilitation Administration (UNRRA) camps, the prevalence of TB was much lower than one had expected: the death rate about 70, the incidence of significant TB in the neighbourhood of 2%. These people were literally the survivors of a veritable holocaust; all those who were in the least susceptible must have succumbed in the camps. [72]

The UNRRA was founded in 1943 as an international relief agency representing 44 nations, and became part of the United Nations in 1945. It played a major role in helping displaced persons return to their home countries in Europe in 1945–1946.

The French doctor, Henri Rosencher, who survived 8 months in the concentration camp in Dachau, describes in a horrifying report (translated in an abbreviated version from French into English) that 40% of autopsies at Dachau showed TB, and that about 20% of the internees died of TB. He assumed that the high TB incidence was much more closely related to malnutrition than to crowding, since some favored internees in a special area (Block 16), who received food far above the average, remained practically free from TB. He continued:

All the clinical types were to be seen. Acute forms appeared as miliary TB under the spur of typhus, but the characteristic form at Dachau developed slowly, was usually bilateral, and radiologically had a floccular appearance. So slowly did it develop among the really cachectic that they did not appear to die any sooner than those with simple cachexia. Pleural effusions were very common, and some were even cured, mirabile dictu! On the whole it was surprising that not more than an average of 20% of the internees in each block died from TB. [74]

A report from a Swiss hospital in Herisau and a sanatorium in Davos quoted that, in the spring of 1945, again a terrifyingly high number of inmates of German concentration camps suffered from TB: of 243 inmates, 112 had active and 25 inactive TB. On the basis of their patient statistics, the authors estimated that the incidence of active TB was 200 times and that of inactive TB 13 times higher than in the normal population [75].

TB in Displaced Persons

Between 11 and 20 million people were displaced from their homes in the course of WWII. The majority were inmates of Nazi concentration camps, labor camps, and prisoner-of-war camps that were freed by the Allied armies [76]. Many had serious health problems. Displaced Jewish persons represented only a small group: in the British Zone, there were about 15,000 Jews in camps; there were many more, around 140,000, in the American Zone, to which about 100,000 Poles had fled after the pogroms at Kielce in Poland [77]. How many suffered from TB is not known, but it can be assumed from the above reports that a huge number were afflicted. In a report from 1944, a continuous increase in TB in foreign workers was described, particularly among workers from the East and Poland; as mentioned above, the total number was estimated at 8–10,000 [49]. A further report by a civil servant with the German Foreign Ministry described in 1943 that TB was the largest scourge in the camps and that the patients were not isolated from other workers but were forced to work by beating [78].

As Allied troops liberated France in 1944 and crossed into Germany they encountered thousands of refugees or "displaced persons" – escaped prisoners from Nazi concentration camps, exhausted and terrified Jews, slave laborers, political prisoners, Allied POWs, and other victims. The Nazi camps that held these people served as incubators for diseases such as TB and typhus, and the frightened, sick, and starved refugees inundated Army hospitals in late 1944 and early 1945. Theodore Badger reported "one of the first waves that arrived on December 18, 1944 when 304 men, most of them Russians, came to the 50th (US Army General Hospital) in Commercy, France." They had been in the Nazi labor camps in the mines and heavy industry, where thousands had died, and the survivors were malnourished and sick. All 304 had TB, 90% with moderate or advanced disease. Four were dead on arrival, eight more died in the first week, and one third of the patients would die by May. Alarmed, General Hawley, Chief Surgeon of the European Theater of Operations, ordered that all displaced civilians and recovered military personnel be examined for signs of TB "to establish the gravity of the situation". [70]

As mentioned earlier, Daniels in 1947 concluded that it was not surprising that among the displaced persons the prevalence of TB was much lower (about 2%) than the expected 70%. He explained that "these people were literally the survivors of a veritable holocaust; all those who were in the least susceptible must have succumbed in the camps" [72].

Inhuman TB Experiments Performed by the Nazis during the War

During WWII, a number of Nazi doctors conducted painful and often deadly experiments on thousands of concentration camp prisoners (for more details, see chapter 4). TB experiments were also performed. In some of the concentration camps, it was usually new treatments that were tested. During the period from 1941 to 1945, several large-scale TB experiments, mainly in Buchenwald, Dachau, Neuengamme, and Sachsenhausen were documented [47]. The people used as guinea pigs did not always have active TB, but were sometimes artificially infected, as in the particularly horrific experiments by Kurt Heissmeyer, senior physician at the TB sanatorium Hohenlychen. In addition to Russian and Serbian POWs, he experimented on 20 Jewish children delivered from Auschwitz. He intended to prove the already disproven hypothesis that the injection of live TB bacilli into subjects would act as a vaccine. Following the experiments, he murdered the children in April 1945 to remove any evidence. Heissmeyer worked undetected after the war as a pulmonary specialist in Magdeburg in the German Democratic Republic (GDR), and was sentenced only in 1966 to life-long imprisonment [79].

Horrifically cruel experiments were also performed in physically and mentally disabled children to test the methods of TB vaccination. Infected and uninfected children were vaccinated with BCG in special pediatric departments in Vienna, Kaufbeuren, and Berlin-Wiesengrund, then again infected with virulent TB bacteria and finally killed and autopsied to investigate whether or not the vaccination was effective [80].

TB in Germany after the War

Upon the defeat of Nazi Germany in WWII, the victorious Allied powers asserted their authority over all the territory of the German Reich that lay west of the Oder-Neisse line. The country was divided into 4 occupation zones from 1945 to 1949. The American, British, and French zones together made up the Western two thirds of Germany, while the Soviet zone comprised the eastern third (Fig. 4).

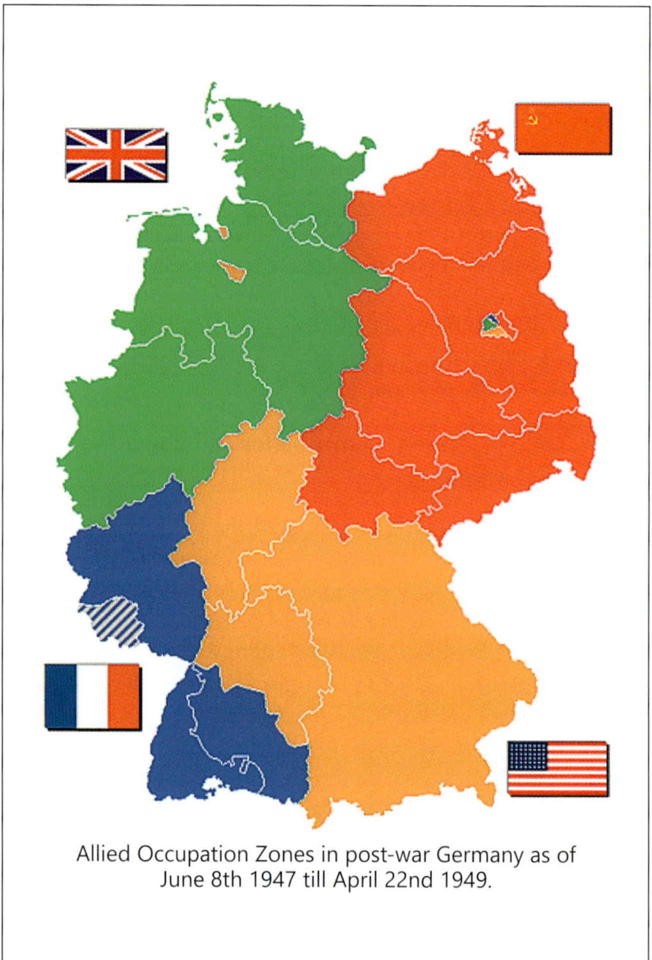

Fig. 4. The 4 occupation zones in Germany after WWII. Wikipedia.

The American zone consisted of Bavaria and Hesse in Southern Germany and the northern portions of the present-day German state of Baden-Württemberg. The ports of Bremen (on the lower Weser River) and Bremerhaven (on the Weser estuary of the North Sea) were also placed under American control because of the American request to have a foothold in Northern Germany.

The British zone consisted of Schleswig-Holstein, Hamburg, Lower Saxony, and the present-day state of North Rhine-Westphalia.

To facilitate German economic self-sufficiency, the United States and British occupation policies soon merged, and by the beginning of 1947 their zones had been joined into one economic area, the Bizone.

The French were apportioned the Länder of Rhineland-Palatinate, the southern half of Baden-Württemberg, and the Saarland, which later received special status.

In May 1949, the British, French, and American zones were joined to form the Federal Republic of Germany (the Saarland became a member only after a vote in 1957).

The Soviet Occupation Zone incorporated Thuringia, Saxony, Saxony-Anhalt, Brandenburg, and Mecklenburg-Vorpommern. On October 7, 1949, the GDR, which became commonly referred to as East Germany, was established in the Soviet Occupation Zone.

Berlin, the former capital, which was surrounded by the Soviet zone, was placed under joint 4-power authority, but was partitioned into 4 sectors for administrative purposes.

Epidemiology

According to Franz Redeker, TB mortality in Germany at the end of the war was estimated to be between 100 and 150/100,000 on average, representing an increase of 160–240% compared with pre-war figures. The lowest TB mortality was registered in Bavaria, at 90/100,000 and the highest in Berlin, at 316/100,000 (see below). For Austria, in 1945, he quotes 155/100,000 or an increase of 162% [7]. However, for several reasons it was difficult or even impossible to collect reliable statistical data directly after the war (see also chapter 2).

The reasons for this were explained in detail by the US Commission [6]. First, the mass migrations at the end of the war made it very difficult to estimate populations. As of 1944, masses of refugees (altogether more than 12 million) left the Eastern parts of the German Reich, including national expellees from Czechoslovakia and Poland. Official statistics started only in summer 1945, with the distribution of food rationing cards to the whole population. Second, large numbers of German POWs (Wehrmacht) were repatriated (of the approximately 11 million German POWs, 5 million were discharged soon after the end of the war); third, there was a great influx of displaced persons: at the end of the war, thousands of inmates of the different concentration camps, where TB was rife, were released, and many wandered at will about the countryside, furnishing further opportunity for chance infection [77]. This mass immigration produced a considerable net increase in the population of the occupied zones of Germany. Furthermore, "data on TB mortality were also subject to several errors. While official death registration figures have been used almost entirely, it should be noted that in some areas death certificates were often signed by laymen [6]". Other reasons were the changes in the boundaries of the provinces (Länder), which made comparisons with earlier data difficult or even impossible. In addition, members of the military were excluded from both population and mortality statistics until the end of the war. Many POWs who returned from Soviet imprisonment suffered from open TB.

There were 2 registration methods for TB mortality, which may explain some of the differences in the published data: one gave figures collected by the Public Health Services (Fürsorgestellen), while for the other the figures came from the civil registry offices (Einwohnermeldeämter) and were higher than the former. A further element of uncertainty is that in Germany, autopsies were (and are still) not obligatory.

Reports, largely based on the rise in morbidity reported by health departments, that TB was epidemic and uncontrolled in Germany directly after the war were much disputed by the TB experts of the British and American occupying powers and the German TB experts [5, 6, 81–83]. The latter claimed that serious malnutrition was responsible for this development, which allegedly did not occur until the final months of the war. The TB experts among the Allies argued that the rise in TB morbidity should be followed by a corresponding rise in TB mortality. As this was not observed, it was assumed by some experts that TB was not such a great epidemiologic problem in Germany. Two reasons may have contributed to the rise in TB morbidity:

The first of these is the fact that TB cases are authorized to receive supplementary food rations. This would appear to create an incentive for physicians to report borderline cases and for patients to seek medical care. The second, and more important factor, is the greatly increased employment of case finding techniques. During and immediately after the war the Fürsorgestellen (public health services/dispensaries) were unable to operate effectively; but during 1946 and 1947 their case finding activities have been greatly intensified. Fluoroscopy is very widely used in Germany as a diagnostic procedure, the use of roentgenograms being often reserved for cases in which fluoroscopic examination has given positive or suspicious findings, and German physicians are highly skilled in this technique. Records are kept of the number of fluoroscopic examinations per month made by the Fürsorgestellen, and the use of the procedure has increased greatly during the past two years. The larger the number of persons examined, the higher will be the yield of new cases of TB, although the yield per 100 examinations may diminish. [6]

In addition, the classification of active TB cases employed at that time in German public health practice was rather elaborate, having 3 categories of respiratory TB and 2 categories of extrapulmonary TB. The 3 respiratory categories may be briefly described as:

Table 2. Total TB mortality in the German Reich (1939) and in the area of FRG (1946–1950) and for pulmonary, extrapulmonary and all forms, separately for males and females [84]

Year	Pulmonary TB			Extrapulmonary TB		All forms		Total
	male	female	all	male	female	male	female	
1939	64	47	55	9	9	73	56	64
1946	94	47	68	17	13	111	60	83
1948	75	40	57	11	10	87	50	67
1950	45	22	33	7	7	52	29	39

(a) Active respiratory TB, with demonstrable tubercle bacilli; (b) active respiratory TB, without the demonstration of tubercle bacilli but with lesions which are regarded as 'open' or infectious. Terms sometimes used for this group are 'clinically open' or 'facultative open'.

(c) Active 'closed' or 'noninfectious' respiratory TB. This group includes stationary infiltrations, hilar and bronchial node enlargements, miliary strand-like lesions of lungs, exudative pleurisy, productive cirrhotic lesions, and infants with positive tuberculin reactions.

Most of the types of disease in group (c) would not ordinarily be reported in the United States. In the absence of knowledge of how large a proportion they constitute, it is felt that this group is best excluded from consideration in the analysis of morbidity.

However, the American experts stated:

morbidity figures from Germany are based upon reports rendered by the TB clinics or Fürsorgestellen, in which nearly all known cases are registered and where most of the diagnoses are checked and confirmed. In this respect they are more reliable than American data.

In 1946, the first year after the war, TB mortality of all forms in the Western occupation zones (from 1949 known as the Federal Republic of Germany [FRG] – without the Saarland, which became a member of the FRG only in 1957) was estimated at 83/100,000 (an increase of 30% compared with 1939), 111/100,000 in males and 60/100,000 in females (Table 2). For pulmonary TB, it was 68/100,000 (94 in males and 47 in females), and for extrapulmonary TB it was 1.5/100,000 (1.7 and 1.3, respectively) [84]. In the following years, mortality decreased substantially, and by 1950 it was below pre-war levels.

Lydtin [43] explains the rise of TB in wartime by the changes in living conditions, and 2 main aspects: first, an increase in infections due to population movement, living in barracks, progressive increases in density of dwellings, poor sanitation, loss of beds for sick persons – in particular, for isolation – and poor registration of infectious sources due to shortages of medical personnel, particularly doctors; and second, the reduced resistance of the population caused by physical and mental stress due to general misery, mainly caused by quantitative and qualitative malnutrition.

Milk was an important source of infection due to *M. bovis* TB bacteria. It was estimated that about 10% of all TB cases were caused by *M. bovis*. General pasteurization of milk was introduced only in 1947. The culling of infected cattle was started in the FRG in 1952 and in the GDR in 1955, at first on a voluntary basis, and then from 1959 as an obligatory measure. By 1961, 99.7% of all cattle herds in the FRG were free of TB (in 1952, more than 90% had been infected), while in the GDR 99% of herds had been cleared of TB by 1971 [85].

The development of the TB situation differed in the 4 occupation zones (American, British, French, and Russian), which will be described separately. As Berlin itself was divided into 4 occupation sectors and had the highest TB mortality, the situation there is described first.

Berlin

TB mortality in Berlin reached its peak in the months following the capitulation in May 1945. In 1945, it was estimated at 291/100,000 (compared to 162/100,000 in 1944) [42]. From June 1946 onward, these figures gradually decreased to 223 in 1947, 173 in 1948, 131 in 1949, and to 65/100,000 in 1950 for the whole of Berlin. In the districts of West Berlin, which comprised approximately two thirds of the population, it was 52/100,000 in 1950, almost reaching the presumptive secular curve of the drop in TB mortality that would have been expected without the war. About 70,000 people died from TB during the war, and it has been estimated, referring to the secular curve, that without the impact of the war about 36,000 individuals would not have died. However, Meyer puts these figures into perspective, pointing to the fact that other diseases, such as cardiac disease or cancer, also showed a substantial increase during the war. Males had a TB mortality rate that was 3 times higher than females. Meyer opposes the opinion that this male preponderance is explained by malnutrition. He assumes as one potential reason a selection process by the war, by which healthy males had been drafted to the army, were killed or returned sick – in particular, after internment in a POW camp – whereas in non-drafted males TB was more prevalent.

Why Berlin suffered so heavily from TB is not entirely clear [6]. Sartwell et al. [6] list several reasons:

Berlin had a higher rate than other large German cities before the war; bombing was continuous rather than sporadic; food shortages were presumably greater because of the difficulty of a large city in procuring food from the surrounding farmland; and Berlin was cut off from the use of its sanatoria to a greater degree than other places (most were outside the city). Berlin's population is older than in other parts of Germany; with the present age distribution of deaths, this in itself would tend to make the crude death rate somewhat higher.

In contrast to the slowly falling TB mortality rate, morbidity rose until 1948. During and immediately after the war, the dispensaries/public health offices (Fürsorgestellen) were unable to operate effectively, but during 1946 and 1947 their case finding activities were greatly intensified by using fluoroscopy and, in cases with suspected TB, roentgenograms. An additional reason may have been that, from August 1946, TB patients received supplementary food rations, which attracted more TB patients who would not otherwise have been registered at the dispensaries. In the last 5 months of 1945, 6815 new TB cases were registered, corresponding to an incidence of 469/100,000, which increased during the following years: to 563 in 1946 (17,779 new cases), to 833 in 1947 (26,788 new cases), and to 889/100,000 in 1948 (28,996 new cases). In 1948, the total number of TB patients rose to 84,450 compared to 34,605 cases in 1934. This increase was also partly due to the new classification by which non-infectious (closed) but active pulmonary TB cases, mainly diagnosed by fluoroscopy/roentgenogram, were included. 1949 was the first year in which the number of new cases declined (25,781) [42]).

In children, milk shortages may have been an important factor that caused the death of newborns and small children, in particular. More than 50 cases of tuberculous meningitis were seen in Berlin each year. A dramatic cure – described by some as a miracle – was observed in these children after the application of streptomycin. This was provided to the newly founded Heckeshorn Chest Clinic (Lungenklinik Heckeshorn) by the Americans in 1947 [86]. Other treatment centers in the US zone, in Munich, Frankfurt, Stuttgart, Heidelberg, and Bremen also received streptomycin. The indication for streptomycin was later extended to miliary TB [87].

United States Occupation Zone
Among the 4 occupation zones, the American Zone is the best investigated, and this includes TB [82]. In her book entitled "Democracy as remedy. Health, disease and politics in the American Occupation Zone 1945–1949" [Healing Democracy – Demokratie als Heilmittel. Gesundheit, Krankheit und Politik in der amerikanischen Besatzungszone 1945–1949], Dagmar Ellerbrock gives a very detailed analysis of the post-war situation in the US Zone. The book also contains a long chapter on TB (On wasting strengths in dire straits [Vom Schwinden der Kräfte in schweren Zeiten, pp 324–444).

According to a comprehensive overview of the TB situation in Germany (and other countries) [88], there were very few mortality data for 1945, except for Berlin, as described above, and Bavaria (see below). In 1946, TB mortality in the US Zone was estimated at 76/100,000 (12,507 deaths) in a population of 16.37 million. Mortality dropped in the following years to 69 in 1947 and to 61/100,000 in 1948.

The post-war situation in the US Zone is also described in depth in 2 publications provided by members of a commission that was appointed by the Secretary of the US Army. The commission consisted of 5 members; the chairman was one of the leading US TB experts, Esmond R. Long [6]. The task of the commission was "to investigate the incidence of and recommend control measures for TB in the German civilian population." Long described the situation in 1948 [5] on the basis of his early visits to Germany since April 1945 and of the studies performed by the commission:

When Military Government was set up in the spring of 1945 (observations here apply to the US Zone), the German TB control program was found badly disorganized. City hospitals and TB clinics had been destroyed and their functions were being carried on in highly inferior quarters with inadequate equipment. Sanatoria outside of the city were occupied in large measure by wounded soldiers, POW and non-German displaced personnel. Widespread disruption of transportation was doubly injurious to the program, preventing patients from going to clinics for diagnosis and treatment, making it very difficult for public health nurses and social workers to go to the homes of patients to give advice and home care. As a result, patients who once would have received prompt hospital and sanatorium care, remained at home. This was soon recognized by German public health authorities as a grave threat to the health of the population.

Long [5] then stated that the data on the prevalence of TB mortality were untrustworthy in the first months after the war, one of the main reasons being "an almost complete change in the German public health authority. Most of the officials in control had records of Nazi affiliation disqualifying them for further service." Therefore

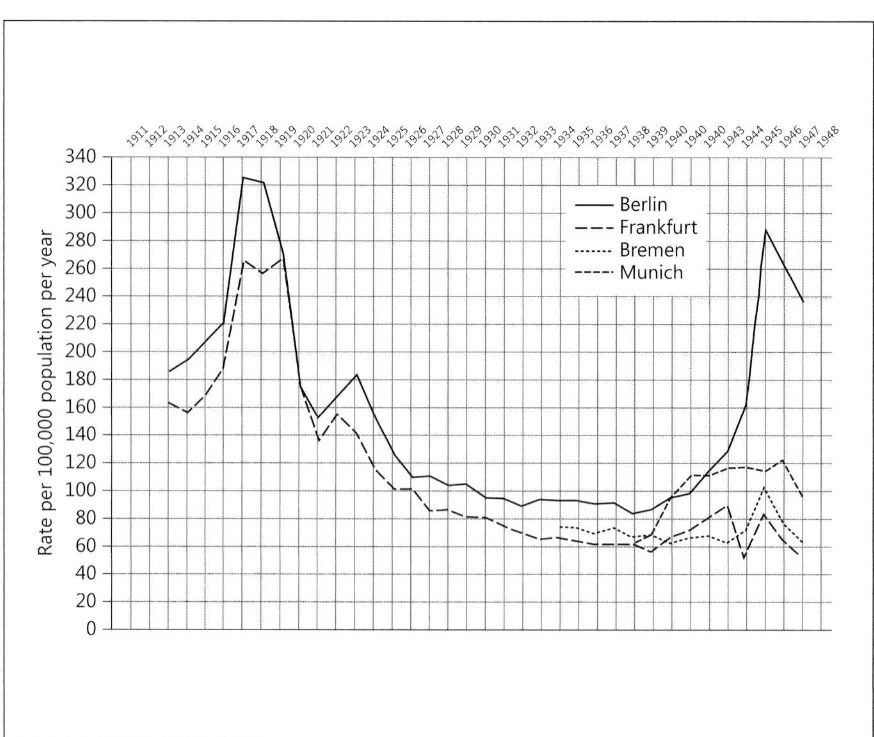

Fig. 5. Tuberculosis mortality in selected large cities in Germany (Berlin, Frankfurt, Bremen, Munich). Death rates for all forms of tuberculosis, 1913–1948 [5].

an immediate essential step was restoration of a German official TB control authority in each department of health. Qualified men were hard to find. Data, which once went promptly to a centralized authority in Berlin, after the war could go no further than an inferior health department in a Land. Frequently they did not get that far. Remarkably, essential data were in general preserved at the source, and in time became again available.

The Military Government started the reorganization of TB control through its Public Health Branch by establishing

politically acceptable, professionally qualified personnel in responsible positions. As Army combat forces released beds first used for POW and the housing of displaced personnel, Military Government officers gradually secured more beds for the care of TB. German barracks which had been made into reasonably effective hospitals during the war become TB hospitals. Attack on the housing problem by newly constituted German officials, effecting urgently needed repairs in usable buildings, reduced the crowding in homes to some extent and thereby decreased opportunity for contagion. Material assistance was given to the new German economy from available Army stocks. In some German TB sanatoria a principal source of food was boxed Army K rations. Outpatient clinics were restored to function, although in considerably reduced number. Gradually the sanatoria reverted to their original use, as POW were released and other provision was made for displaced personnel.

Long then concluded:

Within a surprisingly short time a remarkably effective TB control program was again in operation. The total number of beds available for the treatment of TB, which had reached the low level of less than one per annual TB death at the end of the war, has approximately doubled since that time and now is not far from the accepted ideal standard ratio of 2 and a half beds per annual TB death, with one outstanding exception. In Berlin, a quadripartite-governed city, existing as a municipal island in the Russian Zone, there is a great deficiency in beds for the care of TB. In former times the sanatoria for Berlin patients were outside the city. This is still true and now they are generally unavailable. An attempt is being made to create an additional supply of suitable beds in the city, but thus far the program is very far short of the success obtained in the US and British Zones. Coincidentally with the restoration of a good TB control program a significant drop in TB mortality had occurred. Full data on this development are included in the official report of the commission to which reference has been made. These will be the subject of later exhaustive analysis and report. For present purpose it will suffice to refer to Fig. 5, which shows the rise and fall of mortality in a representative group of cities, including Berlin and the 3 largest cities in the US Zone. (Fig. 5)

Long further noted that "the actual levels of mortality reached in the WWI rise were not reached in WWII, but the percentage increase in mortality over the prewar rate was quite as great".

Finally, he stated that the drop in mortality since 1945 was encouraging, and that it was to be hoped that the worst phase was over. However,

German public health authorities themselves lay less stress on the apparent improvement in death rate than they do on an officially recorded great increase in reported cases of active disease. In the opinion of the commission to which reference has been made this rise in reported cases does not have the full significance attributed to it by some of the German authorities. It appears in large part due to a greatly expanded case-finding program, and is believed to be in some and perhaps large degree affected by the incentive to case reporting furnished by the food supplements granted to persons diagnosed as tuberculous.

Regarding the debate on deficits in food supply being the main cause for the rise in TB cases, E.R. Long remarked that

according to statements made by German authorities serious impairment of nutrition did not occur until the final months of the war. Indeed, the statement has been made by Germans that it did not occur until after the war, when the reversal of authority, the extra provision for the millions of displaced personnel in the country, and the removal of men suspected of Nazi adherence from productive enterprise, sharply curtailed the German civilian ration.

However, this statement has been questioned particularly by the British experts (see below) [81, 82].

The report by E.R. Long was followed in 1949 by a second report by 3 members of the commission [6]. They described in detail the development in Bavaria as a largely agricultural state in the south, where there were few territorial changes after the war. Relatively good statistics were available there, with the limitation that changes due to extensive post-war migration were not taken into account. The other Lander in the US Zone have experienced rises and declines in TB mortality, quite similar to those of Bavaria. The evidence indicates that mortality was highest in 1945 and has steadily fallen since then. Figure 6 shows the mortality rates for pulmonary TB in Bavaria for the years between 1894 and 1947.

Interestingly, the rise in TB mortality in Bavaria between 1937 and 1947 is almost completely due to pulmonary TB, while there is only a very small increase in extrapulmonary TB, which is illustrated in Figure 1 (in chapter 3). The relative frequency of pulmonary and other forms of TB as causes of death showed no remarkable variation in the areas studied, with pulmonary TB ranging from 91% of all TB deaths in Berlin down to 82% in Hesse in 1947. For the 3 principal Lander in the U.S. Zone, 85% of mortality was ascribed to pulmonary TB and 15% to TB of other organs (see

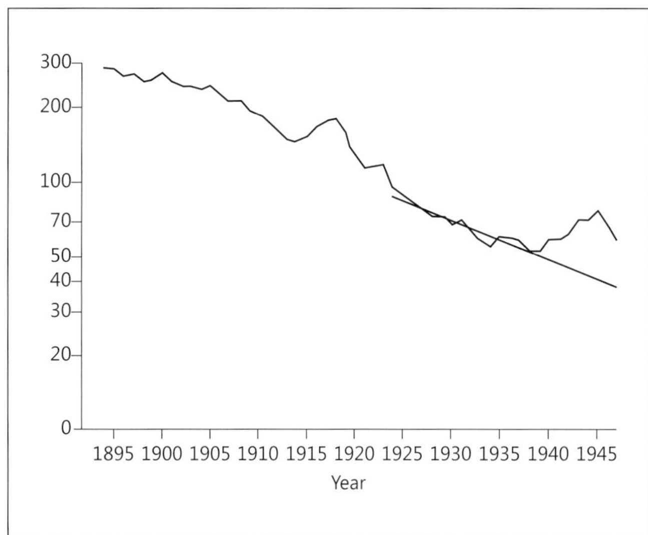

Fig. 6. Mortality rates for pulmonary tuberculosis, Bavaria, by year, 1894–1947 (logarithmic scale) [6].

also chapter 3). These proportions are identical with the figures for whole Germany over the 3 year period 1935–1937 [6].

Age-specific rates for each sex in Bavaria are compared with those in the USA in Figure 6 (in chapter 3): In 1946, the mortality for males was greatly increased in infancy and in all adult age groups. The most marked excess was in the 20–34 year age span. Among females, on the contrary, the only population groups showing an increase in 1946 as compared with 1938 were infants and young children, among whom a rise similar to the male rise was recorded (see chapter 3).

Data from Bavaria confirm that the TB mortality is generally higher in cities than in rural districts, and increased markedly during the war (Fig. 2 in chapter 3).

With American assistance, the TB control program was restructured: The number of hospital and sanatorium beds was substantially increased (except in Berlin), approaching the conditions in the US; case finding and case supervision by the local public health organizations were intensified; a BCG vaccination program was undertaken under the supervision of the Danish and Swedish Red Cross; and food supplements were authorized for tuberculous persons and many essential materials in addition to food, ranging from soap to X-ray film were provided. Sartwell et al. [6] concluded with the general remark that "only general economic recovery can help this situation, and indeed the whole TB problem is closely linked to the economic state of the country."

British Occupation Zone

According to the already mentioned overview by Kröger and Reuter on the TB situation in Germany (and other countries), TB mortality in the British Zone was estimated at 89/100,000 in 1946 (19,336 cases in a population of 21.7 million) [88]. Then, in 1947, mortality dropped to 77 and in 1948 to 62/100,000, almost reaching the lower TB mortality in the US Zone. The much higher mortality in 1946 and 1947 was assumed by some to be related to the differing food supply during these years.

A report on certain aspects of the TB problem in the British Zone of Germany was prepared by the Medical Research Council on the suggestion of the Ministry of Health and published in March 1948 [81]. The opinion expressed in this and other reports by Daniels [72, 89–91] is much more critical than the American one. They compare the German figures with corresponding figures in their own country and come to the conclusion that the overall German TB situation is less severe: "The corresponding figures for London in the same 2 years were 87 and 70. The rates for Hamburg in fact are considerably less than those obtained in Glasgow and Liverpool (and in Paris, Warsaw, and Rome)".

The authors mention that during the post-war period, the death rate from pulmonary TB in Hamburg declined, while in the 3 other regions the figures showed little evidence of change. The death rate from non-pulmonary TB also declined slightly in Hamburg, remained stationary in Schleswig-Holstein, and increased somewhat in the other 2 Länder (provinces). The 1946 death rates were higher than pre-war rates, but the main rises occurred during the war period. The authors underlined their assessment by citing further figures:

The proportionate TB mortality, the number of deaths which occurred from this disease expressed as a percentage of annual deaths from all causes, also confirms the view that TB does not figure more largely among health problems in the British Zone of Germany than in Great Britain. The figure for England and Wales for 1945 was 4.8% as against 4.2% in Niedersachsen and 4.5% in Schleswig-Holstein in 1946. The figure of 5.7% in Hamburg in 1946 may be compared with the 1945 figures for London 5.5% or for Manchester 6.4%. [81]

The British authors mention, like the Americans, that

the rise in morbidity was almost entirely due to a change in the methods of notification and, therefore, the recent steep rise in pulmonary TB case notification rates represents largely a 'paper increase' and has allowed the notification of many equivocal cases that would not be notified in British practice.........We must state categorically that we attach no significance whatever to statistics of pulmonary case notifications as an index of current TB trends in the British Zone.

At the end of 1946, there were 200,000 cases on the TB dispensary registers of the British Zone. For comparison, the report points out that at the end of 1946 there were 244,000 definite cases of TB on the TB dispensary registers of England and Wales, with a population nearly twice as large. The British total, however, is based on criteria that would exclude the German category (c), in which there were 122,000 among British Zone cases.

Two further points are made in the report on the British Zone:

The fact that TB mortality increased more among males than among females during the war is ascribed partly to a selective factor – healthy young men were enlisted and the statistics relate, therefore, to the remaining male population and partly to the greater strain of wartime conditions borne by males. The increase in the mortality from non-pulmonary TB and in the incidence of new cases is probably due to a failure of efficient pasteurization. Much of the pasteurization plant was damaged during the war and it has since then been subject to general deterioration and reduced efficiency. Fuel shortages have also made pasteurization difficult.

The British report ends with the somewhat sardonic comment

We must refer here to the regrettable fact that German officials (some non-medical) have repeatedly during the past year issued to Allied journalists and other visitors misleading and sometimes even false information regarding the TB situation in Germany. These statements have had the effect of putting TB in Germany unjustifiably on the level of a sensational news item. Moreover, since it is generally known that TB figures are a sensitive index of social conditions, sweeping conclusions as to these conditions have been drawn from erroneous data.

Nevertheless, the British allowed, as they had first done in 1947, the re-foundation of the German Central Committee against TB (DZK) in their zone – and together with the Americans the re-foundation of the German Tuberculosis Society – for the whole 3 western zones were permitted in 1949. This finally allowed the reorganization of the TB control program on a broad basis.

French Occupation Zone

TB mortality in the French Occupation Zone resembled in 1946 those of Bavaria. The development in the following years until 1950 was also very much alike, both being mainly a largely agricultural state without many big cities (in Ref. [7], Table page 484).

Jessica Reinisch states in her book entitled "The perils of peace: the public health crisis in occupied Germany" that "it was Germans" dissatisfaction with the French that dominated reports. In the contemporary press, the French zone was described as "the step-child among the 4 zones" run by a country "which, itself, has come out of the war impoverished and diminished in importance [83]".

From the moment they set foot on German soil, the needs of the French occupation troops appeared to come into conflict with those of the occupied population. In contrast to the British and American zones, but like the Soviet zone, the territory occupied by France had to provide much of the occupation troops' upkeep. The burden on each inhabitant, F. Roy Willis has calculated, was proportionately heavier in the French zone than in the British or American. The high density of military government officers and the fact that families of occupation staff were encouraged to settle in the zone, added bodies to be housed and mouths to be fed. One report from 1946 estimated that around 17,000 French people lived in the town of Baden-Baden alone. It thought that the 'amounts of food stuffs used by the occupying forces throughout the zone must be considerable, especially if it is remembered that the rations accorded them are far superior to those given out to the average person. To the number of administrators accompanied by their families must be added numerous mobilized troop contingents, which are rationed in Germany.' Some French reports observed that German rations during the first occupation year were in the region of 1,000–1,300 calories per person per day, and rose to at least 1,400 calories in 1947 and 1,869 in 1948. [83]

And Jessica Rheinisch continues:

German doctors assumed the roles of spokesmen for the German population at large. Food shortages had a direct impact on German public health, they argued. Members of the University of Tübingen's medical faculty produced a series of 4 memoranda on the food situation from August 1945 until summer 1946, which contained reports from various medical specialists about the physical effects of the food shortage. They painted a picture of a town on the verge of a hunger catastrophe. For the Germans real hunger had come with the occupation army; the physical destruction, lack of transport, and disruption of trade with the lost eastern territories were all exacerbated by the French living off the fat of the zone. One of their recommendations was the reduction of the population's working day to between 4 and 6 h, 'to save calories.' Throughout the first years of the occupation, German health officers insisted that lack of food was directly linked to rising rates of TB, the diminution of the population's physical and mental capacities, and the declining health of children. [83]

Rheinisch proceeds:

And yet, by 1949, the initial goals and priorities of the French project had been largely overturned by the French zone's growing proximity to the American and British zones, and its integration into 'Trizonia,' the future Federal Republic of Germany. It was only through political and material support that the persistent conflicts and confrontations in the French zone could be resolved. By then, France itself had already been a beneficiary of substantial amounts of Marshall aid. The new alignments had immediate and visible effects in the zone. In the French sector of Berlin food rations increased markedly during the Soviet blockade. Or, according to Desplats's history, the twelve months from June 1948 to June 1949 saw a complete transformation of the German economy, a currency reform, and the arrival of Marshall aid for imports of both food and medical supplies. Thereafter, drugs such as penicillin, streptomycin, and insulin could be imported, and pharmaceutical supplies in the zone soon reached or even exceeded pre-war levels. By the time the nutrition surveys were terminated in December 1948, health officers reported 'very noticeable improvements in the nutritional state of population' in the wake of the currency reform. By then, too, the sanatoria in the Black Forest, which the French military government had acquired for use by French children, POW, and concentration camp survivors, were returned to the German authorities, because of, as Desplats put it, 'a change in orientation' by the military government. [83]

Soviet Occupation Zone (Since 1949 GDR)

In the Soviet occupation zone (from 1949, officially the GDR), the situation was worse due to the influx of many refugees from the former Eastern provinces of the German Reich which were lost after the war. In 1945–1946 alone, 56,780 cases with infectious pulmonary TB were recorded (excluding Berlin), of whom 23,600 died. In 1947, TB mortality was estimated at 163/100,000, but it is possible that a high number of cases was not reported [92]). More reliable statistics were available only after the stabilization of the health care system with the foundation of the GDR in 1949, when mortality was estimated at 107/100,000 [93]) Thus, mortality was more than twofold higher than in the Western zones, with only 50.9/100,000. According to the official statistics [9], TB mortality in 1950 dropped to 78.5/100,000 (14.439 deaths) and an estimated incidence of 504.5 (92,760 new cases), compared to a mortality of 39.4 (25,345 deaths) and an estimated incidence of 257.1 (130,080 new cases), respectively, in the Western occupation zones (mortality 39.4). These high figures decreased substantially during the following years. In 1955, TB mortality in the GDR was reduced by about two thirds to 25.5/100,000, and the number of new cases more than halved (47,015), with an incidence of 262/100,000 (in the FRG 20.3 and 185.5/100,000, respectively).

To improve TB control, the Soviet military administration issued in 1946 a command (Befehl No. 297) that the TB control should be strictly governed by the principles of Robert Koch [45]. This detailed command then formed the sol-

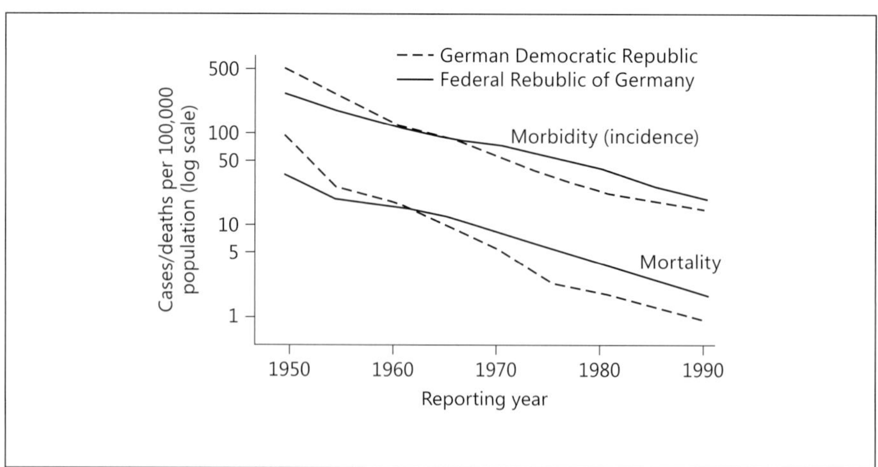

Fig. 7. Tuberculosis case and deaths rates (log scale), German Democratic Republic (GDR) and Federal Republic of Germany (FRG), 1949–1990, modified from [94].

id foundation for all measures against TB in the GDR. Hospitals and sanatoria, and the network of TB dispensaries had to be restored and, within 2 years, approximately 30,000 beds for the isolation and treatment of infectious TB patients were provided.

In the following years, the almost catastrophic situation in the GDR developed in terms of morbidity and mortality rates, an even better position than the western parts of Germany (Federal Republic of Germany [FRG]; Fig. 7). This development was most probably related to the introduction of systematic control measures with strict observation of all TB cases including their treatment, regular mass roentgenography screening introduced in some regions already since 1949 (and as obligatory in the whole country since 1962), and possibly the obligatory BCG vaccination of newborns, repeated at the end of school time which started partially in 1949 and in the whole country from 1961. However, other reasons may have been that TB mortality in the Soviet zone (GDR) was during the first years 2-fold higher than in the Western zones (FRG) by which infectious sources were eliminated faster, thus reducing the spread of the TB bacilli to the population. In addition, the FRG had less favorable conditions due to the substantially larger proportion of foreigners (immigrants and asylum seekers) from countries with high TB incidence [94].

Conclusions

Not only that Germany (together with Austria) started WWII, the Nazi regime also introduced a partially inhuman dictatorial system. This can be shown explicitly with the example of TB. The main health-related motto became "Public interest ahead of self-interest." This edict also changed the existing concepts of TB control in many ways as new control measures were decreed by new laws. The most intrusive was the law for the "Unification of Health Affairs," decreed in July 1934, thereby transferring decision-making power to the central government, with potentially significant consequences for the individual TB patient. The most intrusive laws for the individual were the "Law on the prevention of genetically diseased offspring," followed by the "Law for the protection of the genetic health of the German Volk" (Marriage Health Law) on the basis of which a marriage could be forbidden. The "Regulation on the control of communicable diseases" enabled the compulsory isolation of so-called "anti-social" TB patients in closed TB institutions. Possible consequences for these patients were that they were purposefully undernourished, and ran the real risk of dying of starvation. Furthermore, compulsory isolation of the so-called "anti-social" TB patients was enabled and the "Decree on labor of tuberculous persons" allowed that with very few limitations even patients with open (infectious) TB were considered capable of working.

Worse still and almost unbelievable was the terrible persecution of Jews and other unwanted persons, their accommodation in concentration camps under horrifying conditions, the inhuman medical experiments, also in TB patients, and the so-called "final solution", ending in the holocaust with the murder of millions. It only can be hoped that the lessons have been learned to avoid similar developments in the future.

References

1 Grass H (ed): Der Kampf gegen die Tuberkulose in Deutschland [The fight against tuberculosis in Germany]. Berlin, Reichs-Tuberkulose-Ausschuss, 1939.

2 Murray JF: A century of tuberculosis. Am J Respir Crit Care Med 2004;169:1181–1186.

3 Koch R: Epidemiologie der tuberkulose [epidemiology of tuberculosis]. Zeitschr Hyg Infektionskr 1910;37:1–18.

4 Brügmann E: Die Bewegung der Tuberkulosesterblichkeit im I. und II. Weltkrieg und ihre Ursachen [Fluctuation of tuberculosis mortality in World War I and II and their causes]. Beitr Klin Tuberk 1947;101:94–104.

5 Long ER: Tuberculosis in Germany. Proc Natl Acad Sci U S A 1948;34:271–277.

6 Sartwell PE, Moseley CH, Long ER: Tuberculosis in the German population, United States Zone of Germany. Am Rev Tuberc 1949;59:481–493.

7 Redeker F: Epidemiologie und Statistik der Tuberkulose; in Hein J, Kleinschmidt H, Uehlinger E (eds): Handbuch der Tuberkulose, Vol I of IV, ed 1. Stuttgart, Georg Thieme, 1958, pp 407–498.

8 Berg G: Statistik über Tuberkulosemortalität in Kriegszeiten [Statistics on tuberculosis mortality in wartimes]. Beitr Klin Tuberk 1951;106:1–9.

9 Pöhn HP, Rasch G: Statistik Meldepflichtiger Erkrankungen [Statistics of Notifiable Diseases]. München, MMV Verlag, 1994.

10 Walter O: Die Tuberkulosebekämpfung als politische Aufgabe [The fight against tuberculosis as political task]. Beitr Klin Tuberk 1935:414–424.

11 Proctor R: Racial hygiene. Medicine under the Nazis. Cambridge, Harvard University Press, 1988.

12 Kayser-Petersen J: Das Gesetz zum Schutze der Erbgesundheit des deutschen Volkes vom 18.X.1935 und seine Bedeutung für die Tuberkulosekranken [The law for the protection of genetic health of the German Volk of 18 October 1935 and its impact on tuberculous patients]. Beitr Klin Tuberk Spezif Tuberkuloseforsch 1937;89:736–748.

13 Kayser-Petersen J: Richtlinien für die ärztliche Tätigkeit auf dem Gebiet des Ehegesundheitsgesetzes [Guidelines for medical activities in the field of the marriage health law]. Beitr Klin Tuberk 1937;89:748.

14 Hahn S: Ethische Grundlagen der faschistischen Medizin, dargestellt am Beispiel der Tuberkulosebekämfung [Ethical basis of fascistic medicine, represented by the example of the fight against tuberculosis]; in Thom A, Spaar H (eds): Medizin im Faschismus [Medicine in facism]. Berlin, VEB Verlag, 1985.

15 Seiffert E: Ehegesundheitsgesetz und Tuberkulose [Marriage health law and tuberculosis]. Tuberkuloseblatt 1935/1936(9/10):240–246.

16 Koester F: Lungentuberkulose und Schwangerschaft [Pulmonary tuberculosis and pregnancy]. Tuberkuloseblatt 1939(13):309–317.

17 Kröner H-P: Von der Rassenhygiene zur Humangenetik [From race hygiene to human genetics]. Stuttgart/Jena/Lübeck/Ulm, Gustav Fischer, 1998.

18 Diehl K, von Verschuer O: Zwillingstuberkulose I [Twin tuberculosis I]. Jena, Fischer, 1933.

19 Diehl K, von Verschuer O: Der Erbeinfluss bei der Tuberkulose. Zwillingstuberkulose II [The genetic impact in tuberculosis. Twin tuberculosis II]. Jena, Fischer, 1936.

20 Redeker F: Tuberkulosevererbung und Eugenik [Tuberculosis inheritance and eugenics]. Zeitschr für Tuberkulose und Eugenik 1931;62:25–34.

21 Lange L, Pescatore H: Bakteriologische Untersuchungen zur Lübecker Säuglingstuberkulose. Arbeiten a d Reichsges-Amt 1935;69:205–305.

22 Ulrici H: Über die Bedeutung der Erblichkeit für die Entwicklung und den Verlauf der Tuberkulose [The relevance of heredity for the development and course of tuberculosis]. Med Klinik 1934;10:324–326.

23 Binding K, Hoche A: Die Freigabe der Vernichtung lebensunwerten Lebens: Ihr Mass und ihre Form. [Allowing the Destruction of Life Unworthy of Life: Its Dimension and Form]. Berliner Wissenschaftsverlag 1920.

24 B. P. Ideologie und Mord. Euthanasie bei >lebensunwerten< Menschen (Ideology and murder. Euthanasia in humans <unworthy of life>. Hürtgenwald, Pressler, 1986.

25 Mitscherlich A, Mielke F: Medizin ohne Menschlichkeit. Dokumente des Nürnberger Ärzteprozesses [Medicine without humanity. Documents of the Nuremberg trial against physicians]. Frankfurt a. M./Hamburg, Fischerbücherei, 1949.

26 Aly G: Die Belasteten. >Euthanasie< 1939–1945. Eine Gesellschaftsgeschichte [The burdened. >Euthanasia< 1939–1945. A society story]. Frankfurt a M, Fischer, 2013.

27 Kloos G: Die Zwangsunterbringung von rücksichtslosen Offentuberkulösen [The compulsary isolation of inconsiderate patients with open tuberculosis]. Dt Tuberkulose-Blatt 1942;222–229:42–46.

28 Ferlinz R: Die Tuberkulose in Deutschland und das Deutsche Zentralkomitee zur Bekämpfung der Tuberkulose. Pneumologie 1995;49:617–632.

29 Griesbach R, Holm J: Der Anteil boviner Infektionen an der Lungentuberkulose Erwachsener [Proportion of bovine infections in pulmonary tuberculosis of adults]. Tuberkulosearzt 1948;2.

30 Redeker F: Zentrale Lenkung der Röntgen-Reihenuntersuchung [Central control of roentgenologic mass screening]. Die Gesundheitsführung – Ziel und Weg 1939(12):90–98.

31 Griesbach R: Die Kleinbildschirmphotographie [The miniature photofluorography]. Z Tuberkulose 1939;82:81–89.

32 Beese HJ: Über Röntgenreihenuntersuchungen auf Lungentuberkulose in Reichsheer, Reichsmarine und Schutzpolizei [About radiographic mass screening for pulmonary tuberculosis in the army, navy and defense police]. Beitr Klin Tuberk 1934;85:1–8.

33 Möllers B: Die Bekämpfung der Tuberkulose durch die Gesetzgebung [The fight against tuberculosis by legislation]; in Grass H (ed): Der Kampf gegen die Tuberkulose in Deutschland [The fight against tuberculosis in Germany]. Berlin, Reichs-Tuberkulose-Ausschuss, 1939.

34 Holfelder H: Der erste Grosseinsatz des Röntgenreihenbildners im SS-Lager zu Nürnberg [The first large scale operation of photofluorography in a SS camp at Nuremberg]. Münch Med Wschr 1938;38:1465–1467.

35 Holfelder H, Berner F: Atlas des Röntgenreihenbildes des Brustraums auf Grund der Auswertung von über 900,000 Röntgenreihenschirmbildern [Atlas of photofluorography of the chest on basis of more than 900,000 photofluorographies]. Fortschr Röntgenstr 1939;suppl (59):5–95.

36 Blasius D: Die Tuberkulose im Dritten Reich [The tuberculosis in the Third Reich]; in Konietzko N (ed): 100 Jahre Deutsches Zentralkomitee zur Bekämpfung der Tuberkulose (DZK). Der Kampf gegen die Tuberkulose [100 years of the German Committee for the fight against tuberculosis (DZK). The fight against tuberculosis]. Frankfurt a. M., Pmi Verlagsgruppe, 1996.

37 Lange B, Thon H: Das Ergebnis von Tuberkulinreihenprüfungen bei jugendlichen Erwachsenen; ein Beitrag zur Epidemiologie der Tuberkulose [The result of tuberculin mass investigations in adolescents; a contribution to the epidemiology of tuberculosis]. Dtsch Med Wschr 1939;65:884–888.

38 Lange B: Untersuchungen zur Klärung der Ursachen der im Anschluss an die Calmette-Impfung aufgetretenen Säuglingserkrankungen in Lübeck. Zeitschr Tuberkulose 1930;59:1–18.

39 Moegling A: Die "Epidemiologie" der Lübecker Säuglingstuberkulose. Arbeiten a d Reichsges-Amt 1935;69:1–24.

40 Rieder HL: Die Abklärung der Lübecker Säuglingstuberkulose [Clarification of the Luebeck infant tuberculosis]. Pneumologie 2003;57:402–405.

41 Auersbach K: Zur Einführung der Calmette-Impfung in Deutschland. Ärztl Wschr 1946;1:314–317.

42 Meyer C: Die Entwicklung der Tuberkulose in Berlin. Beitr Klin Tuberk 1951;105:408–428.

43 Lydtin K: Übersicht über das Tuberkulosegeschehen in Deutschland während des 2. Weltkrieges und in der Nachkriegszeit. Beitr Klin Tuberk 1950;102:487–502.

44 Federhen L: Die Lungentuberkulösen eines Bevölkerungsgebietes von 350,000 Einwohnern während eines Zeitraumes von 1928–1951. Beitr Klin Tuberk 1955;114:110–120.

45 Klesse M: Beitrag zum quantitativ-exogenen Tuberkuloseproblem und Wege zur Feststellung des wirklichen Tuberkuloseverlaufs im zweiten Weltkrieg. Dtsch Gesundheitswesen 1946;1:688–695.

46 Schenck EG: Allgemeine und ärztliche Indikationen für die Gewährung von Nahrungsmittelzulagen für Kranke [General and medical indications for the permission of supplementary food for sick persons]. Dtsch Ärztebl 1943;5/6:50.

47 Wolters C: Tuberkulose und Menschenversuche im Nationalsozialismus [Tuberculosis and human experiments in national socialism]. Stuttgart, Franz Steiner, 2011.

48 Nicol K: Die Wiedereingliederung der Tuberkulösen in den Arbeitsprozess [The reintegration of tuberculous persons into the working process]. Dt Tuberkulose-Blatt 1940;14:94–99.

49 Kelting K: Das Tuberkuloseproblem im Nationalsozialismus [The tuberculosis problem in national socialism]. Kiel, Diss Med, 1974.

50 Holm J: Tuberculosis in Europe after the second World War. Am Rev Tuberc 1948;57:115–128.

51 Schrag E: Das Röntgenschirmbild in der Tuberkulosebekämpfung [The roentgenphotofluorogram in the fight against tuberculosis]. Beitr Klin Tuberk 1953;108:107–120.

52 Reichs-Tuberkulose-Ausschuss. Tuberkulose-Lexikon 1943.

53 Enarson DA, Rouillon A: History of the IUATLD. CDC TB Notes 2000;(No. 1):33–37.

54 Steinmeyer O: Formen der Tuberkulose bei Frontsoldaten [Forms of tuberculosis in front-line soldiers]; in Handloser S (ed): Bericht über die Arbeitstagung Ost der beratenden Fachärzte vom 30. November bis 3. Dezember 1942 in der Militärärztlichen Akademie Berlin. VIII. Tuberkulose [Report on the workshop East of the consulting specialists from 30 November to 3 December 1942 in the military medical academy Berlin. VIII. Tuberculosis]. 108–110.

55 Handloser SE: Bericht über die Arbeitstagung Ost der beratenden Fachärzte vom 30. November bis 3. Dezember 1942 in der Militärärztlichen Akademie Berlin. VIII. Tuberkulose [Report on the workshop East of the consulting specialists from 30 November to 3 December 1942 in the military medical academy Berlin. VIII. Tuberculosis]. 107–13.

56 Zimmer AE: Wehrmedizin. Kriegserfahrungen 1939–1943. Vol III. Interne Medizin und Neurologie. Lungenkrankheiten, einschliesslich der Tuberkulose [Military medicine. War experiences 1939–1943]. Vol III. Interne Medizin und Neurologie. Lungenkrankheiten, einschliesslich der Tuberkulose [Lung diseases, including tuberculosis]. Wien, Franz Deuticke, 1944.

57 Szerreiki W: Die rechtzeitige Auffindung der Tuberkulose im Felde [The timely discovery of tuberculosis in the field]; i: Handloser S (ed): Bericht über die Arbeitstagung Ost der beratenden Fachärzte vom 30. November bis 3. Dezember 1942 in der Militärärztlichen Akademie Berlin. VIII. Tuberkulose [Report on the workshop East of the consulting specialists from 30 November to 3 December 1942 in the military medical academy Berlin. VIII. Tuberculosis]. 110–111.

58 Kreuser F: Die Versorgung tuberkulöser Soldaten beim Feldheer [Care of tuberculous soldiers in the army]; in Handloser S (ed): Bericht über die Arbeitstagung Ost der beratenden Fachärzte vom 30. November bis 3. Dezember 1942 in der Militärärztlichen Akademie Berlin. VIII. Tuberkulose [Report on the workshop East of the consulting specialists from 30 November to 3 December 1942 in the military medical academy Berlin. VIII. Tuberculosis]. 111–112.

59 Mayrhofer H: Die Lungentuberkulose als D.U.-Leiden [Pulmonary tuberculosis due to war circumstances]; in Zimmer A (ed): Wehrmedizin. Kriegserfahrungen 1939–1943 [Military medicine. War experiences 1939–1943]. Vol III. Interne Medizin und Neurologie. Lungenkrankheiten, einschliesslich der Tuberkulose [Lung diseases, including tuberculosis]. Wien, Franz Deuticke, 1944.

60 Weidinger E: Tuberkulosebekämpfung im Wehrkreis XVII [Fight against tuberculosis in the military district VIII]; in Zimmer A (ed): Wehrmedizin. Kriegserfahrungen 1939–1943. Vol III. Interne Medizin und Neurologie. Lungenkrankheiten, einschließlich der Tuberkulose [Military medicine. War experiences 1939–1943]. Vol III. Interne Medizin und Neurologie. Lungenkrankheiten, einschliesslich der Tuberkulose [Lung diseases, including tuberculosis]. Wien, Franz Deuticke, 1944.

61 Liebknecht W: Zur Frage der Absonderung Offentuberkulöser [About the question on isolation of patients with open tuberculosis]. Tuberkulosearzt 1948;2:275–277.

62 Streit C: Keine Kameraden. Die Wehrmacht und die sowjetischen Kriegsgefangenen 1941–1945 [No comrades. The Wehrmacht and the Soviet prisoners of war]. Bonn, JHW Dietz, 1997.

63 Nicol K: Die Bedeutung der Tuberkulose der sowjetischen Kriegsgefangenen für die deutsche Zivilbevölkerung [The impact of tuberculosis of Soviet prisoners of war on the civilian population]; in Handloser S (ed): Bericht über die Arbeitstagung Ost der beratenden Fachärzte vom 30. November bis 3. Dezember 1942 in der Militärärztlichen Akademie Berlin. VIII. Tuberkulose. 107–108.

64 Burleigh M: The Third Reich – A New History. New York, Hill and Wang, 2000.

65 Aronson JD: The occurrence and anatomic characteristics of fatal tuberculosis in the U.S. Army during World War II. The Military Surgeon 1946;99:491–503.

66 Roloff W: Über Tuberkulose fremder Kolonialtruppen [About tuberculosis of foreign colonial troops]; in Handloser S (ed): Bericht über die Arbeitstagung Ost der beratenden Fachärzte vom 30. November bis 3. Dezember 1942 in der Militärärztlichen Akademie Berlin. VIII. Tuberkulose [Report on the workshop East of the consulting specialists from 30 November to 3 December 1942 in the military medical academy Berlin. VIII. Tuberculosis]. 112–113.

67 Leyton GB: Effects of slow starvation. Lancet 1946;2:73–79.

68 Cochrane AL: Tuberculosis among prisoners of war in Germany. Br Med J 1945;2:656–658.

69 Cochrane AL: Sickness in Salonica: My first, worst, and most successful clinical trial. Br Med J (Clin Res Ed) 1984;289:1726–1727.

70 Byerly CR: Camp follower: tuberculosis in World War II; in (U.S.) AD, (ed): "Good tuberculosis men:" the Army Medical Department's struggle with tuberculosis (TB). Fort Sam Houston, TX, Office of the Surgeon General, Borden Institute, 2013, pp 273–314.

71 Ley A: Zwischen Erbleiden und Infektionskrankheit: Wahrnehmung und Umgang mit Tuberkulose im Nationalsozialismus. Pneumologie 2006;60:360–365.

72 Daniels M: Tuberculosis in post-war Europe. An international problem. Part II. Tubercle 1947;28:233–238.

73 Lipscomb FM: Medical aspects of Belsen concentration camp. Lancet 1945;246:313–315.

74 Rosencher H: Medicine in Dachau. Br Med J 1946;2:953–955.

75 Zuppinger A, Labhart A: Gestalt und Frühverlauf der Tuberkulose bei Patienten aus Konzentrationslagern. Schweiz Med Wochenschr 1947;77:144–146.

76 Wyman M: DPs: Europe's displaced persons, 1945–1951 (reprinted). New York, Cornell University Press, 1998.

77 Königseder A, Wetzel J: Lebensmut im Wartesaal. Die jüdischen DPs (Displaced Persons) im Nachkriegsdeutschland [Courage to face life in the waiting room. The Jewish DPs (Displaced persons) in post-war Germany]. Frankfurt, Fischer, 1995.

78 Herbert U: Fremdarbeiter. Politik und Praxis des "Ausländer-Einsatzes" in der Kriegswirtschaft des Dritten Reiches. [Foreign workers. Policy and practice of the "assignment of foreigners" in the wartime economy of the Third Reich]. Berlin/Bonn, 1985.

79 Waltrich H: Dr. Heissmeyer und die "Tuberkuloseforschung;" in Aufstieg und Niedergang der Heilanstalten Hohenlychen (1902–1945) [Dr. Heissmeyer and "tuberculosis research"; in Rise and fall of the sanatorium Hohenlychen]. Blankensee, Strelitzia, 2001.

80 Dahl M: "…*deren Lebenshaltung für die Nation keinen Vorteil bedeutet.*" Behinderte Kinder als Versuchsobjekte und die Entwicklung der Tuberkulose-Schutzimpfung ["…. sustaining their lives has no advantage to the nation." Handicapped children as research subjects and the development of preventive tuberculosis vaccination]. Med Hist J 2002;37:57–90.

81 Anonymous. Tuberculosis in the British Zone of Germany. Report of an enquiry (by Drs. M. Daniels and P. D'Arcy Hart) Br Med J 1948;1:508–509.

82 Ellerbrock D: Kapitel 5. Tuberkulose: "Vom Schwinden der Kräfte in schweren Zeiten;" in: "Healing Democracy" – Demokratie als Heilmittel. Gesundheit, Krankheit und Politik in der amerikanischen Besatzungszone 1945–1949 [Tuberculosis: [On wasting strengths in dire straits. In: "Healing Democracy" – Democracy as remedy. Health, disease and politics in the American Occupation Zone 1945–1949]. Bonn, Dietz, 2004.

83 Reinisch J: The perils of peace: the public health crisis in occupied Germany. Oxford, UK, 2013.

84 Statistisches Bundesamt: Statistik der Bundesrepublik Deutschland, Band 61. Gesundheitswesen, Statistische Ergebnisse 1946–1950 [Federal Office of Statistics. Statistics of the Federal Republic of Germany. Volume 61. Public health, Statistical results 1946–1950]. Stuttgart Köln W, Kohlhammer, 1954.

85 Schliesser T: Die Rindertuberkulose im Wandel der letzten 100 Jahre (1882–1982) [Cattle tuberculosis in the course of the last 100 years]. Prax Klin Pneumol 1982;56:151–156.

86 Auersbach K: Die Wirkung des Streptomycins auf die Tuberkulose des Menschen [The effect of streptomycin on human tuberculosis]. Ärztl Wschr 1948;3:428–433.

87 Hessisches Staatsministerium. Der Minister des Inneren. Streptomycin. Tgb. No. 4895. 1948.

88 Kröger E, Reuter H: Entwicklung und gegenwärtiger Stand der Tuberkulose in deutschen und anderen Ländern. Dtsch Med Wochenschr 1949; 74:721–725.

89 Daniels M: Tuberculosis in post-war Europe; an international problem. Tubercle 1947;28:201;passim.

90 Daniels M: Tuberculosis in Europe during and after the second World War. Br Med J 1949;2: 1065–1072.

91 Daniels M: Tuberculosis in Europe during and after the second World War. Br Med J 1949;2: 1135–1140.

92 Wiesner B: Kapitel 7. Tuberkulosebekämpfung und Entwicklung der Pneumologie in der DDR (1945–1990); in Dierkesmann R, Konietzko N, Kropp R, Loddenkemper R, Seehausen V, Wiesner B (eds): 100 Jahre DGP – 100 Jahre deutsche Pneumologie. Berlin/Heidelberg/New York, Springer-Verlag, 2010, pp 49–58.

93 Landmann H: In Berlin begann der Kampf gegen die Tuberkulose [In Berlin started the fight against tuberculosis]. Berlinische Monatsschrift 1998;12:12–20.

94 Ferlinz R, Schicketanz KH, Ferlinz C: Die Tuberkuloseentwicklung in Deutschland – ein Vergleich zwischen der ehemaligen Bundesrepublik und der ehemaligen DDR. Pneumologie 1994;48:160–163.

Prof. Dr. Robert Loddenkemper
German Central Committee against Tuberculosis
Hertastrasse 3
DE–14169 Berlin (Germany)
E-Mail robert.loddenkemper@pneumologie.de

Murray JF, Loddenkemper R (eds): Tuberculosis and War. Lessons Learned from World War II.
Prog Respir Res. Basel, Karger, 2018, vol 43, pp 86–93 (DOI: 10.1159/000481476)

Tuberculosis in Austria before, during, and after World War II

Kunrad Wolf[a] · Ermar Junker[b]

[a]Verein Heilanstalt Alland, and [b]Vienna, Austria

Abstract

The tuberculosis (TB) epidemic in Austria followed a similar pattern to that in major European countries, but evolved a century later than in London. In 1871, the TB death rate in Vienna was 910/100,000. Before World War II (WWII), poor living conditions were ubiquitous throughout Austria. Although mortality from TB had declined since the late 19th century, morbidity was still high, and infection and disease were raging. WWII fed new fuel to the epidemic. From 1939 to 1950, in the capital Vienna, 29,000 persons died from all forms of TB. Hunger, physical, and psychological stress accelerated the disease course. The war tended to even out differences between rich and poor. The post-war years were marked by a high prevalence of infectious cases, which retarded the end of the epidemic. Large migratory movements during and after the war favored new infections and disease, as did the presence of troops, refugees, prisoners of war, and forced laborers. Housing conditions in destroyed towns were poor, and the aftermath of the WWII was recognizable until the end of the 1950's. Improved identification of active cases in risk groups and implementation of effective chemotherapy led to a final turning point.

© 2018 S. Karger AG, Basel

Tuberculosis and World War II in Austria

The tuberculosis (TB) epidemic in Vienna followed a similar pattern to that in all major European cities, but took place 100 years later than in London. In Vienna, the peak of the epidemic was around the year 1871, with a death rate from TB of 910/100,000 inhabitants. For the rest of Austria, as defined by its current borders, this peak level was reached some years later. Following this peak, Vienna experienced a steady decline in mortality from TB, while implementing measures with only minimal effect on the dynamics of the epidemic. This trend also applies to the rest of the country, albeit with significant differences between industrialized regions and rural areas. The decline in TB mortality was most pronounced in Vienna. However, both world wars led to a sudden increase in TB mortality that persisted for several years afterward. After WWI, the period from 1921 was marked by a steep and sustained drop in the mortality curve. After the pronounced rise in TB death rates during and immediately after WWII, the natural course of the epidemic was influenced from the 60s onwards by the introduction of chemotherapy.

With regard to the respective form of government, this topic can be examined over 3 periods:

Period 1. 1918–1938, German Austria, the first Republic, the corporative state.

Period 2. 1938–1945, the Ostmark in the "Deutsche Reich," the Second World War.

Period 3. 1945–1968, the second Republic up to the TB Act of 1968.

The intensity of state and local TB control, the legal situation and different economic and social conditions signifi-

Ermar Junker is a former Director of the Public Health Department of the City of Vienna.

cantly distinguished these 3 periods from each other. Because of the high levels of infection in the 19th century and the significant population movements before, during, and after WWI and because of the autonomous social democratic health policy in the interwar period, Vienna played a special role. In the Constitution of October 1920, Vienna was separated from Lower Austria and established as an independent federal province. At that time, about a third of Austria's population was living in the capital. The available data for Vienna are in some parts more detailed than for the rest of Austria.

German Austria, the First Republic, the Corporative State
After the end of WWI, higher rates of mortality from TB lingered at first: the incidence in 1919 was 482/100,000 inhabitants. However, from 1920 there was a dramatic decrease in mortality from TB. From 1920 to 1937, the proportion of TB mortality to total mortality in Austria had halved. In Vienna, this decline was even more pronounced: the proportion of TB in the overall death rate in 1937 was one third of the percentage of 1920 (Table 1). This rapid decline occurred despite the unfavorable economic situation in the interwar period. Until the decrease in 1920, the markedly higher mortality rate of civilians suffering from TB and of the soldiers returning home was certainly due to the poor nutritional conditions and the hardships of WWI. The considerably higher proportion of women at the peak of this mortality was interpreted differently, but may be partly explained by the large number of soldiers whose causes of death were not known. Another explanation considers the poorer nutritional levels of women and young girls compared with the provisioning for the troops [1]. A significant migration of young women from the former crown lands during WWI has also been cited as a partial cause for the doubled mortality of the female sex [2]. In general, a proportion of young women of up to over 50% can be found in this high incidence of TB.

The rapid decline in mortality after the war and its consequences had not been expected. Due to the violent death of soldiers already diseased and the premature death of many in the civilian population, the sources of infection and the risk of infection for children decreased. In addition, the population structure changed significantly due to a decline in birth rates starting from 1926 and continuing until 1938 [2]. In analyzing death rates from TB in 1923 and 1939, one must consider surviving contemporaries in their respective cohorts. For Vienna, the following statements can be made: among infants and children under 15 years, rates dropped by 1939 to a quarter of the value they were at

Table 1. Mortality from tuberculosis in Vienna and Austria as a whole, 1919–1938 (given as incidences and as proportions of all deaths)

	Vienna incidence/ 100,000	Vienna proportion of all deaths, %	Austria incidence/ 100,000	Austria proportion of all deaths, %
1919	482	26	303	14.9
1920	405	22	277	14.5
1921	283	19	219	12.8
1922	298	18	231	13.2
1923	248	18	206	13.5
1924	221	16	186	12.4
1925	196	15	173	11.9
1926	204	15	178	11.7
1927	204	14	169	11.1
1928	187	14	163	11.0
1929	180	13	154	10.3
1930	159	12	142	10.2
1931	158	12	142	9.9
1932	140	11	134	9.5
1933	134	11	124	9.1
1934	121	10	111	8.8
1935	114	9	109	8.0
1936	106	8	102	7.7
1937	107	8	100	7.5
1938	102	7	–	–

The table shows the dramatic decrease in mortality from TB that occurred despite poor living conditions in the interwar period. The decrease was even more pronounced in Vienna than in Austria as a whole [16].

the 1923. Teenagers older than 15 and young adults experienced decreases from 30 to 50%. From the age of 40, the differences were not as marked; the high point of TB death rate shifts to higher ages [1]. On the contrary, large migratory movements contributed to the spread of TB. Temporarily, 100,000 German-speaking refugees resided in the area of present-day Austria. Austrian citizens from the crown lands were expelled or returned voluntarily. Others, like the Czech population of Vienna returned to their country of origin. The civil war in Austria ended with the installation of the Austro-fascist state and marked the definite end of the First Republic. The social democratic movement was outlawed. This induced, from 1933, an exodus of Social Democrats to the Czech Republic and further on to the Soviet Union. These people however, returned in part and subsequently lived as stateless persons in Austria. Illegal Nazis moved temporarily to Germany [3]. Given these changes in the resident population and the changing age structure of the post-war population, the raw data of the mortality rates from TB are not sufficiently informative. However, a clear trend developed, both in the number of TB deaths and the proportion of these to the overall mortality. The prevalence of infection as an indicator of the dynamics of the epidemic provides a reliable picture in this situation. While there had been a rate of about 50% TB infection among a random sample of 5–6 year-olds before the first war, only 30% were found with a positive tuberculin skin test in the same age group in 1923. This trend continued through the 1920s and into the 1930s. In Vienna's schools in 1934/1935, only 23% of the 5–6 year-olds reacted to tuberculin. In 1948/49, the figure was 13.4% [4].

Institutions and Measures to Combat TB
Before and during WWI, people began to realize that the prospects for cure in a sanatorium had only a limited impact on the TB epidemic. In addition, the construction and operation of sanatoriums was expensive. So, in the 1920s, the emphasis was put on the health care system for selected TB patients. Emphasis was placed on sanatorium treatment of promising cases in the early stages of the disease. These benefited from improved living conditions during the cure and treatment with collapse therapy. Only part of the patients could be helped by these measures. Sanatorium care managed to delay the progression of the disease and allowed patients a working life. However, follow-up provided by the care system was always necessary because of the ongoing threat of recurrence.

The TB care system in Vienna was characterized by its widespread coverage and central organization from 1923 onwards. From a decree of 1917, the tasks of the health care system had been defined [5]. Support from federal funds was provided for what were at the time private-aided organizations. By 1937, 11 community care centers had been created in Vienna. Twelve centers were run by associations and health insurance companies. The municipal area then was almost completely covered. In the outskirts, however, where settlements had grown in an unregulated way, the care system could not be as effective as it should have been. In these areas, patients suffering from TB tended to die early because of the rapid progress of the disease. This was probably due to the precarious living conditions and not because of a change in the virulence of the *Mycobacterium tuberculosis*, as was feared [1].

By 1937, 92 care centers for TB had been created in Austria. The coverage for the population affiliated with those centers was very different, however. For example, in Vorarlberg no such institution existed; Upper Austria and Styria had a comparatively concentrated density of care; of the major cities, Graz and Linz were well equipped thanks to local efforts.

The social improvements that had already been enshrined in law since 1919 and were valid throughout Austria failed beginning the 1930s due to inflationary developments and political disputes between parties. In terms of reducing the workload, the 8 h day, holiday law, the collective contract law, night work prohibitions, and maternity leave had all been introduced. Arbitration offices, Chambers of Labor, and unemployment benefits had been established [3]. Falling state social expenditure due to the economic crisis and subsequent stagnation led to the ineffectiveness of these social regulations. The aftermath of the Great Depression continued in Austria until the end of the 1930s, when the social budget was needed to care for the poor.

Statutory Provisions to Combat TB in the Years Up to 1938
During WWI, an obligation to report cases of infectious TB, both deaths and infectious respiratory TB, was first required by the army administration, then by the Chief Medical Officer. The same bodies founded the Austrian Association for the Control of TB in 1916. Subsequently, the Ministry of the Interior took over the responsibility of the TB care system following the decree of 16 February 1917 [5]. Health insurance providers, insurance companies, and state governments were asked to participate in the construction of the health care system. The tasks of the system were defined as: data collecting, reporting to the health administration, tracing TB patients, contact tracing, housing surveys, training in hygiene measures, counseling, and allocating treatment. But it was not until 1919 that the State Office of Public Health required by law that in addition to deaths, the disease of contagious pulmonary TB and laryngeal TB were also legally notifiable [1]. The circle of those required to report was very broad and went beyond the doctors. However, many people who were addressed were not prepared to comply with the obligation. Therefore, it was not possible to achieve the expected benefit, namely the protection of uninfected children. During the time of the Corporative State (from 1934), there were no changes in laws and theoretically no change in health policy. In practice, however, the ideas of National Socialism slowly prevailed.

The Time of the Ostmark and WWII

With the annexation of Austria to the "Deutsches Reich" on 13 March 1938, the economic situation improved noticeably. This was attributed to industry and primarily to the defense industry. The previously oppressive rate of unemployment fell rapidly. In 1937, 22% of the labor force was still unemployed. By 1939, this figure had dropped to 3% [3]. The housing shortage in Vienna was reduced by, among other things, the Aryanization of homes previously owned by Jews. In the federal provinces, a building boom developed.

However, the expulsion of the Jews and the arrests of political dissidents began immediately. Vienna lost 70% of its registered doctors, and 60% of the teaching staff in the medical faculty of the university were dismissed, forced to retire, arrested or expelled [6].

The public health sector was reorganized. TB control was transferred to the health authorities as a mandatory task. The existing care locations of the associations, the Red Cross, and the health insurance providers were gradually attached to the health authorities. "Deutsches Reich" laws became the basis for the work of the TB care system. The third regulation implementing the law on the unification of health care was decisive in this respect. Health policy became Nazi party politics.

The obligations of the health authorities, as applied by the law, along with the TB care system, did not differ to any great extent from the measures in the interwar period, but the implementation and enforcement was intensified. New approaches included monitoring by the care system of those at risk of TB, collecting details of professional relationships and personal contacts, as well as general assessment in the public interest. This was initially in line with the thinking of the TB doctors and social workers. However, repressive measures emerged increasingly clearly, such as compulsory hospitalization of sick people unwilling to submit to therapy. These people were seen as intransigent and as asocial. Also, marriage bans for those who had contracted TB but were wishing to marry, stood in stark contrast to the intentions of the welfare associations out of which the TB care system had developed. On the contrary, the introduction of TB Relief (1942) that enabled treatment for an uninsured patient and a livelihood for the family were welcomed. The sanatoriums were fully occupied again. During WWII, treatment places were also required for the Army. Thus, emphasis was placed on the reintegration into the work life of patients who were getting better. The funds necessary for all these measures were provided by the TB relief organization of the National Socialist People's Welfare (Tuberkulosehilfswerk der Nationalsozialistischen Volkswohlfahrt). In an attempt to standardize, all institutions of the state and municipalities that had already been involved with TB, as well as insurance companies and private-aided organizations were included in a joint venture under the party leadership [1].

People's welfare was aimed at the defense capacity and the working capacity of the population. A healthy national population, in a utilitarian sense, should be encouraged. This idea had also been discussed in the period before WWI, and given the poor health of the working population, it matured during the interwar years. However, to this practice were added the ideas of racial purity and superiority of the Nordic race. The branding of people as asocial and "useless," which also found its way into medicine and health care, characterized the ideology of the Nazis. In Vienna, human experimentation was practiced on children with disabilities as part of the evaluation of a TB vaccine [7, 8]. For further details on TB in concentration camps and on inhuman TB experiments performed by the Nazis during the war, see chapters 4 (Nazi Medicine, TB and Genocide), 5 (Germany), and 7 (Poland). Nazi propaganda was based on indoctrination and training to deal with infectious patients in a disciplined manner. To this end, leaflets were launched, photo series and films presented, lectures held, and events conducted in schools. These steps were not only planned in terms of a prophylactic measure, but also branded the sick as posing a risk to the public health (for more details, see also Chapter 5 on Germany where identical measures were introduced by the Nazis).

The available methods of examination, radiography, and *M. tuberculosis* detection were made use of too sparingly, in the opinion of the new rulers [9]. To make better use of these methods, necessary facilities were created. The obligation to report became the "duty of disclosure." Hospitals were also required to report a case, on discharging the patient. The sanatoriums and hospitals were required to collaborate with the employment offices. As long as they were youthful and not infected, workers were protected from hazardous working conditions. TB was listed as an occupational disease. People in teaching profession were examined to check if they were free from TB [10]. Tuberculin skin tests were carried out in schools as screening tests. An X-ray survey of the population was supposed to put an end to the disease. However, because of the war, this was not carried out fully. Screening tests by means of radiography have been, however, carried out on a large scale. X-ray micro photography was introduced [11]. In Vienna alone, 126,345 radiography tests were carried out between 1942 and 1945. One active TB case was found in 91 cases investigated. In the last 2 years of the war, some projects had to be abandoned because all available energy had to be channeled into the war effort. However, the benefits of the TB care system remained free of charge.

The mortality rate from TB began to increase in the first year of WWII. Since this was a planned and prepared war, supplies for the civilian population were initially sufficient. Therefore, this early increase in mortality was a surprise. In Austria, the recording of deaths and cases of the disease (Tables 2, 3) had been significantly improved due to the enforcement of reporting obligations. This could explain the early increase in mortality. A clarification in the drafting of the Annual Report, published by the Imperial TB Committee, defines the diagnostic groups: F. a-c respiratory TB, F. d extra-pulmonary forms and F. e bone and joint TB, extrapulmonary glands, and lupus vulgaris. In this context, inactive TB means clinically cured TB and is reported under II a. and II b. Those who were or had been exposed are listed under II c. Detailed rules for check-ups were required for all groups. Diagnostic transition from F. a to F. c was allowed only 2 years after the last detection of *M. tuberculosis*. The counting of deaths included those dying outside the home parish but not the non-locals. At a time of involuntary migration, including military, paramilitary groups, labor service, prisoners of war as forced laborers, this form of counting made sense. By contrast, the massive migratory movements during and immediately after the war influenced the course of the TB epidemic. However, the situation remained totally unclear in the armed forces and paramilitary organizations during the course of the war [1]. Initially, ill soldiers were moved to sanatoriums, and if their condition improved the employment offices switched them to lighter work. With the expansion of the military fronts and ever-increasing losses, even the so-called slightly ill were drafted. Whether these soldiers who were suffering from TB died in the war, on the front or in captivity is unknown. Prisoners of war and forced laborers from the occupied territories died of TB at an above-average frequency.

The Second Republic

The direct effects of WWII on the civilian population were more profound than in WWI. The air raids from 1943 onwards had destroyed or rendered unusable 187,305 homes in Vienna alone. The effects of war had caused 11,305 deaths among the urban population. But beyond that, in the period of Nazi rule 120,000 Viennese men and women had been killed at the fronts, by violence in street fighting, in prisons and concentration camps. The entire infrastructure of the city had been destroyed. The water supply, energy, and transportation had collapsed. There was lack of food and fuel. Food donated by the Soviet Union prevented famine.

Table 2. Mortality from tuberculosis in Vienna 1937–1946 (civilians only)

Year	Inhabitants	All deaths	Deaths from tuberculosis (%)	Incidence/ 100,000
1937	1,875.667	24.453	2.004 (8)	107
1938	1,876.436	25.932	1.910 (7)	102
1939	1,942.458	31.133	2.360 (7)	121
1940	1,875.906	31.222	2.546 (8)	136
1941	1,806.304	28.811	2.328 (8)	129
1942	1,752.487	29.510	2.676 (9)	153
1943	1,759.815	29.176	2.690 (9)	153
1944	1,754.430	35.151	2.978 (8)	170
1945	1,572.376	62.335	4.213 (7)	268
1946	1,572.639	28.329	2.800 (10)	178

The death from TB, as a proportion of all deaths, first increased because of improved reporting. In the last years of the war, the number of violent deaths also rose in civilians. The absolute numbers of mortality from TB show a continuous increase [6].

Table 3. Mortality from pulmonary, extrapulmonary tuberculosis, including miliary tuberculosis and meningitis in 1942

a With respect to the division of the territory in the Nazi era

Reichsgaue*	Pulmonary	Extrapulmonary	All cases
Wien	2,337	339	2,676
Niederdonau	1,445	222	1,667
Oberdonau	784	155	939
Steiermark	828	152	980
Salzburg	180	27	207
Kärnten	230	41	271
Tirol, Vorarlberg	375	78	453
Austria	6,179	1,014	7,193

b With respect to the time course

Pulmonary	Austria/year	Extrapulmonary	All cases
5,904	1938	794	6,698
6,179	1942	1,014	7,193
9,276	1945	1,262	10,529
5,377	1947	1,047	6,424

The increase in mortality numbers may be the result of improved reporting. The consequences of the war became apparent only in the end and years after the war. Compiled from the scarcely accessible statistical data of Statistic Austria, "Statistisches Amt für die Alpen- und Donau-Reichsgaue", from 1945 "Österreichisches statistisches Zentralamt". The Austrian territory was divided into areas called "Gaue".

The lack of clean water and the partially destroyed sewerage system led to outbreaks of typhoid and dysentery. Altogether, 3,700 people died of these infectious diseases, although rigorous disinfection measures were carried out [12]. First, the acute infectious diseases had to be combated. However, an outbreak of epidemic TB was feared. The TB wards of hospitals were occupied down to the last bed. Many TB sufferers died a premature death because of inadequate nutrition and other hardships.

TB after WWII

Baumgartnerhöhe, the biggest sanatorium in Austria at that time, reported the deaths of 10% of the 600 patients every month throughout 1945. The care centers helped with the distribution of food donations, extra rations, clothing, and counseling. Nearly all humanitarian aid came from abroad. The reconstruction of the health care system took place surprisingly quickly. In 1946, there were already 2,258 beds available to treat TB of all forms in the city of Vienna. The 18 community TB care centers in Vienna had become operational again. However, the TB mortality rate in the capital remained high until 1947, but afterwards reached the pre-war figures of 1937. The figure for 1945 (4,213 deaths) cannot be relied upon for various reasons, as after WWI, a higher mortality rate can be clearly seen. In 1946, 2,393 Viennese men and women died of pulmonary TB. In addition, 407 deaths due to extra-pulmonary TB occurred. That made up 10% of all deaths. The proportion of female deaths had increased to 40% during the war, but declined again to a third. The number of children (under 14 years-old) dying from TB in Vienna fell quickly, whereas in Austria as a whole the rate of decline was retarded. Since 1954, detailed data have been available due to a newly published survey form. In the same year, the incorporation of some of the surrounding areas into Vienna, that had been carried out during the Nazi era was revoked, such that the territorial area of Vienna shrank.

Viewed over a longer period, the death rate from TB in Vienna dropped rapidly after the war – at 10.1% annually from 1946 to 1950 – and subsequently – at 8.5% per year from 1950 to 1960. The number of reported new cases of all forms of TB fell slowly. In part, these high figures until 1950 can be ascribed to the charitable impulses of the TB nurses [13]. Food allowances and other gifts to the needy certainly played a role in the classification of active non-infectious forms of TB. The numbers for qualified contagious forms of TB in Vienna are more reliable (Table 4). Within 10

Table 4. Contagious pulmonary tuberculosis in Vienna (1946–1960), absolute numbers and incidence, listed for male and female patients

Year	Male	Incidence	Female	Incidence	Both sexes	Incidence
1946	1,512	210	1,054	107	2,566	151
1947	1,485	200	909	92	2,394	138
1948	1,437	189	940	94	2,377	135
1949	1,158	165	755	82	1,913	118
1950	871	124	636	69	1,507	93
1951	855	121	603	65	1,458	90
1952	860	122	553	60	1,413	87
1953	857	111	530	53	1,387	78
1954	700	91	395	39	1,095	62
1955	634	90	300	33	934	58
1956	555	78	276	30	831	51
1957	493	68	251	27	744	45
1958	470	64	241	26	711	43
1959	468	63	198	21	666	40
1960	433	58	185	20	618	37

The high incidence of contagious pulmonary TB in females after the war was followed by a steep decline, but it took 10 years to reach the ratio of one third of all cases. The overall reduction in contagious cases was decelerated [6].

years, the incidence of infectious cases had fallen to a third (1948–1958) of the numbers at the start of this period. It was only in 1955, that is, 10 years after the war that the proportion of women had returned to that of peacetime. The distribution of infectious cases showed a peak among people of working age. What is striking is the high prevalence of infectious cases. (In 1956, there were 14, 782 cases in Austria, of which 5,765 were in Vienna). Between 1951 and 1970 in Vienna, the ratio of new infectious cases to the prevalence of infectious cases was consistently at an unusually high range: 1–5.1 to a maximum of 1–7.6. In addition, from 1961, the decline in infectious cases stagnated due to an appreciable number of TB cases brought in by guest workers.

Outside Vienna, severe damage had also been caused by bombing, which included railway stations, rail hubs, and industrial facilities: virtually all had been destroyed by the Allies. Residential areas had also been rendered uninhabitable by bombing and fire. Therefore, in the cities living space was scarce, food and fuel were often only available on the black market. Under these conditions, the TB mortality rate throughout Austria reached very high levels in 1947 with 6,424 cases, corresponding to an incidence rate of

110/100,000; the mortality figures for all forms of TB were higher than before the war, but not nearly as high as in Vienna (178/100,000).

From the 1950s onwards, the work of the TB care system had to be adjusted to deal with the significantly changed courses of TB disease under chemotherapeutic treatment. Many patients were considered cured after 2 years of therapy, but had to stay under observation of the care system. However, there were also a relatively high number of recurrences after therapy – up to 16% – and cases of clinical deterioration under continuous therapy. The diagnostic transitions towards contagious TB from the groups of healed, cases under observation (contacts), and those suffering bacteriological deterioration under therapy were estimated for Austria at 1,753 cases in 1956. With the addition of 3,043 new cases of contagious TB, this resulted in 4,796 infectious cases that required hospitalization. A further 2,601 were successfully treated and 1,757 deaths occurred. The reduction in the numbers from the diagnostic groups of infectious cases was thus around 438 people fewer than those being added, which at this time was also a result of a constantly high prevalence of contagious TB [13]. A special class of contagious TB, which at that time was known as chronic TB, included patients with extensive residual findings, with optional *M. tuberculosis* positivity, and those that refused therapy or abandoned it. The fact that resistance to the available drugs frequently occurred in these cases was known. One of the causes for repeated discontinuation was highlighted as being alcohol abuse among men.

Professionals leading the fight against TB expected the discovery of previously unknown cases of TB by X-ray screening. There were screening tests in companies and discussions about a systematic examination of the whole population. No decision could be made about the latter. Following the example of the examination of teachers, fluoroscopic imaging examinations for those working in medical professions and certain cosmetic professions had been proposed (1958). As expected, studies targeted on risk groups revealed very high numbers of cases in Vienna. In the years 1961–1967, one case of active TB was found in each of the risk groups by screening 51 guest workers, 38 homeless people, and 30 nursing home residents [6]. In the TB Act of 1968, mass screenings were then stipulated in risk groups. It emphasized a sufficiently long period of hospitalization for infectious patients, when the disease had already manifested itself. Maintaining the economic survival of families of ill patients was recognized as essential for the success of the treatment in the face of a long-stay in a sanatorium. TB Relief paid for the cost of treatment if no health insurance existed. The problem of full treatment of difficult and undisciplined patients, especially alcoholics could not be solved by the already mentioned approaches [14]. Screening measures proven ever since the interwar years, such as contact tracing, teaching, counseling, assigning therapy places, and social assistance were maintained.

What was new, however, was the BCG vaccine. As early as 1948, a team of the Danish Red Cross had begun to vaccinate school children in Vienna [15]. This was part of the "International TB Campaign." At that time in the preliminary PPD testing, 9.3% of 5-year-olds and 14.3% of 6-year-olds had reacted positively. The children reacting negatively were vaccinated. By 1966, a total of 1,861,719 persons had been vaccinated against TB in Austria. From 1953 onwards, infants were also vaccinated. The vaccination was offered on a voluntary basis. In newborns, high immunization coverage was reached. From the morbidity statistics, however, no clear effects of vaccination on the dynamics of the TB epidemic were revealed. When comparing Vienna and the rest of Austria, Vienna showed a more rapid reduction in children's TB. Children's TB caused by *M. bovis* was not of great importance because already before WWII cow's milk was pasteurized. But in areas outside towns, it was only the culling of infected cattle that brought about a change after war. In Vienna, school leavers (on average 10-years old) were vaccinated a second time, which it was hoped, would have an impact on the morbidity of adolescents and young adults (recruits) [6]. The benefit to the individual was not in dispute. However, the relative efficiency and duration of protection achieved remained under discussion. The role of re-infection remained unknown.

After the war, the TB wards of hospitals were initially hopelessly overcrowded. By 1947, however, the number of beds had been increased and the sanatorium at Alland had been reopened. Further sanatoriums were created in Austria, adding to those that already existed, and these were largely similar to the hospital departments in terms of their equipment and facilities.

Due to the low availability and high costs of use, the beginnings of chemotherapy of TB with streptomycin (SM) around 1946 were dedicated for treating meningitis, miliary TB, and TB of the larynx. Soon, however, recurrences and the development of resistance were observed. Polychemotherapy, especially "triple therapy," to treat TB was developed at the international level and began to be used in Austrian treatment centers soon after 1952. In addition, pneumothorax, pneumolysis, pneumoperitoneum, thoracoplasty, and lung resections continued to be performed until the end of the 1950s [6].

In the TB Act of 1968, the obligation to report the disease was finally extended to non-contagious forms, the obligation to receive treatment and also the obligation to tolerate the examination of contacts was included. The tasks and duties of the TB care system and the administrative authority were listed. The definition of risk groups was given to the provincial authorities. A broad scope was allowed for the provisions dealing with recalcitrant, infectious patients. In this way, the provisions of the Epidemic Act and all existing regulations from the Rechtsüberleitungsgesetz (Transition of Legislation Act), from the period before 1945, were replaced.

Conclusions

Compared with the usual 19th century time-course of the TB epidemic in most Western European countries, the epidemic was delayed in Austria by almost a century: the death rate from TB peaked in 1871 in the capital Vienna. Several years later, this was observed in the rest of the country. Then TB began a slow, roughly 40-year decline that suddenly spiked upwards in 1914 at the beginning of WWI, which lasted through the war and the overlapping influenza pandemic. Once again, the subsequent decline in TB mortality between wars was interrupted by another exacerbation in death rates lasting though the end of WWII. But unlike the decrease in TB mortality that many belligerent countries experienced within 3 years after wartime, high TB mortality persisted a decade after the armistice in May 1945. The Allied bombing raids destroyed railway stations, rail hubs, all known industrial facilities, and vast residential areas. In 1946, TB mortality and incidence figures were higher than before the beginning of the war in 1939. The number of new cases of post-WWII TB fell slowly: in Vienna, the yearly TB mortality decreased 10.1% from 1946 to 1950, then at 8.5% annually from 1950 to 1960. Enormous involuntary movements of military personnel, homeless people, forced laborers, prisoners of war, Jews liberated from concentration camps, and unrecorded others died of TB in "above average frequency."

In Austria, mass X-ray screening and the widespread use of tuberculin and BCG led to the identification of new cases of *M. tuberculosis* infection and disease, and widespread vaccination to prevent TB in the late 1940s. After a cautious beginning in the use of SM after roughly 1947, then para-aminosalicyclic acid and finally isoniazid (INH) in 1952, the long sought after cure for TB, "triple therapy" (SM + para-aminosalicyclic acid + INH), became available for routine use. All of the pre-WWII legal regulations governing TB in Austria have streamlined and greatly improved the current means of diagnosing, treating, and ensuring follow up of candidates who have TB.

Dr. Kunrad Wolf
Verein Heilanstalt Alland
Sieveringerstrasse 41/8
AT–1190 Wien (Austria)
E-Mail wolf.alland@a1.net

References

1 Dietrich-Daum E: Die "Wiener Krankheit." Eine Sozialgeschichte der Tuberkulose in Österreich; in Cerman M, Eder FX, Ehmer J, Landsteiner E (eds): Sozial- und wirtschaftshistorische Studien. Verlag für Geschichte und Politik Wien, Oldenburg Wissenschaftsverlag München, 2007, vol 32, pp 239–240, 267–268, 249–251, 306–309, 316.

2 Weigl A: Demographischer Wandel und Modernisierung in Wien; in Kommentare zum Historischen Atlas von Wien; Wiener Stadt und Landesarchiv, Verein für Geschichte der Stadt Wien, Ludwig Boltzmann Institut für Stadtgeschichtsforschung (eds) Pichler Verlag 2000, vol 1, pp 246, 366.

3 Hanisch E: Der lange Schatten des Staates, Österreichische Gesellschaftsgeschichte im 20. Jhdt. Wien, Carl Ueberreuter Verlag, 1994.

4 Junker E: Die jährlichen Tuberkuloseinfektionsraten in Wien in den Jahren 1902–1958. Prax Pneumol 1972;26:115–121.

5 Decree from February 1917 die Errichtung von Fürsorgestellen Das österreichische Sanitätswesen, 1917, vol 29, p 110.

6 Junker E, Schmidgruber B, Wallner G: Die Tuberkulose in Wien, Literas-Universitätsverlag Wien, 1999, p 76.

7 Czech H: Forschen ohne Skrupel, Die wissenschaftliche Verwertung von Opfern der NS-Psychiatriemorde in Wien; in Gabriel E, Neubauer W (eds): Zur Geschichte der NS-Euthanasie. Wien, Böhlau Verlag, 2002.

8 Dahl M: "Deren Lebenshaltung für die Nation keinen Vorteil bedeutet." Behinderte Kinder als Versuchsobjekte und die Entwicklung der Tuberkuloseschutzimpfung. Med Hist J 2002;37:57–90.

9 Report of Hermann Vellguth, Leiter des Gesundheitsamtes in Wien von 1938 bis 1945. Archiv der zentralen TB Fürsorgestelle des Gesundheitsamtes der Stadt Wien.

10 Schulseuchenerlass des Reichsministers des Inneren vom. April 30, 1942.

11 Vossen J: Handbuch Tuberkulose für Fachkräfte an Gesundheitsämtern, Akademie für öffentliches Gesundheitswesen in Düsseldorf (ed).

12 Temmel CH: Entwicklung der Gesundheitsvorsorge nach Ende des 2. Weltkrieges, Literas-Universitätsverlag, Wien, 2001.

13 Fischer A: Mitteilungen des Volksgesundheitsamtes Heft 10, 1959.

14 Merkel KL, Merkel I: Der tuberkulöse Alkoholiker; Wiener Zeitschrift für Nervenheilkunde und deren Grenzgebiete, Sonderdruck, 1959, vol. 16.

15 World Health Organization: Mass BCG Vaccination Campaigns, 1948–1951. Copenhagen, World Health Organization, 1954.

16 Haider L, Lukesch R: Die Tätigkeit der Tuberkulosefürsorgestellen in Österreich im Jahre 1937. Sonderbeilage zu Mitteilungen der Unterabteilung Gesundheitswesen im Ministerium für innere und kulturelle Angelegenheiten Wien 1938.

Murray JF, Loddenkemper R (eds): Tuberculosis and War. Lessons Learned from World War II.
Prog Respir Res. Basel, Karger, 2018, vol 43, pp 94–102 (DOI: 10.1159/000481477)

Tuberculosis in Poland before, during, and after World War II

Anita Magowska

Department of the History and Philosophy of Medical Sciences, Poznan University of Medical Sciences, Poznan, Poland

Abstract

This chapter presents the mortality rates and the evolution of the tuberculosis (TB) epidemic in the Polish territories during the Second World War, mainly those occupied by the Germans. The Germans divided the occupied Polish territories into 2 parts, the Reichsgau Wartheland *(Warthegau)* and the *Generalgouvernement*. The Nazis considered the *Warthegau* to be definitively incorporated into the Third Reich and resettled nearly one million Poles to the *Generalgouvernement*. In their place over half a million people of German origin from Baltic states were relocated. The Nazis locked Jews in ghettos, where the TB epidemic spread to an unprecedented scale. In addition, people were starved to death or taken to concentration camps. Nazis and only those Poles who had to remain in contact with Germans were treated for TB in the *Warthegau*. The TB epidemic was particularly deadly among Jews in the ghetto of Lodz. The Germans used registers of TB patients as the basis of extermination by methods previously practiced on Jews. After the war, Poland had one of the highest morbidity and mortality rates from TB in Europe. Thanks to international humanitarian aid, the epidemic was eradicated within a few years post-war.

When Marc Daniels, a medical officer and representative of the United Nations Relief and Rehabilitation Administration (UNRRA), came to Poland in spring 1945, he was shocked not just to see thousands of emaciated people camping out in the shells of buildings, but also by the fact that most of them were suffering from tuberculosis (TB) at a time when the epidemic was supposed to have been declining [1]. In 1944, the death rate from TB was 500/100,000 inhabitants in Warsaw and 371/100,000 inhabitants in Lodz. In the following year, the figure for Warsaw dropped to 297/100,000 and that for Lodz to 288/100,000, while the figure for other cities was even lower, for example, 278/100,000 for Krakow [2].

TB before World War II

A TB epidemic was nothing new to Poles. The disease spread first in the 19th century when the country's territory had been annexed by Austria-Hungary, Prussia, and Russia. The invaders did not care about the standard of living and the health of Poles. Poverty-linked malnutrition and absence of hygiene created favorable conditions for the development and spread of *Mycobacterium tuberculosis* infections and disease. The epidemic grew to a record-breaking scale in Lodz, where at the end of the World War I (WWI), the death rate from TB was 970/100,000 [3]. An opportunity to overcome the epidemic did not occur until after independence had been regained, after 1919. It was thanks to voluntary organizations involved in the prevention of TB and the city authorities that 450 dispensaries as the basic diagnostic units were opened, the majority of which were equipped with X-ray machines and microscopes. The first surveys were for children, teenagers, and students. Those suffering from TB were sent to sanatoria and offered the treatment that was available at the time [4]. While in 1925, the death rate from respiratory TB alone was 194/100,000, in 1938 it dropped to 150/100,000 [2]. However, a higher death rate from TB of 176/100,000, was still observed in Lodz [3].

TB during World War II

After the outbreak of World War II (WWII), which began on September 1, 1939 by the invasion of Poland by Nazi Germany, all Polish associations and institutions dealing with the diagnoses, treatment, and prevention of TB, both in the territory invaded by the Third Reich (188,700 km^2 inhabited by 22.14 million people, mostly Poles) and by the Union of Soviet Socialist Republics (USSR; 201,000 km^2 inhabited by approximately 13 million people of various nationalities and ethnicities, among whom Poles played a dominant demographic, social, and economic role) had to cease their activities [5]. In the occupied Western territory, German authorities established the so-called Reichsgau Wartheland (also called *Warthegau*), which they regarded as a territory definitively included in the Third Reich and from which Poles were to be eliminated while in the Eastern territory – the *Generalgouvernement*, an administrative unit was intended for the later displacement of Poles. Up until mid-1941, the Nazis resettled about 900,000 Poles from the *Warthegau* to the *Generalgouvernement* and in their place relocated 500,000 people of German origin, mainly from Baltic states. They joined the 600,000 Germans who had inhabited the area before the outbreak of WWII. The planned extension of the displacement operation turned out to be impossible due to the demand of the *Warthegau* economy for labor. Apart from soldiers and members of other uniformed services, there were a total of 1.3 million German residents in the entire territory occupied by the Third Reich. Their health needs became the priority for the German authorities [5].

The pre-war Polish system of (TB) prevention came under the control of German administrative supervision. Polish medical staff were dismissed and patients were expelled from hospitals and sanatoria, while the buildings and their equipment were requisitioned for the army, SS (abbreviation for Schutzstaffel, the "Defence Squadron" of the Nazi party) and police units, or for German civilians. Some Polish phthisiologists, such as Ewa Torosiewicz-Cybulska (1897–1941), were shot. Brutal terror completely deprived Poles of any chance of treatment [6].

The Germans provided healthcare in the occupied territory of Poland under the Nazi law (*Deutsche Gemeindeordnung* dated 1935). At the beginning of 1940, they established

Table 1. Tuberculosis mortality per 100,000 in Lodz, 1940–1944, data from [2]

Year	Death rate for Poles and Germans	Death rate for Poles	Death rate for Germans
1940	244	311	119
1941	316	371	131
1942	363	442	152
1943	401	488	181
1944	371	461	155
Average death rate for five years	331	414	147

city councils with health departments, where they formed units to take care of TB patients *(Tuberkulosefürsorge)*. These were responsible for running obligatory check-ups of the entire German population living in the occupied territory and the Poles, such as waiters, barbers, and maids, who had contact with them due to the work they performed. In May 1943, the German health administration announced a regulation prohibiting the treatment of Poles suffering from TB at the expense of the German state: except for highly qualified workers who were necessary for war-related production [7].

There still remain some fragments of documents containing statistics of the check-ups carried out to detect TB among the inhabitants of the *Warthegau*. In the Poznań precinct *(Regierungsbezirk)*, where the Third Reich governor was based, these were carried out by 25 physicians (including 6 specialists in pulmonary diseases), who had 15 X-ray machines at their disposal [8]. X-rays, lung photofluorograms, and tuberculin tests were usually restricted to Germans, while percussion and auscultation of the chest and microscopic examination of the sputum constituted the principal methods for detecting TB among Poles. Germans suffering from TB were sent to sanatoriums and leisure centers, while the preferred method of treating Poles was by instructing them to remain at home and undergo medical supervision. Seriously ill Germans were hospitalized while Poles with advanced TB, who were sputum-positive and constituted a threat to their surroundings, were sent to isolation homes, which operated similar to hospices in former hospitals [7].

A large number of check-ups were performed in 1943 – when 3,748 Poles (165 of whom died) and 943 Germans (274 of whom died) in the entire *Warthegau* – were found to be suffering from pulmonary and laryngeal TB. TB had an even higher mortality toll among Germans than Poles, many of whom had some protective immunity, thanks to earlier infections (often during the annexation period), which had spontaneously subsided, and were, therefore, symptom-free before relapsing. Moreover, in 1943 six Germans and 52 Poles suffered from cutaneous TB (no one died), whereas 369 Poles, of whom 122 died and 106 Germans, of whom 22 died suffered from disseminated TB. The greatest number of infections and deaths in both groups occurred among those aged 20–60 years, in other words, of working age. Nevertheless, babies also suffered from and died of TB [8].

Statistics for pulmonary TB usually provide the number of deaths per the number of inhabitants in a certain locality or country. However, during the occupation, the number of inhabitants was not known owing to the incessant displacement, deportation or transportation of people for slave labor in the third Reich. Consequently, the number of deaths due to TB was compared to the overall number of deaths due to infectious diseases, which made it possible to determine the percentage share of TB mortality against other diseases [9]. Statistics showed that TB became the principal cause of deaths among Poles and Germans. In 1943 in the Poznań precinct alone, TB caused the death of 1,383 Poles compared to 70 people who died of other causes, and 294 Germans compared to 55 people who died of other causes. In 1943, 78,554 Poles and 90,713 Germans in the precinct were examined for TB to try to keep the "white death" epidemic at bay. In compliance with the aforesaid ministry regulation, free treatment was provided to Germans and selected Poles, which meant that the latter received healthcare sporadically [8].

In the Reichgau Wartheland
The situation was the most dramatic in Lodz, which the Germans renamed Litzmannstadt and separated as an independent precinct in 1941. In 1943, the death rate from TB in the city was 488/100,000 for Poles and 181/100,000 for Germans [2]. Deprived of access to healthcare, receiving insufficient food rations, overburdened with excessive physical workload, and relocated to one-room flats, Poles had high death-rates from TB. The German authorities attempted to bring the epidemic under control. From the beginning of January until the end of September 1941, 16,923 Germans and 21,108 Poles were examined in Lodz, which led to the detection of 1,222 cases of infection among the former, including 423 persons with infectious (i.e., AFB smear positive) TB, and 5,046 cases among the latter, including 2,530 sputum-positive persons [10]. Subsequent examinations performed from September to November 1941 of 3,661 Germans and 4,366

Poles led to the diagnosis of active TB among 1.5% of Germans and 16.4% of Poles. The scale of infections and the multiple threatening manifestations of TB (the greatest number of patients died of disseminated TB) forced the German authorities to establish in Lodz 4 dispensaries for Germans and 2 for Poles, all of which were equipped with X-ray machines. In the case of the Polish population, the dispensaries were not intended to treat but rather to keep records of Poles suffering from TB [11].

In Lodz, the TB epidemic was more widespread among Jewish inhabitants, who constituted one-third of the city's population. The Germans established a ghetto for them, in which there was an autonomous health unit, 6 hospitals, including 2 hospitals for infectious diseases, and a TB section. Hunger and disease decimated the population of the ghetto. Despite the risk of catching dysentery or typhoid, which could have led to death, Jews suffering from TB often reported to hospitals for infectious diseases because they offered modest meals. However, the Germans continuously decreased food rations, as was carried out again in June 1942. Hospitalized patients in the ghetto received only 200 g of bread a day. Seeing malnutrition as a factor in increasing the risk of children and teenagers falling ill with TB, Jewish doctors tried to save them by providing additional food rations – usually potato peelings. The initiative for the prevention of TB in the ghetto was also supported by Jewish pharmacists. Due to limited provision of medications to ghetto pharmacies, they themselves made ampoules with *calcium chloratum*, which was then considered to be the best medication against TB. Even though very few Jews had suffered from TB before the war, nearly one-half of the Lodz ghetto population had active TB in 1942. The death rate from TB in the ghetto was 3 times higher than the figure for Poles living in non-Jewish districts of Lodz and ten times higher than that for Germans. The end of the Lodz ghetto came in August 1944, when German special units transported all of its residents, both healthy and sick, to extermination camps [7].

Poles probably did not realize that the patient records held in clinics could be very dangerous for them. In 1942, the Germans took the first Poles suffering from TB to a labor camp in Gostynin where exhaustive work was the method of slow killing of undernourished prisoners. After a year in the 14 newly built barracks, there were 500 consumptives forming a work squad *(Arbeitskommando)*. Nothing is known about the fate of these people because only the archives of the 1941–1942 survived [11].

In the face of a growing and uncontrollable epidemic of TB, in May 1942, Arthur Greiser, Third Reich governor in the *Reichsgau Wartheland*, sent a letter to Heinrich Himmler, *Reichsführer-SS* and third Reich Commissioner for Strengthening German Culture, asking him to permit the extermination of approximately 35,000 Poles suffering from open TB and residing in the territory which he governed. He proposed the application of methods used for the extermination of Jews. He wrote, among other things:

I have been receiving reports concerning an ever-growing intensity of risk of infection among German children. Many of our active leaders, especially in the police force, have been infected lately and will temporarily be unable to perform military duty owing to the need for treatment…. I am of the opinion, and take full responsibility for what I am doing, that I will be permitted to propose that you destroy cases of open tuberculosis among Polish nationals in Warthegau. It should be understood that such an operation would only cover those Poles who were diagnosed and certified by an official doctor as having untreatable open tuberculosis. [12]

The concept was supported by R. Heydrich and H. Himmler. However, Professor K. Blome, deputy head of the Chief Health Office, had reservations. He warned that it would have been impossible to keep the operation strictly confidential and that the German population might worry that the same methods could be used to fight TB in the Third Reich. He suggested a different solution instead of extermination, namely the establishment of a "reservation" for Poles suffering from smear-positive TB and residing in the Polish territory annexed by Nazi Germany. Poles with active TB were to work in farming and forestry, which would ensure their rapid deaths from exhaustion. To conceal the actual nature of this death camp, Blome proposed hiring a certain number of Polish doctors and nurses. While Himmler approved the operation in 1942 [7], Greiser had already applied these methods of killing Poles suffering from active, infectious TB on his own authority a few months earlier [13].

Further preparation for mass extermination of patients with active TB included the establishment in 1943 in Poznań of the Central Unit for the Fight against TB in the *Reichsgau Wartheland*, which was supervised by the National Socialist German Workers' Party and SS. The institution began to supervise TB dispensaries and hospitals in the entire *Warthegau* as well as in Lodz and took over the records of Polish patients [7]. These showed that in 1943 in the *Warthegau*, there were 1,046,182 Polish and 339,073 German residents, and that 40% of Poles suffering from infectious diseases had TB [8]. Nonetheless, Greiser and Blome's plan was never implemented, probably due to the worsening military situation in the Eastern front, especial-ly the German defeat in Stalingrad, as well as their simultaneous involvement in the Holocaust in the occupied territory [7].

The Generalgouvernement

The situation of patients with active TB in the territory of the *Generalgouvernement* was different. Until mid-1941, the population of this territory of 94,100 km^2 amounted to 12.1 million people, including 11 million Poles, among them thousands of people displaced from the *Warthegau*, who supported each other and organized underground state structures. After the Third Reich's invasion of the USSR, which began in 1941, the territory of the *Generalgouvernement* grew to over 145,000 km^2 with over 16 million inhabitants, including newly displaced Ukrainians and Russians. For the German authorities of the *Generalgouvernement*, they constituted mainly a large pool of labor that the war economy needed. Slave labor, insufficient food rations, and poor living conditions favored *M. tuberculosis* infection and disease. However, no statistics of infections remain.

Nonetheless, the TB epidemic must have been a serious issue in the *Generalgouvernement* because German authorities organized check-ups among Polish railway workers. In 1941, in the railway workshop in Pruszków, Polish engineers managed, on their own initiative, to turn 2 Pullman-type sleeping carriages (named after their American manufacturer, George Pullman) into X-ray units. Appropriately adapted interiors were equipped with the necessary Siemens devices to perform mass miniature radiography surveys. Dr Aleksander Schreiber, a Polish radiologist displaced from the *Warthegau*, worked in one of the carriages from December 1941 until November 1946. He examined 133,055 railway workers, including 120,647 men, who constituted 90.7% of subjects, and 12,408 women, who made up a distinct minority, 9.3% of subjects. He only excluded those who were gravely ill at the time, those who had been sent away from their places of residence or those who were afraid of undergoing medical examination during occupation. The X-ray carriages traveled on all railway routes in the *Generalgouvernement* area, stopping in major cities for a few days to allow Schreiber to make chest photofluorograms of suspects with possible TB. He showed that approximately 3.3% of those examined had suffered a TB infection without being aware of it, because it had spontaneously subsided; 6.5% of the subjects were diagnosed with active TB, 5 times more than had been noted in German statistics. More sick people than anywhere else were found in Krakow, a city with thousands of displaced people, whose standard of living had deteriorated. Schreiber's medical practice showed that factors, especially favoring TB, included both inadequate diet and depressed living conditions in the city. Consequently, the highest number of diseased people were detected among office workers, especially those over 50-years, and the smallest number among unqualified workers [9].

Not many Polish doctors treated TB in the Saint Lazarus Hospital in Krakow. Such treatment was only possible until autumn 1942, when the hospital was taken over by SS officers who ordered Poles suffering from TB to be moved [14]. Other doctors' accounts shed some light on the extermination of Jews with active TB in Krakow. Physicians were surprised by a noticeably increased incidence of TB among Jews in the *Generalgouvernement* territory. Before the war, Jews fell ill with TB 3 times less frequently than non-Jews. However, in the prevailing ghetto conditions, they fell ill 3 times more often than the population outside the ghetto. In October 1942, the Germans began to exterminate inhabitants of the Krakow ghetto. People suffering from infectious diseases, including active TB, were transported to the concentration camp in Auschwitz and gassed [15].

The situation in Warsaw (Fig. 1), also located in the *Generalgouvernement*, was entirely different. In Warsaw, TB patients had been dealt with by the specialist Wolski Hospital. After the outbreak of WWII, a considerable share of its 300 beds was taken over by surgical patients. However, patients with active TB who were severely ill remained in the hospital. In 1940, Dr. Olgierd Sokołowski (1885–1944), a distinguished Polish phthisiologist, came to Warsaw from Zakopane. Soon after, he began working in the Skarbowców Hospital and after the Nazis closed it, he took over a 120-bed ward in the Wolski Hospital. When he introduced operative treatment of TB [16], the German authorities forced him to treat *Volksdeutsche*, meaning Poles who, during occupation, had declared themselves to be of German nationality and whom other Poles detested and treated as collaborators. In the first days of the Warsaw Uprising, Dr. Sokołowski was arrested by the Germans. When they were leading him to his death, he could have testified that he had treated *Volksdeutsche*, which would have saved his life, but he did not say anything, so he was shot near the hospital [17].

Another distinguished TB specialist, Professor Janusz Zeyland (1897–1944), was displaced from Poznań to Warsaw in 1940. He began establishing a microbiological analysis laboratory at the TB ward run by Dr. Sokołowski in the Skarbowców Hospital. After the hospital was closed, the German Warsaw Hospital Service Department commissioned Zeyland to establish a central TB laboratory in the

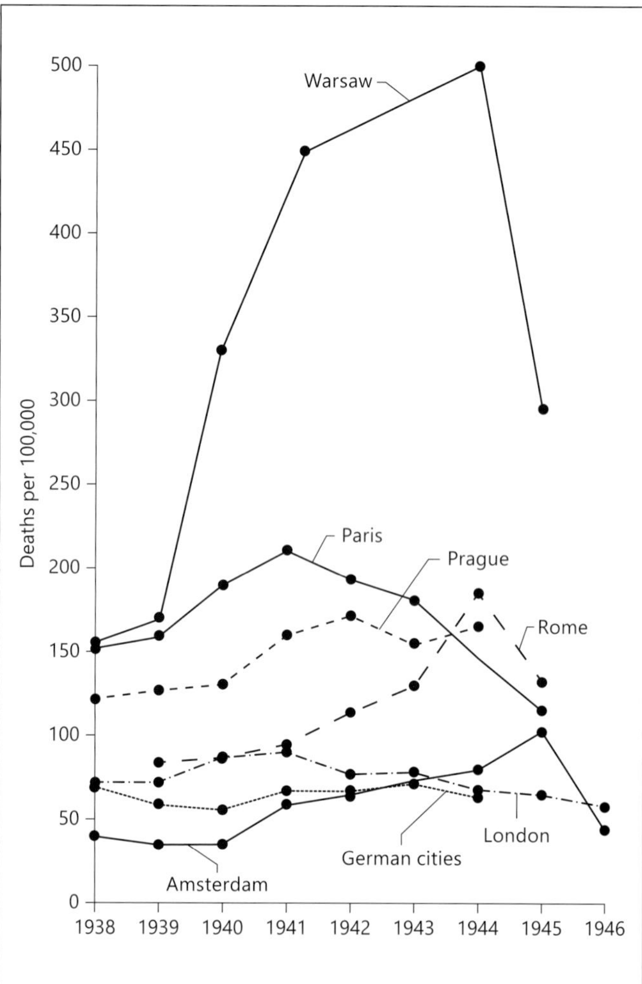

Fig. 1. Tuberculosis death-rates in European cities 1938–1946 per 100,000 population. Data reproduced from [37], with permission from Elsevier.

Wolski Hospital. It was opened in the spring of 1941 and since then served all the TB centers in Warsaw. A few months later, Zeyland established a TB ward for pediatric patients in the Wolski Hospital [18] and remained in the hospital after the outbreak of the Warsaw Uprising. He spoke good German and hoped to be able to negotiate the evacuation of patients and medical staff, but failed. Zeyland was executed by German soldiers in his office. Other TB specialists working in the Wolski Hospital were also killed with him [19].

Physicians who were displaced to Warsaw fought against TB using different methods. Some of them took bank loans to perform check-ups of employees of various institutions and municipal companies, especially in hospital TB wards. Thanks to their effort and the work of a Polish charity called

Miejska Pomoc Lekarska (Municipal Medical Aid) that people diagnosed with TB were sent to sanatoria [20]. Other doctors, like Józef Wolszczan (1900–1946), who were displaced to Warsaw in 1940, established sanatoria for patients with active TB that enabled Poles to be treated there [21]. There were also those who attempted to perform operative treatment of patients with advanced TB. For instance, at the end of 1941, in the Warsaw Child Jesus Hospital, Dr Jan Stopczyk opened a ward for adults suffering from TB and, despite difficult conditions, treated TB cavities using the Monaldi procedure, an early surgical technique to drain accessible TB cavities-abscesses [16]. The hospital also admitted poor and emaciated patients. However, as it did not provide them with proper meals, the doctors and nurses partnered together to provide extra nourishment. Skilled patients with TB did needlework to earn extra money to be able to buy additional food [16].

New Insights about TB

The wartime TB epidemic provided Polish doctors with extensive clinical material and enabled them to draw interesting impressions. These and later observations are of considerable interest, but were never validated by rigorous statistical methods. Before the war, the general opinion was that malnutrition decreased immunity to infectious diseases [22]. However, doctors were surprised to discover that only a quarter of those starving under the German occupation, especially those imprisoned in concentration camps, suffered from TB. Paradoxically, the disease did not develop during hunger but rather when food deficiencies were compensated. Consequently, malnutrition was not the principal pathogenic factor [23]. Furthermore, the most severe form of TB, miliary TB, did not occur in concentration camp conditions and patients infected with the disease did not suffer from meningitis. Physicians concluded that tubercle bacilli's conditions for life deteriorated when people's living conditions were bad, when they suffered from food shortages and avitaminosis. The acidification of the body caused by hunger slowed down the proliferation of TB, which was why TB caused relatively more deaths among the well-nourished Germans than among the starving Poles in *Warthegau*. Additional arguments to support this hypothesis were found after the concentration camps were liberated. The blood of former inmates who then received better food quickly alkalized, which favored the rapid development of TB, leaving doctors powerless [24].

Similar suppositions were drawn by Adolf Zuppinger and Alexis Labhart, who observed 230 former concentration camp prisoners and 296 workers of various nationalities who were transported to work in Germany. External conditions were blamed for a severe outbreak of TB. However, those who had previously suffered an episode of active TB showed an increased immunity to the rampant infection. It was believed that when the malnutrition of emaciated consumptives improved and they were properly fed, the course of active TB became more acute [25].

Physicians realized that TB infections were caused by frequent exposure to *M. tuberculosis*, which explains why the crowds of people exposed to others with active TB, whether or not they had previously been infected – may exacerbate old infections or cause new ones, a situation favored by extreme exhaustion of the immune system. Observation of the course of TB during WWII led to a realization that factors that cause the occurrence and intensification of the disease's symptoms could also include: cold, excessive physical work of malnourished people, lack or insufficient amounts of sleep, psychiatric trauma, and anxiety. In case of prisoners of war, one of the strongest factor leading to the development of TB seemed to be hypothermia. It was to the Ujazdowski Hospital in Warsaw that Germans brought consumptive POWs [23], who, under the Adolf Hitler decree of 1940, worked in mines and quarries or were hired by German farmers [5]. Even though they were well nourished, they lacked shoes and warm clothing, and thus fell ill with TB. Similar observations were made among civilian inhabitants of Warsaw [23].

An entirely different type of interest in the problem was shown by German physicians. In 1942, Dr. Hellmuth Vetter went to the Auschwitz concentration camp. As an associate of the I.G. Farben (Bayer AG), he intended to test a new TB drug, Rutenol, which was an arsenic acid derivative, on the inmates. He easily obtained the approval of the camp doctor, Dr. Friedrich Entress, since most consumptives in the concentration camps were usually the first to be killed for being incapable of working. Vetter began working in block 20, dedicated to infectious diseases. He selected 20 inmates suffering from TB and began experimenting on them in July 1943. For 5 days, he gave them 3 spoonfuls of the drug each, then waited for a week, performed checkups, and administered the pharmaceutical preparation again. After a year of experiments, only 4 inmates were still alive. Vetter later continued his criminal experiments in the Mauthausen-Gusen camp in Austria. After WWII ended, Vetter was sentenced to death and executed in 1949 [26].

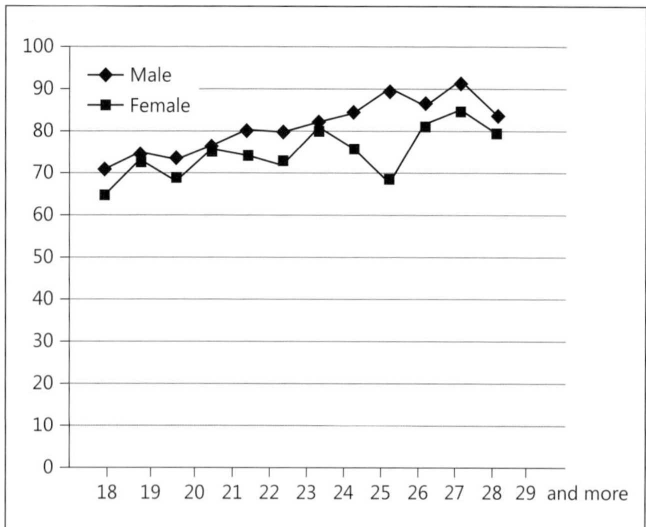

Fig. 2. Percentage of positive tuberculin reactions in students of different ages in Wroclaw, 1945, data from [29], with permission.

TB after the War

There are no archival data concerning the incidence of TB among the Polish population living in the Soviet-occupied Eastern territory of Poland. One may assume that there was also a TB epidemic there. However, the problem is likely to have receded into the background when compared with the immensity of war crimes, including the deportation of about 1 million Poles to Russia in horrendous conditions, few of who survived, and the murder of over 100,000 Poles in Ponary near Vilnius, Lithuania [5].

After the liberation from the German occupation, the Polish Health Ministry did not immediately manage to collect all the data concerning the TB epidemic. In the second half of 1945, the death rate from TB was 240/100,000 people. In the first half of 1946, it was 193/100,000, and in the subsequent 6-month period it was 121/100,000 [27]. Henryk Rudziński, Chief Extraordinary Commissioner for the Fight against Epidemics, considered the TB pandemic of the time to be a social calamity [28]. Nonetheless, it is hard not to note that, had it not been for the significant number of Poles who had been infected before the war and had a positive tuberculin reaction (Fig. 2), thus being somewhat protected against TB, there would have been even more cases of TB during the war [29].

Data collected by the TB Department of the Ministry of Health showed that 120,000 people died of TB in 1946, with 1.2 million people reported as being sick, about 5% of the population. Government statistics showed that the death rate from pulmonary TB in 1946 was 157/100,000, dropping to 120/100,000 in 1949 [30]. The patients included approximately: 100,000 with infectious pulmonary TB; 50,000 with extrapulmonary childhood TB; 40,000 with cutaneous TB; and 30,000 with osteoarticular TB, half of whom were children. Other victims of TB, about 1 million Poles, were carriers of more or less active pulmonary lesions [31]. The data for children were alarming. After WWII in 1946, 0.5% of children aged 6–12-years were diagnosed with active TB and another 70% were diagnosed with "inactive" infections; before the war the value was 40% [28].

The Nazis killed nearly 50% of physicians, including many specialists in pulmonary diseases. They destroyed medical book collections and looted medical apparatus and instruments as well as hospital equipment. Despite such serious shortages, city authorities in cooperation with the Ministry of Health began establishing TB clinics immediately after liberation. They were supervised by provincial clinics, which in turn were supervised by Provincial TB Departments. The highest authority was the Inter-Ministry TB Committee [32]. According to government data, in 1946, there were 639 TB clinics, while there were 312 after the epidemic was brought under control in 1949. This surprising difference meant that many TB clinics had been closed because the condition improved [33].

In Lodz, the city that was most affected by the epidemic, 3 TB clinics were opened soon after liberation. However, they registered only 4,758 patients suffering from active TB [2]. This is a small number when you consider that, in 1945, with a population of 501,551, 9,384 people died in Lodz – including 1,505 from TB – and the death rate from TB was 349/100,000. In the following year, the rate decreased to 170/100,000, and in 1949 to 146/100,000 [34].

By comparison, in Poznań, with a population of 280,000 in 1945, the death rate was 238/100,000, which was significantly greater than before the war: 153/100,000 in 1937, but still lower than in 1944 when it reached 264/100,000 [31]. In 1946, the rate was 175/100,000, and in 1949, it was only 115/100,000 [35]. In the academic year 1945–1946, 6.6% of the students required treatment for TB [35], while in Wrocław the infectious form of pulmonary TB was diagnosed among 0.5% of the city population, and males were more susceptible to TB than females [29].

In Warsaw, a city with a population of 479,000, the TB rate was 158/100,000 in 1946, which dropped to 116/100,000 in 1949. In the same year in Krakow, a city with a population of 300,000, the rate was 156/100,000, which dropped to 131/100,000 in 1949 [34]. In the entire Krakow Province, there were 70 clinics for patients with active TB, but they only registered 9% of the 84,000 inhabitants suffering from the disease [36]. This was because people feared a diagnosis of TB and believed that the disease was untreatable at the time and as stigmatizing as cancer. On the contrary, the clinics that existed at the time only registered patients rather than treated them. As in hospitals and sanatoria, there was a perceptible lack of qualified doctors, X-ray machines, microscopes, surgical instruments, thoracoscopes, needles, anesthetic agents, X-ray films, laboratory reagents, etc. The health insurance system had already been launched in 1946, but it only covered 2,590,300 people, and the Ministry of Health was only able to finance the treatment of 1,000 active TB patients a year. It was necessary to acquire 66,000 hospital beds for consumptives, but, even though only 11,580 were obtained, they were still partially unused due to lack of funds for treatment. For instance, the municipal TB clinic in Lublin registered 1,211 patients, but only 99 of them were sent to a hospital and 9 to a sanatorium. There were still 646 waiting for admission to a hospital and for treatment. Given the high prices of food, patients with TB in hospitals and sanatoriums were given meat or fish no more than twice a week and milk only as an addition to soup. In many sanatoriums, the average daily diet per person was less than 2,000 calories and some meals were only made of vegetables and the UNRRA rice [1].

The Polish government planned to bring the TB epidemic under control within 5 years, which seemed overly optimistic. Nevertheless, they managed to achieve that goal, thanks to the international aid. An important role in the fight against TB in Poland was played by UNRRA, which introduced international standards, provided food for patients, especially children, and equipped sanatoria in Silesia, which had been inherited from Germans [1]. Representatives of UNRRA recognized the key health problems in postwar Poland and quantified them by using registers of patients and deaths as well as information about the number of hospitals and their equipment, and so on. These materials helped other organizations to join the humanitarian aid campaign for Poles. For instance, BCG immunizations were initially dealt with by the Danish Red Cross, and after 1947, by UNICEF in cooperation with both Polish doctors and WHO [37]. Only 5,000 children were vaccinated by BCG in 1946 but by the year 1949, the figure had blossomed to 1.796 million. The epidemic was also brought under control, thanks to 7 X-ray ambulances that Poland received in 1948 as part of international humanitarian aid [38]. Finally, Polish physicians reactivated the pre-WWII TB Association and, working together with the Polish Red Cross and scouts, propagated hygienic principles; these helped prevent TB and other bacillary infections, which needed attention [31]. Nevertheless, until 1967 TB continued to cause the majority of sick leaves and had an immense impact on the polish economy [39].

Conclusion

Poland suffered immense loss of life and countrywide destruction during WWII, proportionally more than any other country. Polish and Jewish doctors were unable to fight the steadily increasing TB epidemic, because it was one of the Nazi strategies of extermination of different ethnic populations in the occupied territories. Full implementation of the Holocaust strategy by the Germans was hampered after their multiple defeats on the USSR Eastern front. Moreover, the course of TB was relatively milder in those poles who were infected by tubercle bacilli during the period of Partitions than the Germans. After the war, international humanitarian aid contributed greatly to the eradication of the TB epidemic in Poland.

References

1 Daniels M: Tuberculosis in Poland. Lancet 1946; 248:537–540.
2 Zierski M: Gruźlica w Łodzi po wojnie [Tuberculosis in Lodz after the war]. Gruźlica [Tuberculosis] 1947;15:329–342.
3 [Anonymus]: Zgony według przyczyn w miastach liczących ponad 100,000 mieszkańców [Mortality by cause in cities with more than 100,000 inhabitants]. Mały Rocznik Statystyczny [Small Statistical Yearbook] 1938;9:292.
4 [Anonymus]: XVI Zebranie Zrzeszenia Dyrektorów Sanatoriów Przeciwgruźliczych [16th session of the Tuberculosis Sanatorium Directors' Association]. Gruźlica [Tuberculosis] 1947;15: 99–107.
5 Eberhardt P: Przemieszczenia ludności na terytorium Polski spowodowane II wojną światową. Dokumentacja geograficzna nr 15 [Displacements in the territory of Poland due to World War II. Geographic documentation No. 15]. Warszawa, IGiPZ PAN, 2000.
6 [Anonymus]: Wspomnienia pośmiertne [Postmortem memoirs]. Gruźlica [Tuberculosis] 1947; 15:382–383.
7 Fijałek A, Supady J: Gruźlica w Łodzi w okresie okupacji hitlerowskiej w latach 1940–1944. Choroba a eksterminacja [Tuberculosis in Nazi-Occupied Lodz 1940–1944. Disease and extermination]. Lodz, Wydawnictwo ADI, 2004.
8 State Archive in Poznan, Record Group 299, Namiestnik Rzeszy w Okręgu Kraju Warty [Third Reich governor in the *Wartheland* precinct], ref. 1920.

9 Schreiber A: Wyniki szeregowych zdjęć rentgenowskich przeprowadzonych wśród polskich pracowników kolejowych w latach 1941–1944 [Results of ordinary X-rays performed among Polish railway staff, 1941–1944]. Nowiny Lekarskie [Medical News] 1946;53:381–389.

10 State Archive in Lodz, Record Group: 221, Zarząd Miasta Łodzi, Wydział Zdrowia [The Lodz City Council, the Health Department], ref. 7.

11 State Archive in Poznan, Record Group: 299, Namiestnik Rzeszy w Okręgu Kraju Warty [Third Reich governor in the *Wartheland* precinct], ref. 3123.

12 Mitscherlich A, Mielke F: Nieludzka medycyna: dokumenty procesu norymberskiego przeciwko lekarzom [Doctors of Infamy: The Story of the Nazi Medical Crimes]. translated by Adam Bukowczyk, Warszawa, PZWL, 1963.

13 State Archive in Poznan, Record Group 1415, Związek Bojowników o Wolność i Demokrację w Poznaniu [Precinct Authority of the Fighters for Freedom and Democracy Society in Poznań], ref. 1525.

14 Kostrzewski J: Państwowy szpital św. Łazarza w Krakowie i kliniki UJ w czasie okupacji i na przełomie [State Saint Lazarus Hospital in Krakow and Jagiellonian University clinics under occupation and afterwards]. Przegl Lek 1946;2:26–39.

15 Nussenfeld J, Bornstein B: Historia wojenna szpitala gminy żydowskiej w Krakowie w okresie 1939–45 r. [The Jewish commune hospital in Krakow during the war, 1939–45]. Przegl Lek 1946;2:39–41.

16 Stopczyk J: O leczeniu jam gruźliczych w płucach sposobem Monaldi'ego [On the treatment of tuberculous cavities in lungs using the Monaldi procedure]. Gruźlica [Tuberculosis] 1947;15:159–187.

17 Madey J: Dr Olgierd Sokołowski w Warszawie w latach wojny (1940–1944) [Dr Olgierd Sokołowski in Warsaw during the war (1940–1944)]. Gruźlica [Tuberculosis] 1947;15:30–33.

18 Jonscher K: Janusz Zeyland (1897–1944). Gruźlica [Tuberculosis] 1947;15:17–27.

19 Misiewicz J: Pamięci lekarzy ftizjologów Szpitala Wolskiego, którzy zginęli jako ofiary terroru i zmarli w latach wojny [In memoriam to phthisiologists from the Wolski Hospital, victims of terror who died during the war]. Gruźlica [Tuberculosis] 1947;15:4–6.

20 Misiewicz J: Zmiany gruźlicze u pracowników Szpitala Wolskiego w Warszawie w latach 1941–1944 [Tuberculous lesions in Warsaw Wolski hospital staff (1941–1944)]. Gruźlica [Tuberculosis] 1947;15:121–133.

21 [Anonymus] Wspomnienia pośmiertne [Postmortem memoire]. Gruźlica [Tuberculosis] 1947;15:382–401.

22 Cegielski JP, McMurray DN. The relationship between malnutrition and tuberculosis: evidence from stuudies in humans and experimental animals. Int J Tuberc Lung Dis 2004;8:286–298.

23 Kucharski T: W sprawie patogenezy gruźlicy płuc u dorosłych [On the pathogenesis of pulmonary tuberculosis among adults]. Nowiny Lekarskie [Medical News] 1946;53:311–315.

24 [Anonymus]: XVI Zebranie Zrzeszenia Dyrektorów Sanatoriów Przeciwgruźliczych [16th session of the Tuberculosis Sanatorium Directors' Association]. Gruźlica [Tuberculosis] 1947;15:99–107.

25 Zuppinger A, Labhart A: Gestalt und Frühverlauf der Tuberkulose bei Patienten aus Konzentrationslagern [The course and symptoms of tuberculosis in patients from concentration camps]. Schweiz Med Wochenschr 1947;77:144–146.

26 Sterkowicz S: Nieludzka medycyna. Lekarze w służbie nazizmu [Inhuman medicine. Doctors in the service of Nazism]. Warszawa, Wydawnictwo Medyk, 2007.

27 [Anonymus]: Zgony na gruźlicę w niektórych większych miastach [Mortality from tuberculosis in some major cities]. Rocznik Statystyczny GUS [Polish Central Statistical Office Yearbook] 1947;11:146.

28 Rudziński H: Konieczność połączenia spraw zwalczania gruźlicy w Polsce z akcją zwalczania chorób epidemicznych w ramach Naczelnego Nadzwyczajnego Komisariatu do Walki z Epidemiami [Necessity to combine the fight against tuberculosis in Poland with the campaign against epidemic diseases under the Chief Extraordinary Commission for the Fight against Epidemics]. Przegl Lek 1946;2:827–829.

29 Skibiński Z, Skibińska J: Gruźlica wśród młodzieży akademickiej we Wrocławiu [Tuberculosis among students in Wroclaw]. Przegl Lek 1947;3:746–753.

30 [Anonymus]: Zgony według przyczyn w niektórych większych miastach [Mortality by causa in some larger cities]. Rocznik Statystyczny GUS [Polish Central Statistical Office Yearbook], 1950; 14:181.

31 May M: Ramowy projekt walki z gruźlicą na terenie stoł. m. Poznania [Framework fight against tuberculosis plan for the capital city of Poznań]. Nowiny Lekarskie [Medical News] 1947;16:115–120.

32 Skibiński Z: Zasady walki społecznej z gruźlicą [The principles of social fight against tuberculosis]. Polski Tygodnik Lekarski [Polish Medical Weekly] 1946;3:1099–1101.

33 [Anonymus]: Poradnie przy ośrodkach zdrowia i punktach sanitarnych według specjalności [Outpatient clinics at health centers and sanitary units according to specialty]. Rocznik Statystyczny GUS [Polish Central Statistical Office Yearbook] 1950; 14:174.

34 [Anonymus]: Zgony na gruźlicę w niektórych większych miastach [Mortality from tuberculosis in some major cities]. Rocznik Statystyczny GUS [Polish Central Statistical Office Yearbook] 1950; 14:183.

35 Schreiber A: Wyniki statystyczne szeregowych zdjęć rentgenowskich, przeprowadzonych w roku akademickim 1945–1946 wśród młodzieży akademickiej w Poznaniu [Statistical results of ordinary X-rays performed in the academic year 1945–1946 among students In Poznan]. Nowiny Lekarskie [Medical News] 1947;53:128–134.

36 Hornung S: Aktualny stan akcji przeciwgruźliczej prowadzonej przez poradnie na terenie wojew. krakowskiego [Current state of the anti-tuberculosis campaign run by clinics in the Krakow Province]. Przegl Lek 1946;2:47–48.

37 Daniels M: Tuberculosis in post-war Europe. An international problem. Tubercle 1947;28:201–222.

38 [Anonymus]: Zakłady leczniczo-zapobiegawcze ruchome i pomocy doraźnej [Mobile medical and emergency units]. Rocznik Statystyczny GUS [Polish Central Statistical Office Yearbook] 1950;14:176.

39 Supady J, Włodarczyk M: Gruźlica w Łodzi w latach 1945–1970. Z dziejów walki z chorobą [Tuberculosis in Lodz in 1945–1970. From the history of fight against the disease]. Łódź, Wydawnictwo ADI, 2006.

Anita Magowska
Department of the History and Philosophy of Medical Sciences
Poznan University of Medical Sciences, ul. Przybyszewskiego 37A
PL–60-346 Poznan (Poland)
E-Mail anitamagowska@yahoo.com

Murray JF, Loddenkemper R (eds): Tuberculosis and War. Lessons Learned from World War II.
Prog Respir Res. Basel, Karger, 2018, vol 43, pp 103–115 (DOI: 10.1159/000481478)

Tuberculosis in the United Kingdom and Ireland before, during, and after World War II

Peter D.O. Davies[a, b] · Rosemary Trafford[c]

[a]Respiratory Medicine, Liverpool Heart and Chest Hospital, [b]School of Medicine, Liverpool University, and [c]Respiratory Medicine, Mersey Deanery, Liverpool, UK

Abstract

The United Kingdom (UK) and Ireland had very different roles in World War II (WWII). The UK was engaged in continuous conflict from September 1939 until August 1945. In contrast, Ireland remained neutral throughout the war. Both countries saw an increase in tuberculosis (TB) deaths and cases during the war. However, cases outstripped mortality in the UK, probably because improved medical services detected cases earlier by screening and medical examination of recruits and industrial workers. Both countries saw an increase in social services and provision for the poorest and most deprived in the land. In the UK, the publication of the Beveridge report in 1942 was probably the single most important event in the fight against disease and poverty during the whole of the 20th century. From that followed the foundation of the National Health Service and the provision of comprehensive social services, including vaccination and screening for TB. Civilian mortality including the mortality of children actually fell during the war years. In spite of the horrific consequences of the war, WWII formed a springboard for improved public and personal health in all aspects of disease, not just TB.

Lenny saw his ghost, the ghost of his lungs. He knew that in this world, the world of his chest, the darkness was healthy tissue and the light patches his illness.

"Ready?"

I could get up and walk out, he thought; I do not have to take this. But he was too tired to stand. He felt the hypodermic enter his chest, an unpleasant sting of pain, then the feeling of being pushed hard, pushed right off the table, and something crunching. Oh God help me he thought he's going to murder me.

Another needle entered him, thicker and attached to the rubber hose.

"You'll start to feel a pulling sensation," the doctor said, "it should feel tight round your neck and shoulder." The dials on the equipment rose and fell.

Lenny received his first induced pneumothorax as lung collapse therapy. An extract from "The dark circle" [1].

The political changes involving the countries and islands that comprise the United Kingdom (UK) over the 20th century need explanation. Had the chapter been about tuberculosis (TB) in the First World War, there would have been no need to consider Ireland as a separate country as at that time it was part of the UK. In 1922, the country we now call Ireland or Eire became a free state and has remained a separate country ever since. The island of Ireland has, henceforth, been divided into 2 countries comprising Ireland or Eire to the South and the 6 counties of Ulster remaining part of the UK, as Northern Ireland.

In 1937, a new Constitution re-established the state as Ireland (or Éire in Irish). In 1949, the state was formally declared a republic and it left the British Commonwealth.

Northern Ireland remained part of the UK through this time such that from 1922 the island of Ireland was politically divided into 2 countries. Northern Ireland keeps its statistics separately from the UK for most things including TB and needs to be considered separately.

England and Wales have politically been a single country since the 14th century and until recently their statistics have been unified. Scotland with its late union with England and Wales (1702) and having separate laws keeps its own statistics for most data, including TB. Investigating any health trend across the islands of the UK and Ireland is, therefore, fraught with problems from the start.

Great Britain (GB) refers to the countries of England Wales and Scotland, but not Northern Ireland.

United Kingdom

The UK declared war on Germany on September 3, 1939, when Germany failed to withdraw its advancing military forces from Poland. Hostilities in Europe ceased with the signing of unconditional surrender by the Germans on May 7, 1945. The UK continued its war with the allies against Japan until it too unconditionally surrendered on August 15, 1945, with the formal signing on September 2. By that time the UK had been continuously at war for just a few days short of 6 years.

Eire remained neutral throughout World War II (WWII), which saved it from much of the horrors of the war, although tens of thousands volunteered to serve in the British forces. Ireland was also impacted by food rationing and coal shortages; peat production became a priority during this time. Though nominally neutral, recent studies have suggested a far greater level of involvement by the South with the Allies than was realized, with D Day's date set on the basis of secret weather information on Atlantic storms supplied by Ireland.

Wartime Civil Measures

Within days of the declaration of war, a number of emergency measures were introduced. Probably the most important as far as spread of infectious diseases was concerned was first the evacuation of children from major cities, particularly London, to the countryside and secondly a planned economy, including the rationing of most food. Contrary to expectations this lead to a more even distribution of food across all socioeconomic classes with the result of improved nutrition among the poorest. The fairness of rationing was one of the major factors maintaining moral in the country. The system was founded on the 3 cornerstones of scientific assessment: of needs, of social justice, and of recommendations for supplying sound special needs [2].

General Health of the Population

Far from a general increase in mortality as a result of wartime deprivation, there was an overall improvement. For example, the annual infant mortality fell between 1938 and 1944 from 74 to 58 per thousand in Liverpool, 71–57 in Nottingham, and 69–54 in Manchester. In greater London, the figures went from 50 to 43 and in Oxford from 23 to 15, showing what scope there was for further improvement across the whole country. In addition, there was a rise in the birth rate to 17.7 per thousand inhabitants.

Measurement of TB

It seems a simple question, but to measure the number of people suffering from TB is not necessarily simple. Basically there are 2 main ways of measuring the impact of the disease: (1) those dying from the disease and (2) those suffering from the disease. Both measures depend on the skill of the doctors to diagnose the disease and also to inform the proper authorities that this has taken place. The law by which a medical attendant had to notify each case of TB came into force in 1919. The medical attendant, usually the doctor, had to notify a case of TB if he or she, "Believed a patient to be suffering from TB." There was no requirement for proof or for the patient to be infectious. Disease at any organ site was sufficient to trigger notification.

Up until the start of WWII, mortality rates and morbidity rates tended to run in parallel, with morbidity rates about twice the rates of mortality. But during the war years, morbidity began to move away from mortality, because better health checks found more cases at an earlier stage of development (see below).

TB in the Pre-War Years

Evidence from the Registrar General's returns available for England and Wales from 1850 show an annualized rate of decline of TB of approximately 1.7% per annum [3]. Darcy Hart has attributed this to a steady improvement in income over the same period [4]. Others have disputed this showing that there was no similar decline in other diseases that might have been poverty related, such as typhoid and cholera. Instead they propose a form of natural selection whereby as the susceptible population died as a result of disease, they gave way to a more resistant population [5].

A graph showing TB mortality for England and Wales from 1900 to 1970 is shown in Figure 1. It clearly shows a steady decline in TB mortality throughout this period with the exceptions of the World War years. There is a sudden spike at the beginning of WWI and a less marked but longer upward trend in the WWII years. [6]. Thereafter, there is a

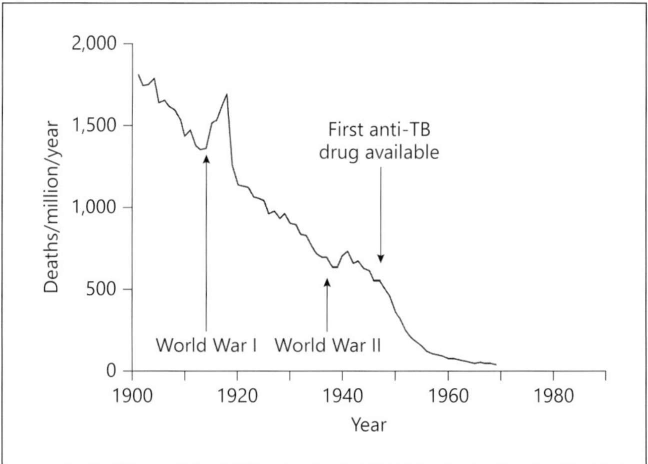

Fig. 1. Decline in TB mortality in England and Wales, and its association in time with the 2 World Wars, and the introduction of chemotherapy against TB [6], with permission.

decline of approximately 10% per annum as the effects of Bacillus Calmette Guérin (BCG) and specific chemotherapy combined to show their effects from the early 1950s onwards.

Russel points out that the decline in notifications leading up to WWII was not uniform across the age groups. He suggests that food deprivation of children during WWI may have led to a cessation of the decline in TB among those aged 25–34 years in the 1930s as remote infection incurred during wartime developed into active disease [7]. Russel also points out that in the pre-war years the ratio of female to male notifications was approximately 1–1.2. This rose to approximately 1–1.4 during the war years. Russel suggests that this may have been due to men receiving more thorough medical examinations as they were recruited into the armed forces than women, who may been more likely to work in factories or in locations where medical services might not have been so rigorous.

What is also apparent from morbidity and mortality statistics is that during WWII there was a more rapid increase in notifications than in mortality. The reasons for this are not clear but perhaps the most likely is that with the increased medical activity, particularly pre-employment screening both in the armed forces and civilian life, early cases of TB were detected that with appropriate rest treatment gave patients a better chance of survival. There may also have been a trend to diagnose TB where there might only have been scarring due to past previously healed infection. By the second and third years of the war, mass miniature X-ray screening of the population was coming into force and became an increasingly common way of detecting the disease.

Bovine TB

Bovine TB was still a real threat to humans in the UK and Eire at the outbreak of WWII. During the 1920s and 30s, various measures had been passed to reduce the level of infection in cattle [8]. The attested Herds Schemes in 1938 provided for tuberculin testing free of charge to the owner of a herd. If the herd was found to have no reactors on 2 separate occasions they were attested as TB free. This gave the herd owners the advantage of selling the milk as Tuberculin Tested or TT milk. By 1939, there were 8,146 attested herds in England and Wales and 2,022 in Scotland, a total of 10,348. The process continued during WWII and by March 1944 there were a total of 16,185 attested herds in GB. However, this still amounted to less than 10% of all cattle.

In contrast, the USA had been much more successful in eliminating bovine TB as it pursued a rigorous policy of slaughter of infected animals. It was felt that the USA had a near surplus of cattle. There would be no real danger of interfering with the milk or meat supply as there might be if similar policies were used in GB. Whereas rates of conversion in USA cattle were below 1%, figures of up to 40% have been quoted for GB with 7% of farms selling TB-infected milk [9]. The author concluded that pasteurization of milk was the best means of protection against bovine infection.

In a tuberculin survey of Cambridge carried out in 1942–1943, on 485 individuals under 30 years of age, it was found that the level of infection in those under 15 years was more than 20% higher in rural areas than in the city of Cambridge. It was concluded that bovine infection was responsible for this high level of positive tuberculin tests in the rural children [10].

Bovine TB, therefore, presented an ongoing threat of morbidity and mortality, especially to children who were more likely to drink milk in larger quantities than adults. WWII would have been likely to slow down the process of herd tuberculin attestation compared with what might have happened under peacetime conditions, thereby increasing the threat of TB in children.

TB in Children

Tuberculin surveys carried out mid-WWII in Cambridge and Hertfordshire [10] showed a very high proportion of converters. Almost 40% of those aged 0–9 years and 55% of those aged 10–15 years among children not known to have had previous TB contact.

Data from a children's sanatorium in the North East of England shows a steady increase in admissions during the war years. In 1940, 4 children were admitted, in 1941 13, in 1942 55, in 1943 173, in 1944 227, and in 1945 117. Thereafter, admissions ranged between 150 and 200. These were children from the poorest areas of the North of England, and the socioeconomic profile did not appear to change throughout the war years [10].

Sir Wilson Jameson, chief medical officer of the Ministry of Education, noted that the nutrition of public elementary school children was probably improved during the war. For example, in London the percentage of undernourished children fell from 4.47 in 1938 to 3.75 in 1945. For England and Wales, the percentage of children whose nutrition was classed as good rose from 88.1 to 90.8%. In most areas where records were kept, there was an increase in height of $^1/_4$ to $^1/_2$ inch and in weight of 1 $^1/_2$ to 2 lbs [11].

TB Mortality

Deaths from TB in children between 1 and 5 years rose in 1941–1943 but by 1945 had fallen to 41/100,000 compared with 45/100,000 in 1938. Those in 5–15 year age groups showed a similar pattern.

Infant mortality also fell over the same period from 53 to 45 per 100,000 [12]. The death rate from respiratory TB rose from 52.2/100,000 in 1939 to 588 in 1940 and 602 in 1941 but by 1942 had fallen to 542, and for the first half of 1946 was 355. The pattern across all ages was, therefore, to see an initial increase followed by a fall below pre-war levels by 1945.

TB Morbidity

In contrast to the figures for TB mortality, which rose and then fell by the end of WWII, figures for morbidity (i.e., notified cases of pulmonary TB for England and Wales) rose throughout the war, as shown in Table 1 [13].

TB in the Armed Forces: In contrast to the entire civilian and armed force populations, figures for notifications among branches of the armed forces show a slight rise towards the end of the war [14].

The British Thoracic Society report points out that because of the emergency at the start of WWII, recruitment for military service was based on the findings from a medical history and physical examination only. No chest X-rays were performed initially. X-ray facilities did become available not long after the beginning of the war for screening of recruits as well as for those who presented later with symptomatic disease. As a consequence, many recruits passed into active service with pulmonary lesions, which is reflected in the number of pensions given in later years on the grounds of "disease aggravated by service." Numbers for pension awards are given after the war as these would have been awarded for "aggravation" while serving during the war.

Table 1. All tuberculosis annual non-military notifications in England and Wales, 1938–1944

Year	Males	Females	Total
1938	21,302	16,577	37,879
1939	19,695	15,235	34,930
1940	20,988	15,163	36,151
1941	23,147	16,352	39,499
1942	23,623	17,006	40,629
1943	24,371	18,039	42,410
1944	24,970	18,824	44,794

Tuberculous in Some English Cities

Birmingham: Geddes, after examining the effect of WWII on TB rates in Birmingham, concluded that the incidence rate was 55.5% above what it would have been had the war not intervened [15]. In contrast, the percentage of deaths per notification fell from an average of 74% for the years 1933–39 but then rose to 93% in 1939 and finally fell again to 56% in 1945.

East Ham: Ellman showed a rapid increase in TB notifications in both adults and children from 1941. The increase was particularly acute in children rising almost 4-fold between 1944 and 1947 [16]. He attributes this to the improvement in screening children with Mass Miniature Radiography (MMR) from 1943 and continuing after the war. Much of this increase was, therefore, due to better case detection rather than a true rise in cases. This must be seen as a benefit of the war to the control of TB.

Rochdale: Rochdale saw little change in TB notifications during the war years; with a rate of 0.90 per 1,000 in 1939 and 0.87 in 1944. Mortality also showed little change being 0.46 per 1,000 in 1939 and 0.48 in 1944 [17].

Fife Scotland: Deaths from TB, both pulmonary and non-pulmonary, roughly paralleled the increase in Scotland from the beginning of the war but with actual numbers roughly one fortieth of the Scottish total [18].

Tuberculin Surveys

Because tuberculin surveys detect the proportion of the population who are infected and involve proactive intervention, which can also be repeated at pre-set intervals and do not depend on the presentation of the patient and the pro-

Time period	Royal Navy	Army	Airforce	Total
Sept 39 to Dec 42	2,115	6,246	1,734	10,095
1943	1,600	3,025	1,358	5,983
1944	2,067	3,878	1,637	7,582
1945	1,929	3,399	1,428	6,766
1946	2,067	3,339	1,473	6,879
1947	2,089	4,117	1,951	8,157

fessional skill of the doctor to diagnose, they can offer a better guide to the rise and fall of the disease than either morbidity or mortality data. One of the most comprehensive tuberculin testing surveys ever undertaken – the Prophit survey – which started in 1935, was underway in the UK at the outbreak of the war [19]. Prospective tuberculin testing was undertaken using the Mantoux test in certain groups of young adults, including nurses, medical students, and naval recruits and also controls not expected to encounter TB in their occupations. Non-reactors were tested 6 monthly.

Control subjects increased their positivity rate to around 50% over a 3-year period, medical students to 75% but nurses up to 95%. Very broadly, the tuberculin positive rate doubled over 3 years across all groups. Contacts who were also included in the study had much higher levels of tuberculin test positivity that were maintained. Because the survey had been planned before the war started and continued through it, no provision was ever made in the protocol for allowing for any changes to occupation, which might have occurred as a result of the war. It is, therefore, not possible to draw conclusions as to what effect the war had on the infection rate in the populations studied.

Individuals who were tuberculin test positive at the outset were evaluated by chest X-rays. The presence of lesions thought to be due to active pulmonary TB was between 1 and 5%.

Wartime Organization of TB Services in the UK
The increase in mortality from respiratory TB in 1940 and a further increase in 1941 brought a staggering increase of 10% in England and Wales and of 18% in Scotland. Additional cause for concern was a sharp rise in deaths from meningeal TB, affecting all age groups up to 45 years. Now acutely alarmed, in 1941 under the auspices of the Medical Research Council, the Ministry of Health appointed a Committee on TB in War-Time with the following terms of reference: "To assist in promoting the investigation of the extent and causes of the war-time increase in the incidence of TB, particularly among young women, and also to advise the Council regarding possible preventive measures" [20].

The committee submitted its report in September 1942 [21]. In this document, stress was laid on the causative factors, of certain circumstances peculiar to WWII, of which the following were the most important: the government policy of evacuating TB hospitals and sanatoria in September 1939 to make way for the feared rush of air raid casualties had resulted in a large number of infectious cases being returned to their homes, while blackout conditions in the home and in the factory had impaired ventilation, increasing cross infection and lowering resistance. The increase in cases of non-respiratory disease was believed to be linked to the large-scale evacuation of town-bred children, who normally consumed pasteurized milk, to country areas where they had to change to raw milk in the absence of pasteurization facilities.

Heaf and Rusby showed that bombing, which began in the autumn of 1940, resulted in the destruction of both sanatoria and homes, resulting in pressure to house TB patients elsewhere. The danger of infection by sharing air raid shelters was to some extent mitigated by getting patients to wear protective masks. There was also an attempt to supply TB affected families with their own Anderson shelters [22].

Recommendations to Reduce the Incidence of TB
Recommendations by the committee began with a clear endorsement to extend pasteurization of milk to all sources as soon as possible. Next the committee turned their attention to the importance of limiting infectivity of cases, of which the most important was early diagnosis. They recommended that responsibility for examination should pass from the patient to the doctor. So instead of waiting for the patient to develop symptoms and seek the doctor, the doctor would initiate the process. This was essentially the first step in an active screening program that was made possible by the rapid expansion of the use of chest X-rays. MMR had begun to be developed in the 1920s and 30s across Europe but had not become widespread by 1942. The goal was to enable X-ray machines to be sent in special vans into the community where patients resided. Thus way, they did not have to attend Hospitals or Chest Clinics.

By 1945, 13 local authorities who were implementing the first recommendation were subject to a report by the Medical Research Council [23]. The second recommendation attempted to counter the prevailing financial disincentive for patients to come forward for screening in case they were found to have TB and be required to leave their work for treatment. The committee recommended that some form of additional financial help should be provided, which, by easing the economic consequences of diagnosis, might encourage the patient to seek treatment earlier. The Committee suggested that such financial provision should ensure an adequate allowance for up to 1 year after notification. The amount was to vary according to the financial needs of the patient and family. At the end of 1 year, the case could be reviewed and the amount of the allowance adjusted to meet the prevailing circumstances.

The fact that both these recommendations were accepted by the Ministry of Health and subsequently implemented is an accurate reflection of the considerable degree of public concern that accompanied the increase in TB in 1940–1941. It is true that the proposed financial benefits, outlined in the official document were initially on a limited scale but did achieve a breakthrough and a more realistic financial provision for TB patients and their financial dependents. Because relatively few women were wage earners at the outbreak of the war, later adjustments were authorized in succeeding years when the benefits of the scheme had proved themselves beyond denial.

Longer Term Consequences of War Time Provision for TB Care

In 1942, the year that the MRC's recommendations for TB control were published, the Beveridge Report was also published [24]. The Beveridge Report offered 3 guiding principles to its recommendations:

1 Proposals for the future should not be limited by "sectional interests" in learning from experience and that a "revolutionary moment in the world's history is a time for revolutions, not for patching."

2 Social insurance is only one part of a "comprehensive policy of social progress." The 5 giants on the road to reconstruction are Want, Disease, Ignorance, Squalor, and Idleness.

3 Policies of social security "must be achieved by cooperation between the State and the individual," with the state securing the service and contributions. The state "should not stifle incentive, opportunity, responsibility; in establishing a national minimum, it should leave room and encouragement for voluntary action by each individual to provide more than that minimum for himself and his family."

In practice, the Beveridge Report laid the ground rules for the Welfare State that was gradually being introduced by the Labor Government in 1945–1951. Of greatest importance was the formation of the National Health Service, which came into being by an act of Parliament in 1948. This provided health care freely to every person in the country paid for out of general taxation.

Administration of Chest Clinics

Different countries had their own ways of managing TB during the 20th century. In the UK, the Chest Clinic was the bedrock of management. These had evolved from the original dispensaries over a generation after the end of WWI. For efficiency, they were equipped to serve a population of approximately 250,000. They tended to operate as a hospital outpatient service but were often more conveniently sited for the patient in the close community. The senior doctor's title was changed from "TB Officer" to "Chest Physician" as it was realized that these physicians had a wider experience over the entire range of differential diagnoses of chest diseases [25].

Staff: In addition to the Chest Physician, there was a need for specialist advisors, usually qualified nurses who would be the link between the clinic and the home. It was appreciated that it was an advantage that these advisors should be working wholly on TB care. There was also a secretary, social worker, records clerk, and short-hand typist.

Equipment: In 1943, mass radiography received official blessing as a method of case finding [27]. First class X-ray apparatus was the most important item of equipment, which should be able to carry out fluoroscopy as well as taking films; it was also suggested that there be a small X-ray apparatus that could do both these functions. It was during WWII that MMR vans first came into general use and were present in most towns and cities by the 1950s and 1960s. These would be based at Chest Clinics where patients would be asked to report if they had an abnormal chest X-ray. There was concern that the workload of reading MMR films might increase up to 400–500 in an hour, which seems impossible [27].

Statistics: The compilation of statistics to supply notifications to local and national levels was essential for TB control. During the war, an alphabetical punch card system was recommended. More sophisticated techniques for the bigger clinics required involvement of outside statistical staff at times.

Notifications: The District Medical Office of Health was required to keep this information but in practice it was important for the clinic to be fully informed – weekly – about notifications of new cases and deaths. A notification should be made if the patient is "suffering" from TB. Notifications by death of patients not known to be previously suffering from TB required special measures to see whether fault might be attached at any time.

Diagnosis: The patients attending a Chest Clinic had usually been referred by a General Practitioner. Ordinarily, Chest Clinic Physicians would be required to carry out a full history and physical examination, probably followed by a chest X-ray, tuberculin test, sputum examination and other investigations suggested by the examination. A prompt reply to the GP's letter within a week would be considered a standard practice.

X-Ray and Fluoroscopy Service: "Case finding is the horse that pulls the cart of the whole TB program," was a line probably coined by Toussaint and Pritchard in 1944 at the Bermondsey and Southwark Chest Clinic. Immediately after it was recognized that the X-ray would detect disease before it became clinically apparent, the process of screening began.

Other Sources of Cases: In addition to contacts, other cases might come from the District Hospital, recruitment boards, and children from infant welfare clinics or other outpatient departments.

Treatment Selection

By the start of WWII, sanatoria in the UK had changed their role from a rustic convalescent home to units capable of major surgery and highly specialized investigation of the respiratory tract. It was the role of the Chest Clinic to separate patients according to what type of management they needed: into sanatoria cases, those who could be managed in local hospital beds, or by "car" outpatients and home (i.e., by car transport to and from home).

More than half the sputum-negative cases were dealt with under home conditions. From home such investigations as gastric and tracheal lavage, laryngeal swabs could be undertaken as well as temperature charted, exercise graduated, and weight recorded.

The management of rest and gradual exercise became central to the treatment of TB both at home and in sanatoria. Advice was given about the detailed construction of garden-based "Chalets" where patients could receive almost sanatorium-like conditions in his or her own back garden, provided it was big enough [28]. Holmes Sellors and Livingstone [25] recorded that only 50% of the sputum-positive group and 25% of the sputum-negative group were suitable for active therapy [26]. There was great pressure for patients to be managed at home rather than in institutional beds. Free treatment was available to many patients and each chest clinic was staffed by an "almoner" to see that no patient endured unnecessary financial hardship [28].

Advanced cases unsuitable for any type of surgical therapy were cared for at home. Specialist TB nurses would visit to advise regarding containment of infection. For example, advise the patient to have a separate sleeping room if this was possible. It was generally believed that such patients had already infected their family or fellow householders but it was desirable to reduce the quantity of exposure to a minimum.

Treatment

The basic principle of treatment was rest, for the patient as a whole and for the affected lung. Bed rest in a sanatorium ensured maximum rest for the patient and, because of greatly reduced activity, a great diminution of lung movement. A good diet was ensured and there was an unsubstantiated belief in the value of open air [29].

Treatment was directed to ensure that tubercle bacilli were sealed in healed or healing fibrous tissue and rendered inactive. Calcified or dense fibrous scars in the lung were welcomed as a sign of healing. The attainment of a sputum negative state was essential as an indication of inactivity of the disease and the removal of infection to possible contacts.

There were a number of ways in which surgery attempted healing of the lung in post-primary TB by reducing the lung volume.

1 Elevation of the diaphragm on the affected side. This was achieved by crushing the phrenic nerve under local anesthesia.

2 Partial collapse of the diseased lung. This could be achieved using several means a. Induced pneumothorax whereby air was introduced in the pleural space (see extract at beginning of chapter) b. Thoracoplasty that involved the removal of some of the uppermost ribs of the chest wall c. Plombage that consisted of the pleural cavity being packed with space-occupying materials, including melted paraffin and plastic packing. Where cavities persisted they could be closed by the technique of apicolysis, which involved the indentation of the lung over the cavity until it was collapsed and then over-sewing the lung to maintain the collapse.

In extensive lung disease, particularly where empyema had destroyed one lung and adjacent pleura, a very radical operation consisted of removing all ribs to leave only skin and muscles attached to the scapula were left to be placed against the rigid mediastinum. Temple describes this operation as being highly successful when carried out radically and long survival was the rule; however, "the patient had the appearance of being chopped in half" [29]. Temple who was working just after WWII, chiefly with sputum-negative patients, gives his own surgical cases a survival of 88% compared with the expected survival of sputum-positive cases of 50%. Early deaths and late deaths after surgery were both similar at around 4%.

Rehabilitation of Patients
During WWII, the debate and supply of facilities for rehabilitation continued. The idea had been to set up whole villages where sputum smear-negative patients could be gradually upgraded in exercise, including gentle manual labor. These came to be referred to as settlements: so-called patient workers who were able to benefit following the Ministry of Labor scheme that developed from the Disabled Persons' Employment Act of 1944 [30]. Such schemes could be pre-paid for up to 2 years and in exceptional circumstance 3 years. Papworth on the Western outskirts of London was one place so designated. The problem was that these village communities were very expensive to set up. If there were too few sanatorium places for the patients who needed them because of expense, there were certainly far too few places for rehabilitation. Plans to increase these were effectively ended by the advent of chemotherapy soon after the war [31]. Heaf points out that 42% of sanatoria that he knew of had established occupational therapy units but regretted that only 3 of these could give the patient work that simulated industrial conditions [32].

Bacillus Calmette Guérin
Scandinavian countries spearheaded the BCG campaign so that by 1948 some ten million individuals across the world had been vaccinated. The UK had long stood in a "posture of tepid approval," so that it was not until 1950 that BCG was submitted to careful statistical survey [33]. BCG played no part in TB control in WWII.

Chemotherapy for TB
Sulfonamides, which had become widely available in the 1930s, were used to treat TB during the WWII years. Gold therapy was also employed, but on the decline. Cod liver oil and calcium preparations were also in vogue but there was no evidence of any efficacy. It was not until the months immediately following the war that the British Medical Research Council began to set up proper clinical trials of streptomycin and then para-aminosalicylic acid plus streptomycin [34].

Relationship of TB to Social Class
There has always been a close association between social class and TB. Cheeseman in 1941 showed that the association continued in the war years [35]. Whereas the Standardized Mortality Ratio for respiratory TB was 61 for males and 52 for married females aged 20–65 years in social class I; the corresponding figures for social class II were 70 and 67; for social class III 100 and 99; for social class IV 104 and 106; and for social class V 125 and 132, respectively: a twofold difference between the highest and lowest social classes.

Occupation and TB
It has long been known that occupations that exposed workers to the dust of free silica (SiO_2) had extremely high rates of TB. Tin and copper mine workers had the highest risk of disease, with a Standard Mortality Ratio (SMR) of over 800. Sandblasters, other metallic mine workers, and slate workers also had very high ratios such as 750, 533, and 340, respectively. More surprisingly, perhaps hatters (218), barmen (212), boot and shoe manufacturers (188), and waiters (178) also had high SMRs. The reason for some of these occupations having a high risk is not clear but knowledge of the higher risk in these occupations provided data leading to better directed screening to detect cases before they became clinically apparent and, just as important, infectious. In contrast, coal miners in general had a lower SMR (78) showing that coal by itself was not a risk factor. However, within the coal mining industry those workers responsible for tunneling into the rock strata on either side of the coal seam were at higher risk because of exposure to silicon.

Screening of Occupationally at Risk Workers
Screening of those at risk from occupational factors (see above) across the country were 3.6 cases per 1,000 of active disease varying from 3.1 to 4.4 across several surveys. One specific area of risk was the boot and shoe trade in the country of Northamptonshire, which showed 5.7/1,000 active cases [36].

Food and TB
Good nutrition was believed to protect against TB just as good nutrition was deemed to be an essential part of therapy. A great deal of research went into the relationship between food and TB. Countries that suffered the greatest extent from nutritional deprivation during the war, such as Germany and Poland, were shown to have much higher rates of disease than others in which nutrition was better

sustained, such as the UK; Clarke showed that among the national populations of Europe, there was an inverse association between death rates from TB and intake of animal protein, although he does not provide statistical analyses to validate his conclusions [37]. Certain foods were deemed to be protective against TB and TB patients were to be encouraged to consume them [22]. These included bread, margarine, sugar, potatoes, meat, eggs, vegetables, and fruit. Milk was very important as were vitamin and calcium supplements.

Medical Student and Post-Graduate Teaching
Concern was expressed that with the chaos of war, teaching about TB might become neglected. TB officers were asked to ensure that TB was included in the undergraduate curriculum in the areas they were responsible for. This might include the use of willing volunteer patients to demonstrate symptoms and signs. Post-graduate courses were arranged by the Joint TB Council [27].

Other Environmental Factors Associated with TB
Physical overstrain among factory workers in heavy industry was said to be a cause of the increase in TB in Glasgow in 1941 [38]. No such increase occurred in the professional or business classes. Whereas only 20% of the commercial classes exceeded the recommended hours of work, among those working over the recommended hours, TB morbidity rose to 40% in medium work industries and 67% in heavy industries.

Working in industry was also believed to be a factor for the increase in TB in women in Northern Ireland from 1938–1947. Rates in women were much higher in Londonderry than Belfast, which employed more women in industry.

Overcrowding: In 1943, a survey of 1,472 pulmonary TB patients in Belfast, Northern Ireland showed that only 330 had a separate bedroom. Not until 1946 was it proposed to provide free sleeping areas [39]. Similar statistics are not available for the other parts of the UK at this time, so comparisons are difficult but clearly conditions for the containment of TB were difficult.

Late Result of the War
One curious fact about mortality from TB was that in the years immediately after WWII there was a sudden and unexpected increase in deaths from TB in men over the age of 64 years. This phenomenon occurred in areas as far afield as upstate New York and Western Europe, including England and Wales [40]. It was believed to be due to the extra strain incurred by men in their 50s from wartime service whether in military forces or in industry. That said, the phenomenon must await further elucidation.

Conclusions

Though it was feared that the UK would experience an increase in TB as a result of WWII, the outcome was better than had been expected. After an initial upsurge in cases and mortality in the first 2 years of the war, rates for both measurements declined such that by 1944 the death rates were 58/100,000 compared with 60/100,000 for 1939. Figures from Poland saw mortality increase from 155/100,000 to 500, Yugoslavia from 95/100,000 to 263, and Austria from 109/100,000 to 257 [26]. Appreciable benefits from the war were a better co-ordinated health service that led to the eventual formation of the National Health Service. Screening for new cases of TB became integral to the control of the disease and gave the medical and nursing professions a special responsibility in becoming proactive in the selection of individuals to be screened.

Ireland

Whilst there were many similar influences in Ireland that affected the TB epidemic around the time of WWI and WWII, there were many differing factors both geographic and political. Mortality rates from TB in Ireland continued to exceed that of England and Wales, and Scotland well into the early 20th century.

Ireland was partitioned in 1922 with Northern Ireland and Eire becoming separate countries. As such Eire remained neutral politically during WWII, although approximately 50,000 young Irish men volunteered to join the British army. Despite Irish neutrality, there were some common war-related factors that impacted the general health of the state, such as food and coal rationing. Although some suggest that food rationing in particular may actually have led to a fairer, more uniform supply of food to the poorest in society.

Industrialization
The early 1900s saw the age of industrialization, with Ireland being no exception to this. The shift away from the majority of young people pursuing mainly rural occupations such as farming saw a change in demographics in the population with many emigrating to more urban areas, particularly to the North East of the country (e.g., Belfast) in the early 1900s.

This shift continued in the 20th century and after the partitioning of the country, also saw an increase in emigration rates of young people out of Ireland, particularly to the industrialized cities of England.

Agricultural production also suffered as raw materials and other imports, such as fertilizers, fell in the war years as they heavily relied on importation via British ships.

During and around WWII industrial production inevitably fell, leading to a fall in average income as a consequence and this continued for some time after the war years. The average working wage failed to keep up with the rate of inflation. As poverty levels increased in Ireland this had an adverse effect on the health status of this group of the population in particular, leading to increasing numbers of TB notifications and mortality rates during the early 1940s [41]. As notification rates climbed, this observation led to a number of vital and radical reforms in Ireland's health policy to tackle the increasing problem of TB.

Health Policy Reforms
In the 1940s, poverty, social deprivation and poor, overcrowded living conditions, compounded by the mass emigration to urban areas, were accepted as major contributing factors to both the transmission of TB and a poor prognosis once it had been contracted.

Using Dublin as an example, Counihan and Dillon's 1943 study corroborated that unemployment and urbanization, in particular, were fundamentally responsible for the increasing TB death rates, or "TBR". They surmised that Ireland's position (with regard to TBR) had "disimproved markedly in recent years." Urbanization and mass emigration, particularly to Dublin, was one of the main causes and main environmental factors leading to this observation [42].

In 1942, the Rockefeller foundation commissioned Dr. Daniel O'Brien to further evaluate the extent of social deprivation in Ireland at the time [43]. His report confirmed what was expected: that social deprivation was rife and still at an unacceptable level.

It was proposed that the government should be held responsible and should come up with a solution for such inadequacies in social and also medical care. Changes were called to address inequalities in the access to health care. The poorest and most vulnerable members of society should be able to receive TB treatment regardless of whether or not they could pay for it themselves. The reforms that were occurring in England – which led to the establishment of the welfare state and ultimately the National Health Service –undoubtedly impacted the changes that were occurring in Ireland. Such drastic changes in health care provision in England put pressure on those in Ireland to similarly address the issue of unequal access to health care [24].

The "Anti TB League" and Subsequent Policy Reforms
No discussion on the reforms in TB provision and policy would be complete without discussing the contribution of the "Anti TB League." Founded in 1942, it consisted of medical professionals, and later, politicians involved or interested in TB and its impact on the population. Their work highlighted TB as a national problem, which in turn needed a coordinated, national attention if a workable solution was to be found and implemented. Improvement in medical and social care with government support was central to their approach as well as raising public awareness.

In the years that followed, a number of significant reforms took place. Groups such as the Anti TB League and growing public dissatisfaction with the situation encouraged change, although at a slower pace than many would have liked or was judged to be acceptable by many.

These included the 1945 Sanatoria Act that outlined plans to

Make further and better provision for the establishment of sanatoria for the treatment of persons suffering from TB and to make provision for matters incidental to or connected with such establishment.

As a result of this Act, 3 sanatoria were planned to be built in Dublin, Cork, and Galway. Furthermore, in 1945 the Public Health Bill was drawn. However, this was not wholly embraced as it was felt to be overly pejorative to TB sufferers, portraying them as "dangerous and in need of control." This was revised more sympathetically in the Bills' restructuring in 1947.

Despite these efforts, there were still significant shortfalls in the number of sanatoria beds available in Ireland. In 1943, there were fewer than 3,000, this had only risen to 3,701 by 1948 [44].

By the 1940s, the Irish public was becoming more vocal about the perceived shortfalls in TB care. Issues included the lack of sanatoria beds and access to medical treatment, but also the services in place for the care of TB survivors. This excerpt from a letter to the *Daily Mail* in July 1944 entitled *"T.B. – Must They Die."* from Dermot Findlater, member of a merchant family originating from Dublin, summarizes public feeling at the time;

We, the citizens of Eire, want immediate action and not a scheme in a year, 3 years' or 10 years' time when the position will be far worse. If you do nothing you are blameworthy. [45]

He also concluded that TB should become a notifiable disease – which was not the case in Ireland at the time.

The "Post Sanatorium League" was developed in July 1944 with their objective being to improve care and conditions for those suffering from TB. One of their main concerns was that even if TB sufferers received medical treatment and survived the disease, they would financially be destitute and more impoverished than before they became unwell. Multiple reports were produced, campaigning to the government to increase allowances for those affected. One of the most influential figures in the league was Noel Browne. He himself had personal experience of the ravages of TB as many of his family had succumbed to the disease. Browne was particularly scathing of the Irish government, judging their response to the TB epidemic as inadequate. He had experienced the effects of the reforms that were taking place in England and was appalled by the lack of progress being made in Ireland in comparison.

Browne was appointed as Minister of Health in February 1948 and during his time in office, the number of sanatoria beds increased from approximately 3,000 in 1944 to 6,857 in 1951 leading to a drop in the death rate from TB in this time [46].

The Catholic Church in Ireland had an influence on social change and policy reforms during and around WWII. There was tension between groups such as the league (who were pushing for government driven change) and the church that advocated reform.

Medical Advances

In addition to developments leading to a more integrated social policy, medical advances were also pushing forward. For example, in 1944 Theo McWeeny (Chief Medical Inspector for TB) investigated registers of deaths from TB since 1922 [47]. Although he conceded that the data he collected was by no means comprehensive, he noted that of the 350 cases of TB deaths he identified, most of them were presenting late in the disease process. It was, therefore, accepted that the earlier a diagnosis could be made, the better the prognosis was likely to be.

The widespread support for the use of BCG vaccines was promoted in Ireland by Dorothy Price, who became head of the Consultative Medical Committee of TB established in 1948. She had traveled widely, researching the use of the BCG vaccination in Ireland. In her book, *TB in Childhood 1941* she emphasized the importance of early diagnosis of the condition in children, outlining strategies and diagnostic protocols. She also challenged the belief that "TB (was) a benign and self-healing condition." Radiological screening and BCG vaccination were 2 of the cornerstones to her suggested approach to discussing the TB epidemic [48].

Mass BCG vaccination was promoted, and by 1949 the National BCG committee was founded and an increase in vaccination numbers was seen as a result. By 1952, rates surpassed those seen in the UK. Compulsory screening and vaccination for Irish emigrants, though heavily encouraged, was not made compulsory – mainly due to the cost and complexity of instituting that approach.

The introduction of chest X-ray screening also contributed to the push for swifter diagnosis and treatment.

Drug Development

The development of effective chemotherapy agents against tubercle bacilli led to the revolution of TB treatment in Ireland, as it did in England (as discussed earlier).

Streptomycin was available for use in Ireland by 1947; however, its usage was restricted due to concerns regarding the development of drug resistance. Therefore, the use was stringently controlled by the Irish government.

It took until the early 1950–1951 for streptomycin usage to become common in sanatoria, then later para-aminosalicylic acid and isoniazid in combination with streptomycin – triple therapy – leading to the remarkable drop in mortality from TB as seen in other countries where these drugs were available.

Deaths from TB (all forms/all ages) per 1,000 decreased from 1.22 during 1945–1947, then to 0.69 during 1950–1952, and even further to 0.24 by 1957 [49].

Bovine TB

Bovine TB remained a significant problem in Ireland in the 1950s. Whilst the UK had a program of attestation with formally declared "eradicated zones" between which free movement of cattle was permitted compared with movement of cattle between "non-eradicated" zones, which was restricted, this was not the case in Ireland. The eradication scheme in UK had started in 1935 and 50% of the herds had been attested by 1954, although there was obviously significant interruption during the war years. Ireland had to act to preserve cattle trading with the UK and maintain its agricultural output, which had already suffered due to the effects of rationing and the impact WWII had had on importing. This led to the "Bovine TB Eradication Scheme" in September 1954. Full attestation of the country was announced on 19 October 1965. Bovine TB rates fell from 17% in 1954 to 2.8% in 1966 as a consequence [50].

TB in Eire; Conclusion

There were many factors unique to Ireland in its fight against TB. However, common themes such as the introduction of drugs effective against the disease heralded control of the epidemic as in many other countries.

The work of politicians and physicians like Noel Browne and Dorothy Price [46, 48] contributed significantly to the era of social change, improved social conditions, and financial incentives for potential sufferers to come forward and be tested and treated. The realization that TB was indeed a transmissible infection requiring prompt diagnosis, treatment and isolation, but that thrived in areas of poverty and social deprivation promoted a mood of change in the way resources were organized to tackle its spread.

The effect of WWII undoubtedly heightened the sense of urgency to find a solution as notifications and death rates increased. In addition to the major social and medical changes around the war years, the widespread attestation of bovine TB with the main objective to secure continued agricultural trade was another positive step taken by the Irish government that in combination led to highly significant lessening of the TB epidemic.

Final Conclusions

WWII was the last period that a non-scientific approach was used in the management of TB. First vaccination, then chemotherapy, the effectiveness of which were both proven by randomized controlled trials, began reducing TB rates dramatically wherever they were applied. WWII proved to be the furnace from which the effective eradication of TB could begin.

References

1 "The dark circle" Linda Grant. Virago 2016, pp 105–106.
2 Stevenson AC: Public Health in Britain. Brit Med Bull 1947;5:72–75.
3 Registrar General's annual returns. HMSO. Years 1949–1946.
4 D'Arcy Hart P, Payling Wright G: Tuberculosis and Social Conditions in England with Special Reference to Young Adults. London, National Association for the Prevention of Tuberculosis, 1939, pp 1–165.
5 Davies RP, Tocque K, Bellis M, et al: Historical declines in tuberculosis in England and Wales: improving social conditions or natural selection? Int J Tuberc Lung Dis 1999;3:1051–1054.
6 Lönnroth K, Jaramillo E, Williams BG, Dye C, Raviglione M: Drivers of tuberculosis epidemics: the role of risk factors and social determinants. Soc Sci Med 2009;68:2240–2246.
7 Russel WT: The Morbidity of Pulmonary Tuberculosis-Statistical Aspects. Tubercle September 1946, pp 138–145.
8 Ritchie JN: The progress of eradication of Tuberculosis from cattle in Great Britain. Proc Nutr Soc 1945;3:180–185.
9 Wilson GS: Report of the tuberculosis association bovine infection and disease. Lancet 1945;252: 779–780.
10 Couts B: Tuberculin surveys and the tuberculin test. Tubercle 1947;28:42–49.
11 Roberts CA Bernard MC: Tuberculosis: a biosocial study of admissions to a children's sanatorium (1936–1954) in Stannington, Northumberland, England. Tuberculosis 2015;95(suppl 1):S105–S108.
12 Anon: Children's health in war time. Lancet 1948; 251:188–189.
13 Anon: Epidemiological Section. Br Med J 1947;1: 362–363.
14 Anon: Tuberculosis in the armed forces and its, control by BCG vaccination; a report to the research committee of the British Tuberculosis Association. Tubercle 1957;38:249–258.
15 Geddes JE: War conditions and tuberculosis in Birmingham. Med Off 1946;76:149.
16 Ellman P: Twenty years progress at a municipal chest clinic. Med Off 1949;81:59–61.
17 Innes J: Pulmonary tuberculosis in wartime. Med Off 1946;75:61.
18 Anderson RW: Tuberculosis and the war. Med Off 1947;78:47–49.
19 Daniels M, Ridehalgh F, Springett VH, Hall IM, Lewis HK: Tuberculosis in Young Adults, Report on the Prophit Tuberculosis survey 1935–44, HKLewis and Co Ltd. London, 1948.
20 Keers RY: Pulmonary Tuberculosis, A Journey Down the Centuries. London, Balliere Tindall, 1978.
21 Medical Research Council: Report of the Committee on Tuberculosis in War-Time London, H.M.S.O., 1942.
22 Heaf F, Rusby L: A review of the present position of tuberculosis. Tubercle 1940;21(suppl):17–33.
23 Medical Research Council. Mass Miniature Radiography of Civilians. London, H.M.S.O., 1945.
24 Beveridge W: Social Insurance and Allied Services. HMSO, 1942.
25 Holmes Sellors T, Livingstone JL: Modern Practice in Tuberculosis. London, Butterworth and Co Ltd, 1952.
26 Williams H: War Time and after, Requiem for a Great Killer. London, Health Horizon, 1973, pp 90–100.
27 Heaf F, Rusby L: A further review of tuberculosis in wartime. Tubercle 1942;23:107–130.
28 Maxwell J: The Care of Tuberculosis in the Home (ed 2): London, Hodder and Stoughton Ltd, 1947, pp 49–63.
29 Temple LJ: Surgery of Pulmonary Tuberculosis; a Historical Approach; in Davies PDO (ed): Clinical Tuberculosis (ed 2): London, Chapman and Hall, 1998, pp 21–33.
30 Trail RR: The Colony and the Tuberculosis Patient; in Holmes Sellors T, Livingstone JL (eds): Modern Practice in Tuberculosis. London, Butterworth and Co Ltd, 1952, vol 1, pp 191–202.
31 McPhail WM: Rehabilitation; in Holmes Sellors T, Livingstone JL: Modern Practice in Tuberculosis. London, Butterworth and Co Ltd, 1952, vol 1, pp 163–167.
32 Heaf FRG: Present trends in tuberculosis. Ir J Med Sci 1946;252:761–773.
33 Williams H: Calmette's Tame Bacillus in Requiem for a Great Killer Health Horizon, London, 1973, pp 59–63.
34 Hart PD: Chemotherapy of tuberculosis; research during the past 100 years. Br Med J 1946;2:805.
35 Cheeseman EA: Comparison between the direct and indirect occupational risk in mortality from pulmonary tuberculosis. J Hyg (Lond) 1941;41: 463–472.
36 Holmes Sellors T, Livingstone JL: Modern Practice in Tuberculosis. London, Butterworth and Co. Ltd., 1952;1:223.
37 Clarke RB: Food and Tuberculosis. Causes and Prevention of Tuberculosis. Livingstone, 1952, pp 91–132.
38 Laidlaw S, Macfarlane D: Factors influencing the increased incidence of phthisis in Glasgow. Br Med J 1942;2:63.
39 Clarke RB: Other Environmental Factors Causes and Prevention of Tuberculosis Livingstone, 1952, pp 133–157.
40 Monk Mary A: Increase in tuberculosis mortality in Elderly men from1940 to 1950. Am J Public Health 1958;48:1020–1030.
41 Deeny J: Tuberculosis in Ireland. The National Tuberculosis Survey. Dublin, 1954.

42 Counihan JE, Dillon TWT: Irish tuberculosis
death rates: a statistical study of their reliability,
with some socio-economic correlations. J Stat Soc
Inq Soc Ireland 1943;17:169–188.

43 Rockefeller Foundation RF 1.1 Ireland 403, Box 1
Folder 2. Daniel P. O'Brien, Report on Conditions
In Ireland 1942, Chapter 8 on Health Conditions
in Ireland, 3.

44 Charles O'Connor, The Fight Against T.B. in Ireland in the 1940. Charles O'Connor, 1994.

45 Findlater. The Story of a Dublin merchant family
1774–2001, Chapter 12 A. Findlater, 2013.

46 Captain of all these men of death. The History of
Tuberculosis in Nineteenth and Twentieth Century Ireland. Greta Jones, 2001.

47 National archives of Ireland (NAI), Department of
local government and public health 1942
D112/38.)

48 Price D: Tuberculosis in Childhood. Williams and
Wilkins Company, 1941.

49 Report on Vital statistics for Ireland 1957. page
xxiv table XVII.

50 Watchorn RC: Bovine Tuberculosis Eradication
Scheme 1954–1965, 1965.

Peter D.O. Davies
Liverpool Heart and Chest Hospital
Thomas Drive
Liverpool, L14 3PE (UK)
E-Mail Peter.davies@lhch.nhs.uk

Murray JF, Loddenkemper R (eds): Tuberculosis and War. Lessons Learned from World War II.
Prog Respir Res. Basel, Karger, 2018, vol 43, pp 116–123 (DOI: 10.1159/000481479)

Tuberculosis in France before, during, and after World War II

Jacques Grosset[a] · Arnaud Trébucq[b]

[a]Professor Emeritus, Johns Hopkins University, Baltimore, MD, USA; [b]International Union Against Tuberculosis and Lung Diseases, Paris, France

Abstract

Tuberculosis (TB) was highly endemic in France at the beginning of the 20th century, with a TB death rate of 250/100,000 at the end of World War I (WWI). TB control progressed considerably between WWI and WWII. Due to a great political involvement, implicating all the different layers of the population, and the support of the "Rockefeller mission to France," the mortality declined to 150/100,000 just before WWII. It increased in 1941 (plus 11%) and stayed high in 1942–1943. Different factors are closely interlinked: (1) huge movements of population, several million people tried to escape the German invasion, and hundreds of thousands of people were sent to Germany for the STO (Compulsory Work Service) or incarcerated in jails and concentration camps; (2) extremely severe food shortages in large or medium-sized cities; (3) negative impact on health services, resulting in lack of available beds in the sanatoria. There were more fatal cases in 1941 than in 1938, not because there were more new patients but because they were affected with more malignant forms of TB. However, as early as 1944, mortality from TB declined to 121/100,000, and again in 1945 (102/100,000), and decreased dramatically in the following years with antibiotic therapy.   © 2018 S. Karger AG, Basel

Tuberculosis in France on the Eve of World War II

Tuberculosis (TB) was highly endemic in France around the time of World War I (WWI). The severity of the epidemic is illustrated by the fact that an estimated 150,000 French soldiers were discharged from military service up to about the middle of 1917, because of active TB disease [1].

To curb the spread of TB throughout France, TB control progressed considerably between the 2 World Wars. Former Prime Minister Léon Bourgeois (1851–1925) played an important role in the development of TB control in France. First President of the "Comité national de défense contre la tuberculose," he was both founder and commander of the anti-TB dispensaries. For his constant promotion of solidarity and involvement in conflict resolution, Bourgeois was awarded the Nobel Peace prize in 1920. During WWI, a first law (1916), reinforced by a second (1919), refined the anti-TB dispensaries. The "Rockefeller mission to France" which was launched in 1919, was also key in pioneering widespread anti-TB campaigns based on 3 principles: forming mobile health education teams, creating anti-TB dispensaries, and training health workers, particularly "visiting nurses" [1]. The results were spectacular. There were 40 anti-TB dispensaries in 1916 and 920 in 1939, covering each of the 90 French departments [2]. The role of these dispensaries was to organize case finding, prophylaxis, and social support for TB patients and their families. They were generally run by charity organizations, and were not very technical due to a lack of medical professionals: in 1939, only 77 medical doctors were working full time in the 920 dispensaries. Similarly, the number of sanatoria increased considerably. In 1923, when the Rockefeller mission completed its mission there were 72 public sanatoria for pulmonary TB, offering 9,910 beds.

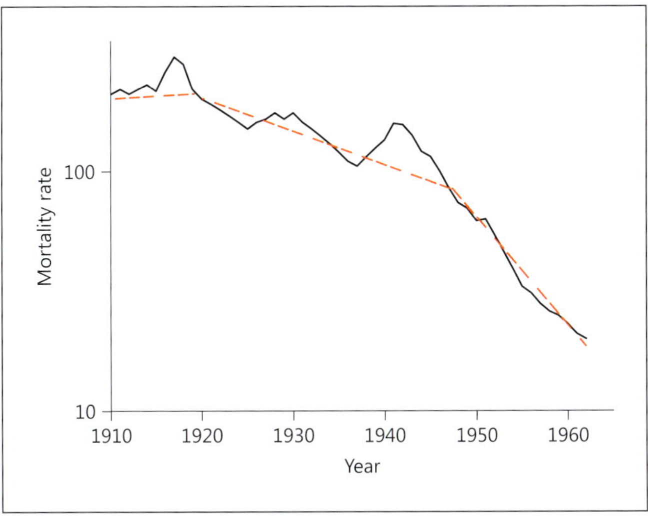

Fig. 1. Mortality from all forms of tuberculosis per 100,000 population in France, 1910–1965. Institut National d'Hygiène, with permission.

In 1925, the first campaign to create and sell TB stamps was organized to attract funds for TB control and – above all – diffusion of educational messages. Each year, a new message concerning hygiene or prophylaxis against TB was chosen. The President of the Republic would open the national campaign while the Prefect (a high authority in the administration) would oversee each department charged with selling the stamps and promoting the educational message. These campaigns were very popular nationwide, with massive involvement of school children. These stamp campaigns were cancelled during the war, but resumed again in 1945.

BCG vaccination was beginning to be used in 1921 [3], however, coverage remained insignificant until the end of World War II (WWII).

Between the 2 world wars, the sanatorium network was extended, and each department had to have at least one sanatorium or a signed agreement with another department to use beds according to their needs (Law Honorat, September 1919). The number of available beds for pulmonary TB increased with time: from 9,910 in 1923 to 19,490 in 1929 and 25,166 in 1939. In 1939, also, there were 11,243 beds in 58 sanatoria for extra-pulmonary TB and 10,418 beds in general hospitals reserved for TB patients, bringing to 46,827 the total number of hospital beds devoted to TB in 1939 [2, 4]. There were 179 sanatoria at this time, 82 public institutions dealing with 59% of the total available number of TB beds, 30 private non-profit institutions associated with the public service and running 23% of the beds, and 67 in the private sector accounting for 18% of the beds. In addition,

there were 117 preventoriums in 1939, run in a similar manner as sanatoria, but welcoming only patients with a mild non-infectious TB disease. Aeriums were institutions that were not specifically dedicated to TB, but which took care of children exposed to TB who needed to be distanced from infectious source(s).

All of the above efforts likely contributed to the decline of the TB epidemic in France. However, in the first half of the 20th century, national data on TB morbidity are rare and much less reliable than those on mortality. The first law on mandatory notification of epidemic illness in France dates back to 1882, but did not include TB. Notification of TB cases was made compulsory only in 1964. Before this date, only estimations are available.

To summarize, the average TB death rate of 250/100,000 at the end of WWI declined to around 150/100,000 just before WWII (Fig. 1) [5]. The peak of TB mortality was estimated to be about 250/100,000 in males between 35–55 years of age and 150/100,000 in females between 20–30 years of age in 1936 [6]. The average TB death rate was associated with large regional variations. In 1938, the TB mortality rate was still superior to 200/100,000 in the city of Paris (specifically, the Seine department), and Brittany and Northern regions, whereas it was between 150/100,000 and 199/100,000 in the Normandy and Alps regions [7]. In a restricted number of departments, mainly in the South-West of France, the death rate was less than 100/100,000.

As the incidence of TB disease was assumed to be double that of TB mortality, it may be considered that on average the incidence of TB in France was around 300/100,000 population in France on the eve of WWII.

TB in France during WWII

Living Conditions

After the fall of the French army in June 1940, the German occupation army divided the country into 2 zones: a free or unoccupied zone "known as Vichy France," because the administrative government was located in the city of Vichy, and an occupied zone (Fig. 2). The division lasted until November 1942 at the time of the Allies' invasion of North Africa, then the Germans occupied the whole country. These events worsened the living conditions in France during the 1940 German invasion and subsequent occupation, and indirectly may have contributed to the early rise in TB [8].

First, there were numerous movements of population. In September–October 1939, many people from the Eastern

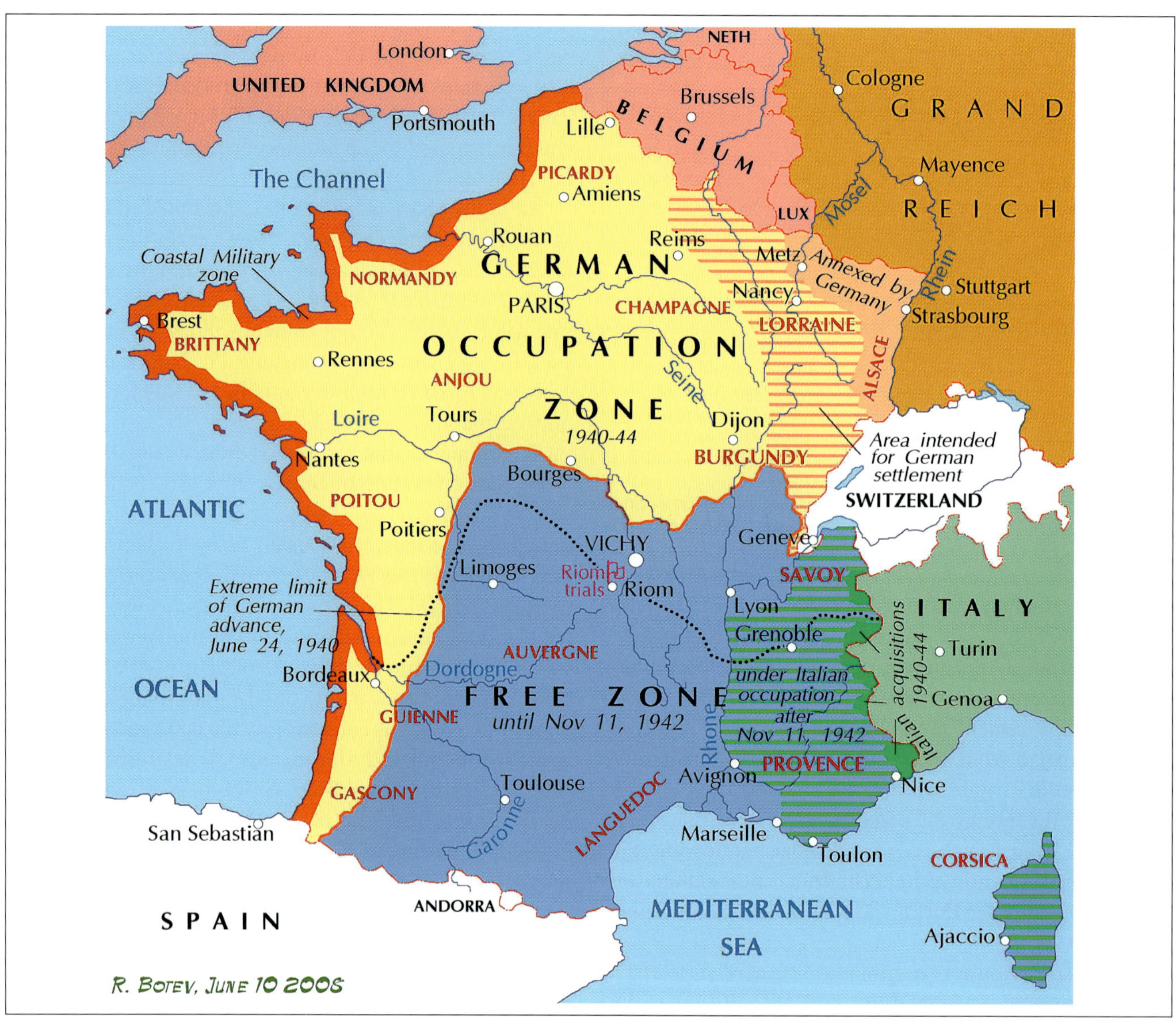

Fig. 2. France occupied by Axis powers, 1940–1944 [17], with permission.

departments of Alsace and Lorraine, close to German territory and historically disputed between France and Germany, were displaced to the West-Central districts of France. In June 1940, several million people from French Northern departments plus those from Belgium, Luxembourg, and even Holland fled South of the Loire River to escape the invasion by German troops. During the occupation of France, between June 1940 and the fall of 1944, hundreds of thousands of people were incarcerated in jails and concentration camps. The STO (Compulsory Work Service) was created under laws and regulations of Vichy France, but was used by Nazi Germany to compensate for its loss of manpower as it conscripted more and more soldiers for the Eastern Front. The German government promised that for every 3 French workers it sent to Germany, it would release one French prisoner of war (POW). Those requisitioned under the STO were accommodated in work camps on German soil. A total of 600,000–650,000 French workers were sent to Germany between June 1942 and July 1944. France was the third largest forced labor provider, after the USSR and Poland, and it was also the country that provided the largest number of skilled workers. In addition 250,000 POWs had to work for the Reich from 1943 onwards, having been "transformed," voluntarily or involuntarily, into civilian workers; during

WWII, French prisoners of war were primarily soldiers from France and its colonial empire who had been captured by Nazi Germany. Although no precise data exist, the number of French soldiers captured during the Battle of France between May and June 1940 is generally estimated to be close to 1.8 million, equivalent to around 10% of the total adult male population of France at the time. After a brief period of captivity in France, most of the prisoners were deported to Germany where they were incarcerated according to rank either in *Stalag* (for non-commissioned personnel) or *Oflag* (for officers) prison camps; not long afterward, the vast majority of Stalag prisoners were transferred to work details *(Kommandos)* working in German agriculture or industry. Colonial prisoners, however, remained in camps in France where living conditions were atrocious owing to Nazi racial ideologies.

Second, during the occupation of France, the food rationing was particularly onerous. The occupied country had to pay more than 20 million Reichmark/day for the 300,000-man German occupational army. Also, the Germans established an artificial exchange rate of 20 francs per Reichmark, which resulted in endemic food shortages and thus malnutrition, especially in young, elderly, and poor persons. Supply problems in stores led to government-created food charts and tickets that could be exchanged for bread, meat, butter, and cooking oil. Manual workers were given more food than the white-collar workers due to the more labor intensive-work that manual workers were forced to do. People living in the country were often better off than those in cities, because they were able to supplement their rations with food from their farms, or with game from hunting. For example, in certain rural areas, such as Normandy, Brittany, and South-Western France, the supply of food was ample. By contrast, in large or medium-sized cities, especially in Paris, Lyon, and other industrial areas, the food shortage was particularly severe. A similar situation prevailed in the South-East of France. Of course, this was associated with a thriving black market. On the positive side, it should be emphasized that patients in sanatoria were allocated a special, more favorable diet (arrêté of 11 December 1940 and circulaires of 19 and 28 October 1942). The circulaire of 19 March 1942 allocated to TB patients in sanatorium the food chart T (for Travailleur/manual worker), allowing them a daily supplement of proteins and lipids. Exceptions included psychiatric patients, who received very little food, and TB was estimated to be the cause of death of 42% of these victims in 1942 [9].

Third, the Nazi occupation had a major negative impact on living accommodations and equipment. Some sanatoria

Table 1. Death rates from all forms of tuberculosis in France from 1938 to 1945, data from [7–9]

Year	Number of departments	Number of deaths	Rate per 100,000	Related to 1938 data, %
1938	90	60,016	143	–
1940	87	53,320	not evaluated	–
1941	87	59,972	158	+10.5
1942	87	57,962	156	+9
1943*	86	53,483	141	–1.3
1944*	82	43,879	121	–15
1945*	86	40,398	106	–26

* Imprecise data (±10%).

were converted into hospitals for the German troops and much delicate and other instrumental equipment deteriorated and could not be replaced. In 1943, due to the war, 13 sanatoria were officially requisitioned for purposes other than TB, occupying 3,889 beds previously dedicated to TB (15% of the beds). Difficulties in maintaining technical equipment (X-ray machines, microscopes, etc.), a lack of basic supplies, such as bed linen and possibility of replacing broken furniture, etc. led to new TB patients being turned away from sanatoria. For example, in the Department du Nord, where all repatriated POWs were systematically screened by radioscopy, only 37% of the active TB cases detected were offered a place in a sanatorium due to a lack of available beds [10].

The TB Epidemic

TB Death Rates (Mortality)

Available information on the evolution of TB death rates in France during WWII is given in Table 1 [7, 8, 11]. No national data are available for the year 1940. For the year 1941, following the occupation of France by German troops and the disturbances related to this event, there was a 10% increase in TB death rates compared to the 1938 death rate. In 1942, the increase continued to remain around 9% but in the following year (1943), there did not seem to be an appreciable difference between the 1938 mortality figure (143/100,000) and 1943 figure (141/100,000). In 1944, the decline in death rate that had been suspected in 1943 turned out to be spectacular at 121/100,000 (43,879 cases), that is, a 15% reduction compared to the 1938 data. This remarkable decline was confirmed in 1945 when the death rate was further reduced to 106/100,000.

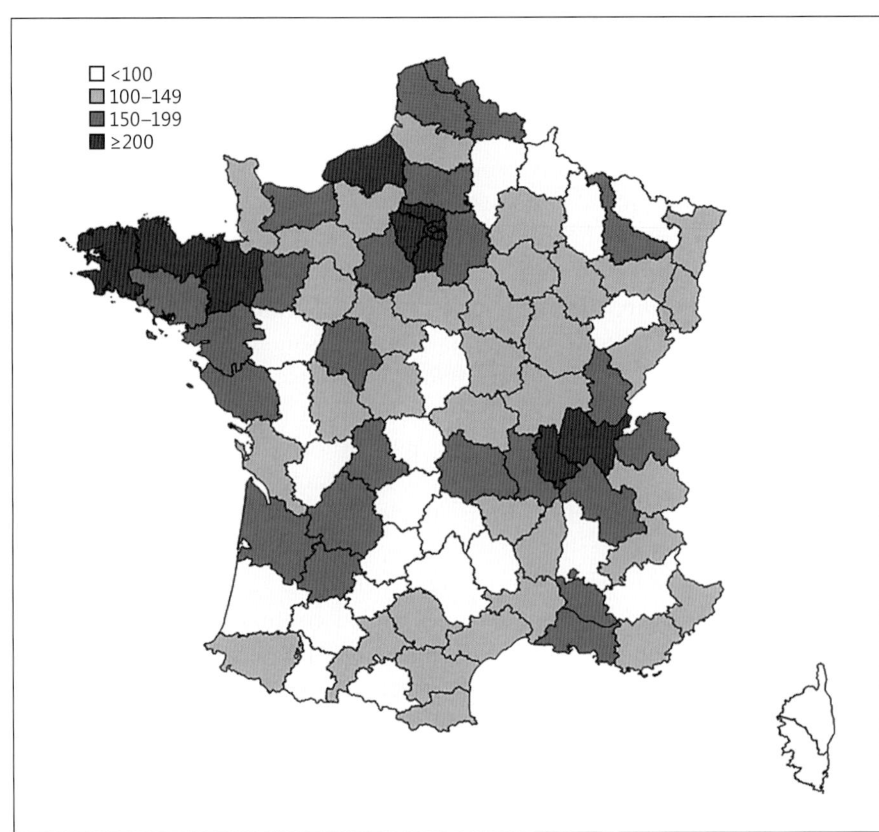

Fig. 3. Death rate from all forms of tuberculosis per 100,000 population, by department, France, 1941 [7].

Age and Sex Analysis of Death Rates

Before WWII, the peak TB mortality lay between 40 and 44 years of age in men and reached more than 250/100,000, whereas it was 150/100,000 in women between 20 and 24 years of age [6]. The rise in TB deaths during the years 1940–1942 was predominantly in men, but there was a slight rise in the female mortality in the years 1939–1941. In males, the initial large increase involved all ages and was followed by a subsequent drop to well below the 1935 rates. It was particularly marked in the 30–50-year age group. Among children below 5 years of age, the death rate of TB declined by almost 55% between 1925 and 1936, but increased by 65% between 1936 and 1941 [7]. After 1943, a noteworthy feature is the remarkable subsequent drop in TB mortality in France that occurred in all age groups except young children and old people.

Regional Differences in Death Rates

There were significant regional variations in the TB death rates in France during the war (Fig. 3). For example, in the *Seine department* (Table 2) a 34.4% increase in the TB death rate compared to the 1938 rate occurred in 1941, which was followed by a 15.5% more modest in-

Table 2. Death rates from all forms of tuberculosis in the Seine department from 1938 to 1945, data from [7]

Year	Cases of tuberculosis		Related to 1938, %
	number	rate	
1938	8 650	174	–
1939	7 934	172	–
1940	7 461	176	–
1941	9 658	234	+34.4
1942	8 224	201	+15.5
1943	7 322	179	+2.9
1944	6 056	149	–14.3
1945	5 424	122	–30

crease in the year 1942. Then in 1943 the increase was almost nil (+2.9%), whereas there were declines of minus 14.3% and minus 30% in the years 1944 and 1945, respectively. Despite the relative imprecision of these data, it is surprising that the 1944 TB death rate was less than that of 1938.

Other Regions of France. Quite different outcomes were observed in other regions of France. In 17 departments, the

Table 3. Differing death rates from all forms of tuberculosis in 4 French departments from 1938 to 1945, data from [7]

Year	Bouches du Rhône		Var		Finistère		Côtes-du-Nord	
	rate	related to 1938, %	rate	related to 1938, %	rate	related to 1938, %	rate	related to 1938, %
1938	133	–	131	–	306	–	257	–
1941	184	+38.3	162	+23.6	297	–3	248	–3.5
1942	212	+59.4	185	+41.2	238	–22.2	208	–19
1943	231	+74.0	221	+68.7	174	–43.1	180	–30
1945	127	–4.5	214	+63.5	147	–52	136	–47

death rate in 1943 was on average 30% higher than in 1938: in Bouches-du-Rhône, which includes Marseilles, there was an 84% increase; in the departments of Var, which includes Toulon, there was a 51% increase; and in Vaucluse, there was an 86% increase. In all these places, the food supply was limited. Conversely, despite high mortality from TB before WWII, the TB death rate decreased from over 250/100,000 in 1938 to less than 200/100,000 in the year 1943 in rural areas, such as in Brittany (Table 3). In this region, like in Normandy and generally speaking the Western part of France, there was ample supply of food from animals and milk, and the mortality rate declined throughout the war. In the South of France, by contrast, especially in the departments of Bouches-du-Rhône, Vaucluse and Var, epidemic TB continued to rise up to 1943 and even later, which can be largely explained by the very severe food shortage.

TB Morbidity

Because of the lack of mandatory reporting and the numerous difficulties related to the war and the Nazi military occupation, it is almost impossible to report precise data on TB morbidity in France during WWII. However, there is complete agreement on the increase of TB death rates during the period 1940–1942. But this poses a question: were these augmented death rates the result either of an increase of the incidence of TB or greater severity of the disease, or both? The data provided by the Leon Bourgeois TB dispensary that took care of TB patients in the 1st, 2nd, and 7th districts of the city of Paris during wartime help to answer this question [7]. Among the smear-positive TB patients taken care of by the dispensary in these 3 Parisian districts, the death rate increased by 15.4% during the period 1941–1944, not because the numbers of new cases were more numerous, but because their lethality increased and they died more rapidly. Indirect data supporting the findings

that morbidity figures went down even in the worst conditions experienced by the city of Paris during the war are provided by 2 studies, the first of TB morbidity among postal workers [12], and the second study of the prevalence of tuberculin infection among students [8]. Among the postal employees, the incidence rate of TB decreased from 263/100,000 in the year 1943 at the acme of WWII to 155/100,000 in the year 1946 just after the end of the WWII. Among the Parisian students, the rate of positive tuberculin skin test results steadily decreased from 56 to 50% for those 19 years of age, 59–56% for those 20 years of age and 62–54% for those 21 years of age between the year 1938 to the year 1943.

The next issue to address is to determine why the TB patients died more rapidly? During WWI (1914–1918), increased numbers of acute forms of TB, especially bronchopneumonia, caseous and miliary TB, were observed. A similar observation was made during WWII [13]. Comparing the 551 patients admitted from March 1935 to November 1935 to the same medical department (La Charité Hospital, Lille) and 531 patients admitted from March 1941 to November 1941, the authors found a similar number of TB patients in both 1935 and in 1941: 143 (26%) and 163 (30%), respectively. The chief point of interest in 1941 was the advanced seriousness of the types of TB disease, which included more acute forms such as 26 (15%) patients with acute TB: 1 miliary, 1 pneumonia, 24 caseous bronchopneumonia (lethal in 4–6 months). The diagnoses in 1935 included mainly milder cases, 10 (7%) patients with acute TB: 1 miliary, 1 caseous pneumonia, and 8 caseous broncho-pneumonia. Moreover, in 1941, there was more rapid bilateral extension in 24 patients versus only 7 in 1935; and more severe extra-pulmonary TB: 10 pleuritis versus 5 in 1935, plus there were 2 additional cases of peritoneal and 2 of bone TB in 1941. The authors considered immune deficiency to be the cause of the higher gravity.

Therefore, it is likely there were more fatal cases in 1941 than in 1935, not because there were more new patients but because they were affected with more malignant forms of the disease. The number of infectious cases – hence, the risk of spreading infection – was diminished because patients died after a few weeks instead of months and years: the early death of an infectious TB patient meant the early suppression of a source of infection!

TB in France after WWII

At the end of WWII, surviving POWs and members of the STO (Compulsory Work Service) were repatriated to France. Because they were all considered to be at high risk of suffering from active TB, a total of 25 medical centers were equipped with 30 X-ray machines for detecting TB among the POWs. Over a period of 2½ months in 1945, a total of 1,402,242 repatriates were X-rayed [14]. In the Bouches-du-Rhone department (specifically, the Marseilles Medical Center), 1.5% of the POWs and 2.5% of the STOs were found to have active pulmonary TB. These figures are similar to those found in the Department of the Nord among the repatriated POWs: they were systematically screened by fluoroscopy, and of 24,693 POWs, 440 (1.8%) had active pulmonary TB [10]. The relatively low prevalence of pulmonary TB among these special population groups surprised the medical teams, but a number of factors had to be taken into account. First, during the course of the war, those POWs and STOs who were diagnosed with TB in Germany and were repatriated to France were not included in the post-war percentages. Second, an unknown proportion of these individuals died from TB during their time away from France and do not appear in the present statistics.

Figures for the political deportees are much higher, and despite the fact that a number of them died before returning to France, or were directly sent to hospital facilities and were not included in the post-war percentages, it was estimated that 12–15% of those who were screened had TB [14].

After WWII, with the arrival of antibiotics, mortality due to TB declined dramatically [15]. Streptomycin and para-aminosalicylic acid (PAS) were both initiated in Europe at the end of 1946 and coverage increased in 1947, but PAS was not widely administered [16]. When isoniazid became available in 1952, standard treatment of TB evolved into combined streptomycin + PAS + isoniazid – or triple therapy – a regimen that lasted well over a decade and began to cure a high percentage of patients with the disease. Its systematic implementation was enhanced by the free-of-charge sanatorium treatment that became the rule for all TB patients following the development of the social security system in France. TB control was high on the agenda of public health authorities, and efficient treatment coupled with very active case-finding through mass radiography campaigns and mandatory BCG vaccination of the children succeeded in reducing the mortality rate by 11% annually, which had already fallen from 106/100,000 in 1945 to around 20/100,000 in 1960, and <1/100,000 in 2015.

Conclusions

Even though the accuracy of the mortality figures during WWII cannot be guaranteed, trends and comparisons among the multiple years are reliable. Furthermore, there has been much conjecture regarding the nature of the wartime increase in TB incidence. Three contributing influences may have played a role. First, additional deaths could include patients who under normal conditions would have lived a little longer. Second, they could also be those patients who would normally have overcome their disease and survived. In both cases, the main factors responsible would be the deterioration of living conditions and lack of adequate nutrition, aggravating the prognosis of patients with established disease. Third, deaths from TB could be among persons who were being infected for the first time in greater numbers than usual, due to increased exposure linked to the huge population movements during that period. In most countries, the increases were no doubt due to a combination of all 3 factors.

If the rise in mortality were due solely to the premature death of patients suffering from the disease, we would expect a steep rise followed by a reciprocal steep or even steeper fall. And it is possible that this would occur where conditions were severe enough to precipitate the death of patients having a poor prognosis, without provoking any great amplification in numbers of patients with the disease. This may partly explain the remarkable fall in TB incidence during the later years of wartime in France, but other factors must also intervene. One possible factor is the fall in consumption of alcohol after the introduction of rationing of wines and spirits in France during WWII. This was followed by a marked fall in morbidity and mortality from diseases attributable to alcohol, a fall not paralleled in any disease other than TB [13].

References

1 Farley J: To Cast Out Disease: A History of the International Health Division of the Rockefeller Foundation, 1913–1951. New York, Oxford University Press, 2004, vol. 47.
2 Poix G, Aujaleu E: La réorganisation de la lutte contre la tuberculose en France. Bull UICTMR 1947;17:249–278.
3 Calmette A, Guérin C, Nègre L, Boquet A: Résultats des essais de prémunition des nouveau-nés contre la tuberculose par le vaccin BCG de 1921 à 1926. Bull Acad Natle Med1926;16:241–242.
4 Voisin C: La tuberculose. Parcours imagé. Tome 2. Regards. Hauts-de-France, (eds) 1995.
5 Beaujeu-Garnier J: La mortalité pour tuberculose en France pendant la guerre. In: L'information géographique 1947;11:28.
6 Henry L, Pressat R: La Situation Démographique; population, 10e année [No. 2], 1955, pp 317–336.
7 Malthete R, Boulanger P: La tuberculose en France depuis 1938. J Société statistique Paris, 1946;87: 243–268.
8 Rist E: Tuberculosis in France during the war. Tubercle 1946;27:13–18.
9 Even R: Les tuberculeux et les restrictions. Rev Tuberc 1941;3–4:215–219.
10 Gernez C, Verhaeghe A, Cartegnie. Bilan statistique, clinique et médico-social de la tuberculose chez les prisonniers de guerre rapatriés du Département du Nord. Paris médical 1945;129: 37–42.
11 Duthoit A, Warembourg H, Bocquet M: Modifications actuelles de la tuberculose de l'adulte et du vieillard. Paris Medical, October 30, 1942, pp 329–332.
12 Lotte A, Coudreau H: Etude de la mortalité tuberculeuse dans une collectivité parisienne (PTT de Paris et de la Seine). Bulletin de l'Institut National d'Hygiène, Tome 6, N°2 avril-juin.
13 Daniels M: Tuberculosis in Europe during and after the second world war. Br Med J 1949;2: 1065–1072.
14 Bourgeois P, Genevrier R, Theil P: Résultats statistiques du dépistage radiologique systématique de la tuberculose effectué au cours du rapatriement des prisonniers de guerre et déportes. Rev Tuberc 1945;9:366–369.
15 Huchon G: Tuberculose. Editions ESTEM, 1994.
16 Gonzales J: Il y a cinquante ans naissait la streptomycine. Hist Des Sci Med 1994;289:239–248.
17 Botev R: Map of Vichy France. Illustration. Wikipedia. https://en.wikipedia.org/wiki/Demarcation_line_(France)#/media/File:Vichy_France_Map.jpg (July 3, 2008).

Jacques Grosset
8 rue Jules Edouard Voisembert
92130 Issy-les-Moulineaux (France)
E-Mail jgrosse4@gmail.com

Murray JF, Loddenkemper R (eds): Tuberculosis and War. Lessons Learned from World War II.
Prog Respir Res. Basel, Karger, 2018, vol 43, p 124 (DOI: 10.1159/000481480)

Tuberculosis in The British Empire before, during, and after World War II

John F. Murray

University of California San Francisco, San Francisco, CA, USA

World War II (WWII) began on 1 September 1939 when Nazi Germany invaded Poland. On 3 September 1939, after a United Kingdom ultimatum directing the Nazis to withdraw their troops was ignored, the United Kingdom declared war against Germany at 11:00 a.m., and then its collaborating partner France declared war at 5:00 p.m.; still later that same day, so did India, Australia, and New Zealand. South Africa declared war on Germany on September 6th and Canada on September 10th. Within 2 weeks, residents living where "The Sun Never Sets on the British Empire" began to empower a military force of nearly 15 million men and woman, which certainly changed the duration and outcome of WWII. After all, the Empire had economic and political control of 25% of the world's population, and 30% of the world's landmass stood strongly behind it.

The British Empire included several crown colonies, protectorates, and India, plus four of 5 independent Dominions, Australia, Canada, South Africa, and New Zealand, which had also declared war on Germany, and Ireland, which chose to remain neutral.

However, the same international clock that ensured that the sun was always shining somewhere in the British Empire and Commonwealth created significant political disagreements and differences of opinion over regional military goals and strategic objectives of newly declared WWII. In addition, competition over hierarchy of control and coordination and deployment of resources may have delayed or thwarted the needed action. Victory over the Axis Powers did not come easy and the cost was high, including the deaths of 150,000 military personnel and over 300,000 civilians.

The British Empire and Commonwealth "defeated, held back or slowed the Axis powers for 3 years," while rapidly creating not only a tremendous fighting machine, but a global economic enterprise that incorporated novel techniques of funding, producing, storing, and distributing material throughout the world. After 7 December 1941, the US became increasingly involved, it took command of several international theatres of war, thereby relieving the Empire forces in other locations, and greatly expanding the size and military might of the joint war effort.

The 2 subchapters – entitled Australia and South Africa – that are included with this brief introduction, illustrate the extremes of the 3 integral factors that control the diagnosis, treatment, and prognosis of tuberculosis (TB): (1) political commitment; (2) an efficacious program; (3) and socioeconomic development of the community. On the one hand, Australia demonstrates that each of these essential components operates at full speed and is staffed with top-notch parliamentary and scientific professionals, all collaborating to reduce TB mortality, case-finding rates, and means of prevention. On the other hand, South Africa continues to provide a wealth of political incompetence and chaos coupled with extreme poverty, poor working conditions, malnutrition, migration, and social disruption. Plus, there has always been fragmentation and lack of co-ordination of health services.

These 2 countries serve as contrasting examples of how to staff and conduct a current anti-TB case-finding, treatment, and prevention program.

Murray JF, Loddenkemper R (eds): Tuberculosis and War. Lessons Learned from World War II.
Prog Respir Res. Basel, Karger, 2018, vol 43, pp 125–129 (DOI: 10.1159/000481593)

Tuberculosis in Australia before, during, and after World War II

Carol Putland

History Department, Flinders University, Adelaide, SA, Australia

Abstract

Australia's history of tuberculosis (TB) before World War II (WWII) was similar to that of many western nations: the overall mortality rate began its decline late in the 19th century. In addition, mortality rates were generally lower than most other nations. Before the late 1940s, public health management of TB rested with each Australian state, making the attack on TB piecemeal and incomplete. The exception was medical repatriation after WWI, when returned tubercular soldiers ultimately received higher pension rates than civilians, which influenced post WWII policy. At the start of WWII, military authorities began screening recruits with miniature X rays. Australia's relatively low TB mortality rate coupled with early screening resulted in battlefield rates that compared favorably with other nations. WWII did not greatly increase TB in Australia, but the social and political changes it wrought shifted health policy dramatically and created a modern national public health campaign against TB. The agenda of post-war reconstruction linked TB prevention with the vision of a just, strong, and prosperous post-war society. The national scheme coincided with the development of efficacious drug therapy, but the wider campaign ensured early detection and largely negated the long-standing tendency to hide the disease.

In October 1945, the Australian Parliament passed legislation creating the first national health campaign to eradicate a disease by committing funds to an anti-TB campaign. This announcement came at a time when the death rate from TB had been declining for decades. At the same time, medical breakthroughs in antibiotics brought the possibility of a long sought after cure closer. This did not reduce long-standing pressure from the medical profession and public health reformers for a prevention campaign, nor did it change the direction the campaign was to take. After years of lobbying by public health physicians, the Commonwealth Labor Government incorporated an anti-TB campaign into its post-war reconstruction policies.

The agenda of post-war reconstruction advanced the national TB policy. By linking TB prevention with the vision of a just, strong, and prosperous post-war society, long standing, but unfulfilled, public health propositions gained potency. This trend had begun before World War II (WWII) as Australia debated how it might improve social welfare policies to avoid a repetition of the hardships of the Great Depression. Then, in the early 1940s, with the outcome of the war still far from certain, policy makers turned optimistically to plan the post-war society. The new post-war social welfare agenda enabled anti-TB campaigners to promote a national prevention scheme within a political context of increasing federal centralism and the ideals of post-war reconstruction.

Tuberculosis before WWII

Australia's history of tuberculosis (TB) before WWII was similar to many western nations in that the overall mortality rate began its decline late in the 19th century [1]. Australia also enjoyed a lower mortality rate than most other nations [2]. Mortality rates presented here are drawn primarily from

Table 1. Five yearly national death rates, all forms of tuberculosis, per 100,000 1891–1970

Year	Per 100,000
1891	111.00
1896	97.80
1901	92.10
1905	80.80
1910	83.00
1915	72.00
1920	68.00
1925	58.00
1930	51.00
1935	42.00
1940	37.00
1946	33.00
1950	20.00
1955	8.00
1960	5.00
1965	3.00
1970	0.20

the official statistics of the Australian Bureau of Census and Statistics, but it must be pointed out that these figures precluded a proportion of the indigenous population. Table 1 shows the steady decline of mortality from all forms of TB from 1891 to 1970. Although these five yearly figures do not reveal nuances and variations in the decline, they demonstrate the steady fall in mortality rates in the decades before WWII, a trend that barely abated during the war years. Official reports did not calculate the yearly mortality values for respiratory TB rates for 1942, 1943, 1945, 1947, and 1949, but the number of deaths rose in 1941 and 1942, fell for the balance of the war years before another rise in 1946 as troops returned home. Thereafter, the decline was continuous.

Before the late 1940s, public health management of TB rested with each Australian state, the federal government being responsible only for quarantine. It was not until 1921 that the national government established its own health department. Even then, it was a small poorly funded department with little or no power. Nevertheless, during the interwar years, a cohort of public health physicians, particularly those employed by the new Commonwealth Department, lobbied for a nationally uniform public health approach to TB, in line with their philosophy of state intervention in matters of health. A fundamental premise was the elevation of preventive medicine.

In 1928, the head of the Commonwealth Division of Tuberculosis and Venereal Disease, Mervyn J. Holmes, investigated each state's TB public health policies. Finding state measures to be inadequate, he produced wide ranging recommendations for nationally consistent measures, but the national government had no power to force such measures on the states and Holmes' report went largely unheeded. Spread as it was across the different states, the attack on TB was piecemeal and incomplete. Nor did Australia adopt the Bacillus Calmette Guérin vaccine as a preventive measure until the end of WWII [3].

One area of TB management that did engage the Commonwealth Government was the treatment of soldiers returning from World War I (WWI) with TB, repatriation being a federal responsibility. The total number of Australian soldiers with TB was fewer than that of European countries but were regarded as a serious post-war repatriation problem. The term repatriation is used in Australia generically to mean reestablishment and rehabilitation of returned military personnel. The Commonwealth Repatriation Department's rather low estimate of 3,000 returned soldiers with TB constituted 32% of cases in the country [4] if the conservative ratio of 3 cases for every death is employed. On their return, tubercular soldiers quickly became self-advocates for special attention in the repatriation system and, in effect, proxy advocates for civilian sufferers, who were more likely to hide their disease than lobby the government for assistance. From 1920 to 1943, tubercular soldiers demanded and gradually received more and more repatriation benefits, notably a higher pension rate than civilians.

TB during the 1930s
During the mid- to late-1930s, public health physicians and some politicians bemoaned the slow progress of public health policy in Australia [5], and TB management was among the areas thought to be neglected. Many doctors believed that their profession had provided the state with all necessary knowledge to manage TB, but their message had not been heeded. Yet, doctors' ability to diagnose and treat the disease remained problematic. The medical profession spoke of treatment, but cure still eluded them. Mortality rates had declined but appeared to be related to fewer new cases than to an improving case-fatality rate.

As the worst years of the Great Depression passed, public health bureaucrats intensified their calls for more comprehensive and uniform TB prevention programs, especially higher pensions. This persistent advocacy for better financial help led the Federal Government to make the invalid pension accessible to more categories of sufferers. Before 1939, only late stage TB victims qualified for an invalid pension, although in reality authorities were applying it more liberally [6]. Even so, this was still less than soldiers' pensions.

Table 2. Age-specific male and female deaths from respiratory tuberculosis 1938–1947

Year	Male, age, years						Female, age, years					
	15–19	20–29	30–39	40–49	50–59	60–69	15–19	20–29	30–39	40–49	50–59	60–69
1938	20 (27)	148 (37)	224 (48)	330 (**70**)	360 (**80**)	258 (**79**)	54 (**73**)	257 (**63**)	242 (**52**)	139 (29)	92 (20)	69 (21)
1939	24 (34)	134 (34)	262 (**54**)	321 (**69**)	396 (**79**)	271 (**80**)	46 (**66**)	264 (**66**)	226 (46)	142 (31)	103 (21)	69 (20)
1940	24 (32)	118 (35)	189 (48)	319 (**71**)	339 (**78**)	223 (**73**)	52 (**68**)	223 (**65**)	206 (**52**)	133 (29)	96 (22)	82 (27)
1941	23 (34)	122 (37)	245 (**53**)	312 (**68**)	384 (**79**)	278 (**76**)	44 (**66**)	206 (**63**)	220 (47)	146 (32)	105 (21)	86 (24)
1942	53 (**55**)	110 (31)	208 (47)	340 (**71**)	390 (**82**)	315 (**76**)	44 (45)	243 (**69**)	236 (**53**)	138 (29)	87 (18)	101 (24)
1943	18 (43)	108 (35)	204 (50)	278 (**67**)	362 (**81**)	298 (**82**)	24 (**57**)	205 (**65**)	207 (50)	138 (33)	83 (19)	64 (18)
1944	17 (39)	110 (36)	178 (50)	266 (**66**)	359 (**83**)	293 (**79**)	27 (**61**)	199 (**64**)	176 (50)	137 (34)	74 (17)	79 (21)
1945	19 (32)	92 (32)	196 (50)	244 (**65**)	347 (**81**)	284 (**81**)	40 (**68**)	192 (**68**)	198 (50)	129 (35)	83 (19)	68 (19)
1946	19 (39)	83 (31)	186 (50)	265 (**68**)	351 (**80**)	303 (**80**)	30 (**61**)	186 (**69**)	188 (50)	127 (32)	88 (20)	75 (20)
1947	6 (16)	87 (38)	153 (46)	272 (**72**)	321 (**78**)	298 (**86**)	32 (**84**)	145 (**62**)	180 (**54**)	105 (28)	93 (22)	50 (14)

Figures in parentheses are percentages. Figures in bold indicate which gender had the higher percentage of deaths in each age group. Compiled from Commonwealth Bureau of Census and Statistics, Demography Bulletins, 1938–1947.

Gender Differences and TB

Of increasing concern in the late 1930s was the higher mortality rate of young women compared with young men. Investigations in the late 1930s revealed a long-standing pattern of disadvantage for young women. A further difference was a steeper decline in male mortality than female mortality and a shift for men to mortality peaks in older age groups than women [7]. The mortality rate of young women was understood but largely ignored until this time. As Alison Bashford pointed out, TB public health policy was seen through the prism of labor and the economy and as such, concentrated on maintaining the health of the male breadwinner [8].

If physicians were aware of the problem, it is pertinent to ask why young women became a greater focus of medical attention at this time. Part of the answer lies with concern about the health of the nation's child bearers in the aftermath of the Depression, first because of Australia's continuing anxiety about increasing the population through a higher birth rate rather than immigration, and second, because maternal mortality finally began to decline in 1937 [9], which drew the medical gaze to other aspects of women's health [10]. Table 2 details the gender differences in age-specific groups from 1938 to 1947, indicating that this trend continued during WWII. The number of male deaths were double that of female deaths, but the pattern for men was higher mortality in older age groups.

Shortly before WWII, a Commonwealth Health Department report stressed two aspects of prevention that was to have an impact on how the post-war campaign was framed. First, the state should provide additional economic support based on findings that families receiving the higher repatriation pension had lower TB incidence rates than those on the invalid pension [11]. Second was the conduct of X-ray surveys of wide sections of the population, particularly in light of the new miniature X-ray apparatus. WWII stalled the campaign but would later assist it as TB found a place on the post-war reconstruction agenda.

TB during WWII

The battlefields of WWII came very close to Australia's northern shores, and the northern city of Darwin endured air raids by Japanese forces in 1942 and 1943, as did other northern towns and bases. Sydney also experienced light shelling from Japanese submarines in 1942, but Australia's home population did not suffer the same privations as citizens in the main theatres of war. Nevertheless, like other nations, inhabitants were drafted into war work at home and subjected to rations and other legal restrictions. Between 1939 and 1945, some 1.5 million men and women enlisted or were drafted into the military, to serve first in Europe and the Middle East, and then in the Pacific.

During WWII, TB lacked the prominence it had had in WWI as the hierarchy of diseases shifted dramatically for Australians. Former medical priorities were overtaken by the demands of managing tropical diseases and the challenges of the hot and humid conditions in the Pacific fields of battle. As Lloyd and Rees noted, TB and shell-shock casualties were replaced with malaria and other tropical diseases [12]. Even so, in 1939 military authorities were aware of the problems TB could present. In 1938, the Australian Military College,

Duntroon, reported active TB among its recruits, which led the army to decide on December 7, 1939 to use the new miniature X-ray technology to screen all recruits. An important consideration in this decision was the cost of medical treatment for tubercular soldiers of the First World War. Exclusion of even a portion of infective cases was seen as a future saving in repatriation costs [13]. TB accounted for 2.87% of rejections, 14th of 19 causes [14], but its significance lay in the fact that it was one of the few air-borne contagions on the rejection list and of course, still a greatly feared disease.

Australia's relatively low mortality rate coupled with early screening resulted in battlefield rates that were generally lower than other nations. Prisoners of the Japanese were most vulnerable because they suffered the greatest privations. Even so, Australian cases were fewer than other nationalities in Japanese POW camps. In Changi, for example, 30 British TB cases arose in the first six months but Australian cases were not detected until 12 months had elapsed. Allied medical officers attempted what treatment they could, specifically artificial pneumothorax, but with little effect because of the conditions in the camps [15].

Unsurprisingly, as the war continued TB cases rose. When sick and injured service personnel returned to Australia, medical services whether military, repatriation or civilian, came under pressure. Major hospitals in the capital cities faced overcrowding and medical expertise was depleted at home as public and private medical officers joined the services, as did nurses. In 1944, most tubercular servicemen and women in all branches of the military were directed to one hospital, the 106th Australian General Hospital at Bonegilla near Albury in Victoria. These patients remained under the care of the military for up to 12 months before discharge. Standard treatments such as pneumothorax were employed. At the end of 1945, a limited amount of streptomycin came into use [16].

On the home front, by 1942, ideas about post-war society gained more attention, and ridding the country of TB became a goal for the Australian post-war world. A Commonwealth Government committee was established to investigate the needs and structure of post-war society and this committee provided a forum for champions of a national campaign against TB. Authors of the Committee report described Australia's attack on the disease as "a reproach to all" those who had not used their knowledge to provide improved facilities, early detection methods, and economic support [17]. The political climate provided an opportunity for anti-TB campaigners to press their case for nationally uniform public health measures and a special pension [18].

In June 1943, State Health Ministers agreed to plan a post-war anti-TB program involving all States and the Commonwealth. In October 1945 and again in August 1946, the Commonwealth passed Tuberculosis Acts, both of which presented administrative and constitutional problems, which were resolved late in 1946 when the Labor Government won a referendum to change the Australian Constitution giving social service powers to the Commonwealth. This allowed the federal government to take control of a special TB allowance. Finally, in 1948 the Commonwealth TB Act 1948 established a national program to fight TB. States would be reimbursed for expenditure on services, facilities, and capital works; the Commonwealth Director-General of Health received powers to establish or take control of hospitals, sanatoria, laboratories, and diagnostic centers; and the Commonwealth would subsidize universities for training and research. Importantly, it provided for direct payment of a TB allowance to sufferers, in addition to other welfare payments [19].

Post WWII Anti-TB Campaign

Before WWII, states had shown little interest in cooperating with each other or the Federal Health Department on TB policy despite the urging of the medical profession dating back to at least 1911. The post-war social and political climate, however, changed dramatically. Between 1949 and 1953, the six Australian States passed enabling legislation allowing them to conduct campaigns against TB and receive Commonwealth reimbursement. This included mass X-ray surveys across the country. A TB allowance for individual sufferers began to be paid on July 13, 1950.

The national program ceased at the end of 1976. The mortality rate for pulmonary TB had declined from 24.8/100,000 in 1949 to 1.1/100,000 in 1976 [20]. This led many commentators to conclude that the post-war campaign had been a success. Fitzgerald, for example, noted of Western Australia that by 1960 most adults had been X-rayed and the goal of controlling and preventing TB in effect had been achieved [21]. Others questioned this certainty. Tyler queried the need for the campaign, suggesting that curative drug therapy accounted for control of the disease rather than the wide scheme of X-ray screening, chest clinics, and sanatoria [22]. Marianna Stylianou [23] pointed to specific inequalities in mortality rates in Victoria, where mortality and morbidity rates remained higher among the indigenous than the non-indigenous population. While we must critically consider the nature of the campaign, given the discovery of drug therapy and the eventual administration of Bacillus Calmette Guérin vaccination, the extensive nature of the anti-TB campaign, particularly mass X-ray and economic support, ensured wide detection of early cases and reduced the long-standing tendency to hide the disease to continue earning a living, or because treatment was protracted.

Conclusion

The doubts expressed about the campaign raise the general question of why some public health campaigns receive support while others flounder. This is not to suggest that any public health campaign about serious health issues is without merit, but as historians of social medicine emphasize, social, economic, and political pressures, as much as morbidity, mortality, and medical science, dictate which diseases generate modern public health movements. Although long discussed, it was the political climate of post-war reconstruction that allowed for a national anti-TB campaign with a preventive imperative in Australia. The campaign was a replication of earlier ideas converted to tangible policy by the injection of federal funds and enthusiasm for post-war reconstruction. The image of TB with its long term invalidism, contagion, and undertones of immorality as a causal factor was the antithesis of the post-war vision of Australia. Post-war reconstruction required a healthy workforce to build the nation and healthy young women for motherhood. In the Australian case, WWII did not greatly exacerbate TB, but the social and political changes it wrought shifted public health policy on the disease dramatically and created a modern and effective public health campaign.

References

1   Cumpston, "Statistical Review of Tuberculosis in Australia". Australasian Medical Congress, 1924, pp 237, 243. Commonwealth Bureau of Census and Statistics, Professional Papers, G.H. Knibbs, The International Nosological Classification, &c., Secular Progress of Pulmonary Tuberculosis and Cancer, Reprinted from the Journal of the Australasian Medical Congress, Sydney, 1911, Sydney, 1913.

2   Australia, Department of Trade and Customs, Committee Concerning Causes of Death and Invalidity in the Commonwealth, Report on Tuberculosis, 19 September, 1916 (J. Mathews, M.P., Chairman), Albert J. Mullett, Government Printer for the State of Victoria, 1916, p 7. Commonwealth Bureau of Census and Statistics, *Official Year Book of the Commonwealth of Australia,* No. 28, 1935, Commonwealth Government Printer, Canberra, p 608.

3   Smith FB, Tuberculosis and bureaucracy. Bacillus Calmette et Guerin: its troubled path to acceptance in Britain and Australia. MJA, September 20, 1993, p 408.

4   MJA, May 1917, p 421.

5   Gaha J: Report of the National Health and Medical Research Council. First Session, 1–3 February 1937. Canberra, Commonwealth Government Printer, Canberra, pp 5–6

6   NAA: A1928/1, 690/13, Memorandum, Commonwealth Director-General of Health to Secretary, Prime Minister's Department, 7 March 1939;Letter, Prime Minister to Tom Playford, Premier of South Australia, 3 May 1939; M.J. Holmes, "Tuberculosis," 19 April, 1940, p 1. NAA: A1928/1, 690/13, Letter, T. Playford, Premier of South Australia, to the Prime Minister, January 10, 1939.

7   Holmes MJ: Tuberculosis in Australia. MJA, November 6, 1937, pp 813–818.

8   Bashford, Alison: "Tuberculosis and Economy: Public Health and Labour in the early Welfare State," Health and History 2002, 4/2, pp 19, 20, 24–25, 28, 29, 32, 34–35, *passim.*

9   Taylor Richard, Lewis, Milton, Powles, John: "The Australian mortality decline: all-cause mortality 1788–1990, Australian and New Zealand Journal of Public Health, 1998, vol 22, No. 1, 27–36, pp 27, 30.

10 McCalman J: "Maternity"; in Graeme Davison, John Hirst, Stuart Macintyre (eds): The Oxford Companion to Australian History. Melbourne, Oxford University Press, 1998, p 416.

11 NAA: AWM 41 [264], M.J. Holmes, Senior Medical Officer, Commonwealth Department of Health, 'Tuberculosis in Australia. Part II. Implications of the Research Work in Australia in Relation to Prevention and Control of Tuberculosis. u.d. circa May, 1940, p 3.

12 Lloyd Clem, Rees, Jacqui: The Last Shilling: A History of Repatriation in Australia, Melbourne University Press, 1994, p 283.

13 Vamplew, Wray, ed: Australians, historical statistics. Broadway, NSW, Fairfax, Syme & Weldon Associates, 1987, p 414.

14 White, Bruce: "Mass Radiography of the Thorax, with Special Reference to its Application to recruits for the Army'. MJA, 1941, p 25.

15 Walker AS: Clinical Problems of War. Canberra, Australian War Memorial, 1952, pp 259, 260.

16 Walker AS: Clinical Problems of War. Canberra, Australian War Memorial, 1952, pp 260–261.

17 Australia, House of Representatives, Debates, 16 March, 1943, pp 1785–1786;17 March, 1943, p 1895.

18 Australia, Parliament, Joint Committee on Social Security (JCSS) 1943, List of Witnesses and Index to Minutes of Evidence from 21st July, 1941 to 2nd June, 1943, Commonwealth Government Printer, Canberra, p 646 (Dr. Calov, witness).

19 Tuberculosis Act 1948 (Cwlth), ss. 5, 5(1), 6, 7, 9.

20 Porter RM, Boag TC: The Australian Tuberculosis Campaign 1948–1976. Melbourne, 1991, p 91.

21 Fitzgerald C: Kissing Can Be Dangerous, The Public Health Campaigns to Prevent and Control Tuberculosis in Western Australia, 1900–1960. Crawley WA, University of Western Australia Press, 2006, p 204.

22 Peter J Tyler: Visualising Tuberculosis – Compulsory Radiography in Australia, 1950–1980, Australian Historical Association 12th Biennial Conference, Newcastle, 5–9 July 2004 pp 3–4. With thanks to the author.

23 Marianna Stylianou, "A Scandal Which Must be Corrected:" Reconsidering the Success of the Australian Tuberculosis Campaign', Health and History, Vol. 11, No. 2, 2009, pp 21–41.

Carol Putland, PhD
History Department, Flinders University
14 Harold Lea Way
Hackham, Adelaide, SA 5163 (Australia)
E-Mail carol.putland@parliament.sa.gov.au and putlaca@tpg.com.au

Murray JF, Loddenkemper R (eds): Tuberculosis and War. Lessons Learned from World War II.
Prog Respir Res. Basel, Karger, 2018, vol 43, pp 130–133 (DOI: 10.1159/000481595)

Tuberculosis in South Africa before, during, and after World War II

Nulda Beyers · Robert Gie

Desmond Tutu TB Centre, Department of Paediatrics and Child Health, Faculty of Medicine and Health Sciences, Stellenbosch University, Cape Town, South Africa

Abstract

Unlike many countries where the trends in tuberculosis (TB) before and after World War II (WWII) can be assumed to be mainly a result of the war, in South Africa there were extreme political and economic changes before, during, and after WWII, making it impossible to separate the influence of these changes from the effects of WWII itself. Before WWII (first wave of TB), early colonization, mainly due to the discovery of diamonds (1867) and gold (1886), resulted in rapid urbanization and migrant labor, which led to huge inequalities among population groups in South Africa. With the onset of WWII (second wave of TB), wartime shortages of manufactured goods became a catalyst for new industries that once again required cheap labor; thousands of Black African families poured into large cities seeking employment. Accordingly, mortality from TB increased. After WWII (third wave of TB), the post-war decline in TB seen in Europe was not seen in South Africa, where there were and still are enormous inequalities in health. A perfect storm developed that currently continues and is now fueled by HIV and MDR-TB.

The factors that were (and still are) responsible for the tuberculosis (TB) epidemic in South Africa were, like in so many other countries, poverty, stressful living, poor working conditions, especially in the mines, poor nutrition, migration, and social disruption. In addition in South Africa, there has always been fragmentation and lack of co-ordination of health services [1]. These conditions originated in the colonial past and have been perpetuated by health policy and legislation and sadly, although legislation has changed, many of these factors are still present today.

Many infectious disease epidemics are aggravated by these conditions, but fortunately many other epidemics like measles and influenza are short-lived (a couple of years), while a TB epidemic lasts a few decades, if not centuries, and the effect of poor TB control at any specific time has a long-term effect. TB in South Africa was not under control at the start of World War II (WWII), and it is therefore not surprising that after the second wave of TB during WWII, TB in South Africa which has now been aggravated by HIV/AIDS, is still not under control.

Unlike many other countries where the trends in TB before and after WWII can be assumed to be mainly as a result of the war, in South Africa there were extreme political and economic changes during this period as well. These political and economic changes affected the health, the health services, and TB trends in South Africa. It is, therefore, impossible to separate the influence of these changes from the effects of WWII, especially as WWII brought an unexpected industrial revolution to South Africa. At the onset of WWII, there was rapid urbanization mainly due to migrant labor in the mines, but housing could not be provided to the rural people streaming to the cities as South Africa's resources were used as South Africa aligned with the allied forces [2].

TB in South Africa Prior to WWII

The First Wave of TB

Since the 1500 and 1600s, South Africa has been a halfway stop between Europe and the East Indies. The effect of early colonization, by especially the Dutch and British, led to huge inequalities in various population groups in South Africa. It is not clear whether TB existed in South Africa before colonization but it is clear that colonization of Southern Africa was responsible for bringing TB to the region, which then spread rapidly among the indigenous populations in South Africa.

South Africa was transformed from a largely agricultural economy to an industrialized economy by the discovery of diamonds (1867) and gold (1886). Massive foreign investment flowed into South Africa with the lure being the generation of wealth through mining [3]. These discoveries resulted in an influx of miners from especially Europe. To successfully mine the diamonds and gold, required a large but cheap labor force and resulted in uncontrolled influx, of especially Black African laborers, which in turn led to rapid urbanization and informal living conditions or squatter communities. These Black Africans became the mainstay of social, economic, and political development in South Africa. The Black African miners lived in squalor, and it was reported that the discriminatory practices produced in Kimberley (the home of the diamond mining) resulted in the highest level of incarceration and lowest living standards for urban Black people in the Cape Colony. This resulted in the first wave of TB in South Africa.

Europeans in the late 18th century and the early 19th century played an important role in the spread of TB in South Africa. They were attracted to South Africa by the promise of a climatic cure for TB. This led to the "selective immigration of TB" [1] and by 1902 half the Europeans dying in South Africa were immigrants [4]. The epidemic spread rapidly within the mixed race population (Coloreds) of the Western Cape who had death rates that were 4-fold those in Britain, ranging from 510 to 1,430/100,000.

As a result of urbanization, the urban population in South Africa grew rapidly as illustrated by the growth in Black African miners. In 1889, there were 10,000 miners, which had grown to 200,000 by 1910 and 400,000 by 1940 [3]. The influx of Black miners of course led to their families also coming to the cities and between 1921 and 1936 the urban Black African population grew by 94% [3]. By the late 1920s, it is estimated that the 90% of Black Africans were infected with TB. This high rate of infection was due to urbanization, a high turnover of the work force and the forced repatriation of sick miners to their rural homes. Black African miners with TB were managed differently to White miners. White miners were admitted to sanatoria that were supported by the mines while Black miners were hospitalized for a week or 2 before being returned to their rural homes [5]. The situation was further perpetuated by the preventative and curative health services, which were segregated by the 1897 Public Amendment Act. The effect of the TB epidemic on the ruling White population in South Africa, even long before the apartheid government came to power, was twofold. First they were concerned about the effect on the health of the White population. The second concern was that TB would rapidly exhaust the reservoir of cheap Black labor. Between 1920 and 1930s, TB control in South Africa was based on building social barriers between populations but in the late 1930 and 1940s these barriers were swept aside causing a new wave of TB [6].

WWII in South Africa: 1939–1945

With the onset of WWII, wartime shortages of manufactured goods served as a catalyst for new industries to develop. The new industries again required cheap labor, which resulted in thousands of Black African men, women, and children pouring into especially large urban areas to escape rural poverty and to seek employment. The rapid rise in the economic growth resulted in the economy's gross output increasing by approximately 250%. The Black population increased in the major industrial cities by an average of 60% with some cities, like Cape Town, having a 130% increase in the Black African population. The number of Black men in the manufacturing industries increased by 60% [2].

The increase in the urban population was not planned for, and it was the Black African population who bore the brunt of the maldistribution of services. The housing shortage resulted in most Black Africans living in squatter communities. In Johannesburg, 66% of Black Africans lived in overcrowded households. For families with children, this was even worse with 80% of children living in overcrowded households in Orlando, Johannesburg in 1948.

During this period of rapid economic growth, the cost to maintain a minimum living standard rose by 87% between 1938 and 1950 and the cost of food increased by 75%. The increases in the cost of living and food were not matched by increases in laborers' wages. This disparity increased the already present poverty and malnutrition.

These factors resulted in the Black African population living in squatter communities surrounding the large cities.

Their health was further compromised by malnutrition due to the increase in food prices far beyond the increases in income, and the situation was further compounded by the fragmented health services which mostly catered for the White population while the Black African population had access to minimal health services. This situation was an ideal springboard for creating a perfect TB storm.

TB during WWII

The Second Wave of TB
During WWII, 32,000 South Africans were deployed to Europe of which 21,1000 were White South Africans. This created a vacuum in the labor force that resulted once again in an influx of Black Africans into the urban areas.

Due to poor quality of data available, it is very difficult to reconstruct an accurate picture of the TB situation in South Africa during WWII. The best illustration of the poor quality of data is illustrated by the data on mortality from all forms of TB. In 1945, there were 758 deaths from TB among White people, while it was estimated that 10,000 Black people died from TB. By 1953, the TB deaths in the White population has decreased to 271 for the year while the estimate for the African Black population remained at an estimated 10,000 [2].

TB mortality rates increased dramatically (88%) between 1938 and 1945. This increase is likely to be an underestimate as TB deaths in rural areas were under-reported. On the mines, the TB incidence increased from 300/100,000 in 1938 to 700/100,000 in 1942, while in the province of Natal, where large numbers of miners came from, the TB incidence of new cases increased from 250/100,000 to 800/100,000 population in1948 [6]. Tragically, the largest increase in mortality was among children younger than 2 years of age where the mortality increased from 550/100,000 to 1580/100,000 [6]. This is, however, not dissimilar to the British experience where pulmonary TB as a cause death in boys and girls under 5 years of age increased by 55% and 105%, respectively [7]. Where the TB epidemic in South Africa differed from the epidemic in Europe was that in those countries in Europe where the TB incidence increased during WWII, it quickly returned to the pre-war levels and continued its decline. In South Africa, this post-war decline did not occur. The second wave of the TB epidemic continued. The post-war decline in TB in Europe is partially attributed to the re-establishment of sanatoria and other TB health services, while in South Africa the health services continued to be segregated and those that needed it most were isolated in the homelands.

Before and during WWII, isolation of infectious TB patients was an essential intervention to prevent new cases being infected. The health policy estimated that 1 bed was required for each TB death per year. During WWII, approximately 750 White patients died from TB per year and there were 610 TB beds available for this population group. In contrast to this, there were 1,850 TB beds available for the more than 10,000 Black Africans who died from TB. This discrepancy was ascribed to a lack of funding. This is just an example of the fragmented and segregated health services that occurred in South Africa at the time.

Initially the high TB rates among the mixed race, Indian and Black African population was ascribed to racial susceptibility. This theory was later replaced by environmental theories with the living conditions, malnutrition, and unhygienic factors resulting in a decreased immunity and increased susceptibility to TB. Later it was realized that liberal capitalism was the driving force for the increase in TB in the Black African population. The need for a cheap labor force working under harsh conditions to generate large profits, was the fundamental cause of the epidemic of TB in South Africa.

TB after WWII

The Third Wave of TB – The Perfect Storm
In 1948, the apartheid government came to power and the injustices of the colonial system were passed into law. Apartheid policy entrenched migrant labor and poverty in the black population and this had an enormous effect on the health of poor people. In addition, Black people were forced to live in Bantustans that were regarded as "separate" countries from South Africa. Moreover, they had to provide their own health services and in addition, the health data did not form part of the official South Africa health records. The South African government took over the mission hospitals, which provided many of the services in the Bantustans. Another consequence of Apartheid on the health of the people was the exclusion from and isolation of South Africa from international scientific world by sanctions [1]. South Africa always had a fragmented health service and in 1994, when the new democratically elected government came to power, there were 14 separate health departments in South Africa and health services were focused much more on hospital services than on basic primary health care provision [3]. These conditions were conducive to the heightened incidence and rapid escalation of South Africa's TB epidemic.

A perfect TB storm had been created and has continued for more than 5 decades after WWII. Since the 1990s, this perfect storm has been aggravated by HIV and MDR-TB. The hope was that the new democratically elected government would improve the situation, especially since the new South African constitution clearly states that the right to health is a progressive right for every person in South Africa. Sadly, 23 years after democracy, there are still enormous health inequities in South Africa. South Africa has one of the highest incidences of TB in the world, a huge TB burden and TB is still a main cause of death in South Africa.

Conclusions

Lessons Applicable to South Africa Today
TB remains a disease that mainly affects the people living in poverty. It will not be possible to eliminate TB without having policies that address poverty and inequality still present in South Africa after centuries of neglect. It is not possible to treat a country out of an epidemic and therefore a comprehensive approach is needed to eliminate TB and other infectious diseases, especially in the era of HIV. The only other option for eradicating TB, is if an effective anti-TB vaccine is discovered and all indications are that this is still decades or longer away.

The situation in present South Africa has probably changed very little since WWII, as stated by Dormer in 1948;

The organisms and disease patterns were just the results of something more potent. Industry, economic need, Western civilization – call it what you will, it is today's social system which was responsible for the death of our patient, as it is for a death rate from TB of 900 per 100,000 of industrial natives in South Africa today – perhaps the highest death rate in the world. [8]

References

1 Van Rensburg D, Janse van Rensburg-Bonthuizen E, Heunis C, Meulenmans S: Tuberculosis control in South Africa: reasons for persistent failure. Acta Academic Suppl 2005;1:1–55.
2 Dormer BA: Tuberculosis in South Africa. Br J Tuberc Dis Chest 1956;50:52–60.
3 Coovadia H, Jewkes R, Barron P, Sanders D, McIntyre D: The health and health system of South Africa: historical roots of current public health challenges. Lancet 2009;374:817–834.
4 Macvicar N: Tuberculosis in Southern Africa. Br J Tuberc 1909;3:101–106.
5 Wilson F: Labour in South African Goldmines 1911–1969. Cambridge, Cambridge University Press, 1972.
6 Packard RM: In White plague, Black death: Industrial expansion, squatters and the Second Tuberculosis Epidemic, 1938–1948. p212. University of Natal Press 1989. Pietermaritzburg, South Africa.
7 Daniels M: Tuberculosis in Europe during and after the World War II. Br Med J 1949;19:1135–1140.
8 Dormer BA: A case of tuberculosis. S Afr Med J 1948;22:82–88.

Nulda Beyers
Desmond Tutu TB Centre, Department of Paediatrics and Child Health
Faculty of Medicine and Health Sciences, Stellenbosch University
PO Box 241
Cape Town, 8000 (South Africa)
E-Mail nb@sun.ac.za

Murray JF, Loddenkemper R (eds): Tuberculosis and War. Lessons Learned from World War II.
Prog Respir Res. Basel, Karger, 2018, vol 43, pp 134–143 (DOI: 10.1159/000481481)

Tuberculosis in The Netherlands before, during, and after World War II

Maarten R.A. van Cleeff[a] · Ernest Hueting[b] · Agnes Dessing[c]

[a]Bussum, [b]Naarden, and [c]Haarlem, The Netherlands

Abstract

For The Netherlands, World War II started on May 10, 1940 and ended on May 6, 1945. Mortality from tuberculosis (TB) had shown a gradual pre-war decline of around 7% annually, reaching a nadir of 41/100,000 population in 1939, then worsened throughout the war. Chief factors were the deteriorating food situation, overcrowding, and psychosocial stress. While the morbidity also rose, the risk of infection kept declining. Treatment included eliminating harmful external immunologic factors, hygienic-dietary treatment, surgery, and personal protection. If possible, patients were admitted to sanatoria or hospitals. Because the Nazi occupiers were afraid of TB, these services were left relatively unaffected; some new controls were even introduced, including pasteurization of milk. Nevertheless, the large increase in patients overwhelmed the system and increasing attention was directed towards home care. Later, particularly during the Dutch famine of 1944–1945, known as the Hongerwinter ("Winter of Hunger"), hunger, exhaustion, poor hygiene, and congested living circumstances in shelters took their toll. At the end of 1944, anti-TB clinics stopped operating, and the crumbling general health care system promoted an increase in morbidity and mortality of TB. In 1945, TB mortality had risen to 85.9/100,000, twice as high as in 1939.

© 2018 S. Karger AG, Basel

Nine months after the beginning of World War II (WWII) (early September 1939), the Netherlands was invaded, on May 10, 1940, when, in the very early morning, the Germans attacked the country in the south-east. Four days later, the Nazi Luftwaffe bombed Rotterdam [1]. After receiving threats to bomb the city of Utrecht as well, General H. Win-kelman ordered the Dutch army to stop fighting. Later in the afternoon, Rotterdam surrendered and the next day, on May 15, Winkelman signed the Dutch capitulation [1]. The Netherlands became an occupied country for the next 5 years, until it was liberated by the allied forces and the Germans signed their unconditional surrender on May 6, 1945. In 1940, the country counted 8,834,000 inhabitants, including 140,000 Jews. Around 591,400 died during the war – with by far the highest peak in 1944 – but this figure excludes the 101,800 Jews who were killed in concentration camps or died from illness, starvation, and exhaustion.

Epidemiology

Before the introduction of anti-TB drugs, analysis of TB mortality data was considered a fair method of examining the epidemiology of the disease [2]. Against expectations, even during the socioeconomic crisis preceding the war, TB mortality showed a gradual declining trend of around 7% per year, from 52.5/100,000 in 1935 to 41/100,000 in 1939. It was therefore thought that TB was under control and that eradication could even be anticipated in the foreseeable future.

The war, however, compromised everything. Figure 1 and Table 1 show that during the first year of the German occupation, mortality had already risen by approximately 45% compared to 1939, and in 1945 the mortality rate was

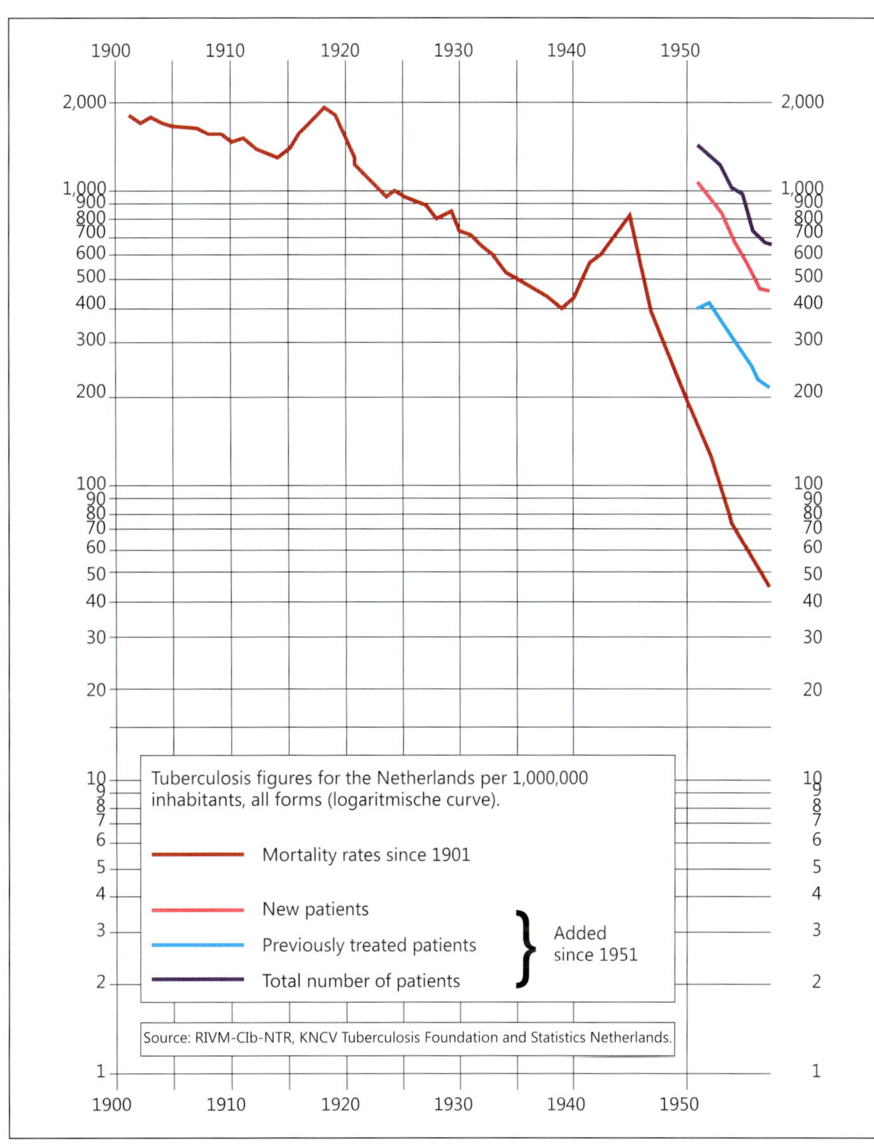

Fig. 1. Tuberculosis in The Netherlands, 1901–1960.

Table 1. Mortality rates per 100,000 in The Netherlands and Amsterdam by year

	1930	1939	1940	1941	1942	1943	1944	1945
Mortality per 100,000; The Netherlands all forms	74.3	41	43.7	59.2	61.2	70	74.3	85.9
Change from previous period, %		−45	7	35	3	14	6	16
Mortality per 100,000, Amsterdam all forms	70	35.2	37	59.1	71.1	76.6	82.7	
Change from previous period, %		−50	5	60	20	8	8	

85.9/100,000 population, twice as high as compared to 1939. In one year, mortality had increased by 35% in Amsterdam and by 37% in The Hague [3].

Both TB mortality and TB morbidity rose. To what extent increased mortality could be ascribed to increased mor-bidity or increased case-fatality is difficult to establish. There was no obligatory national registration system in place in the Netherlands and no mandatory notification for TB [4, 5], although in 1918, notification for TB was compulsory in several countries, including Norway, Sweden, Denmark,

Germany, Hungary, Switzerland, Italy, Spain, Portugal, Brazil, Australia, and most states in the US.

In 1918, to draw lessons from WWI, a special National Committee was established during which the Netherlands explicitly chose not to require mandatory notification. Instead, to guarantee anonymity, they favored the development of a country-wide network of "consultatiebureaus" (anti-TB clinics). The idea was to maximize patient access, unimpeded by the restrictions of medical secrecy, and protection of patients' financial interests (particularly, when they were the breadwinners), and limit the stigma and social consequences of having TB. The arguments mentioned at the time against mandatory notification were the risk of creating social divisions in which one half of the population was opposing the other, and the issue around the difficulty of diagnosing "closed" TB. Notification became mandatory by law only in 1980.

In September 1945, the district of Nijmegen nevertheless reported 2,544 patients with active TB compared to 1,148 by the end of 1941 [6]. Similarly, Amsterdam reported 2,180 new cases in 1943 against 860 in 1939 [7], with a greater increase among men than women. In The Hague, mortality increased from 32 in 1940 to 44/100,000 population in 1941 [3]. For the whole of The Netherlands, the number of registered new patients more than doubled, from 8,840 in 1939 to 18,571 in 1943, as shown in Figure 2 [8].

Due to the lack of sanatorium beds, many TB patients were obliged to remain at home, thus further adding to the transmission of the disease. As in peacetime, it was mainly young adults who contracted TB, but in addition, there was a notable increase in the age group 50–79 years. There were also growing numbers of relapse cases.

It is remarkable that, despite the increase of sources of infection, the risk of TB infection kept declining during the war period. This may have been caused by the rapid and high mortality rate, offsetting the rate of spread of new infections. Van den Berg tentatively suggested that a significant number of new cases during the war could have been ascribed to endogenous reactivation rather than an exogenous reinfection [7].

Styblo estimated a gradual decline in the prevalence of TB infection from 11,310/100,000 average population in 1910, to 6,690 in 1920, 3,920 in 1930, 2,080 in 1940 to 530/100,000 in 1950 [9]. And based on all available data from standard tuberculin surveys conducted in the Netherlands, he estimated an annual decline in the annual risk of infection of 5.4% from 1913 to 1939, while from 1940 to 1966 the annual decline increased even further to 12.9% (Fig. 3). In addition, Styblo ascribed the more rapid decline starting in 1940 to the

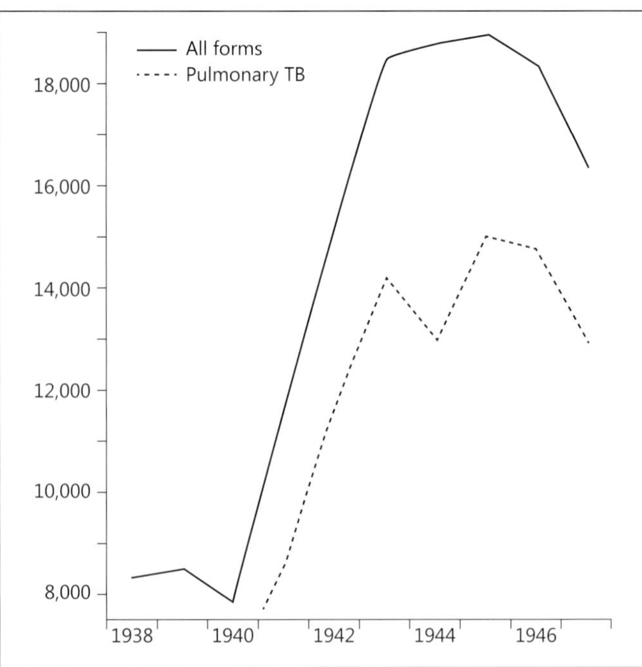

Fig. 2. Number of new cases of active TB, The Netherlands, 1938–1947.

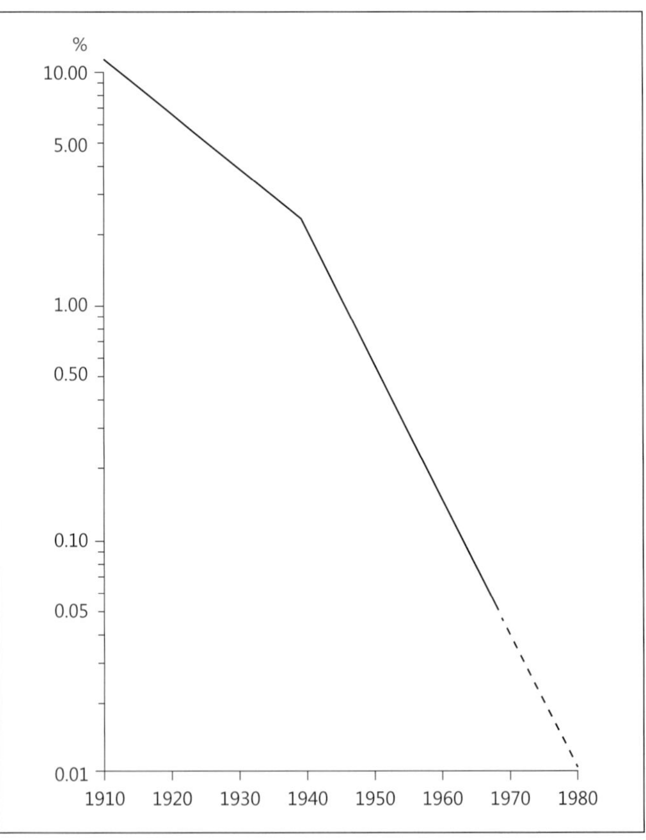

Fig. 3. Annual risk of tuberculosis infection (%), The Netherlands, 1910–1980.

van Cleeff · Hueting · Dessing

pasteurization of milk (introduced by the Germans) as the main cause. Between 1933 and 1939, 10% of pulmonary and 17% of extra-pulmonary TB was due to bovine strains. From 1940 to 1944 this was reduced to 2% and 7% respectively and further reduced to 1% and 0% between 1946 to 1950 [2].

Another study showed similar findings of bovine infection and suggested raw milk and dairy products as the main causes [10]. After a small study on dairy infection, where he isolated viable *Mycobacterium bovis* strains from butter milk (2/15), cheese (1/56), and farmers' butter (2/24), van der Hoeden was already recommending compulsory pasteurization [11]. Finally, on this subject, at the municipal slaughterhouse in Rotterdam, the recorded rate of TB in cattle varied during the period 1934–1938 from 35 to 37%, including TB of the udders [12].

Determinants for the Increase in TB

What were the possible explanations for this aggravation? First was the deteriorating food situation. In June 1940, the first food distribution measures had already been proclaimed, which resulted in a reduction in food quality; in particular, nutrients important for TB (fats and proteins) were difficult to acquire. Reports also mention shortages in vitamin A. However, this explanation is not sufficient. If indeed there was a direct causal link between food supply and TB, the increase in TB would have been less pronounced in the countryside, where food supplies were relatively good. In fact, the opposite was the case: there was an increase in mortality due to TB and a sharp rise in the number of patients, even in rural provinces.

Second, in his report of 1943, the Medical Superintendent suggested another possible explanation for the sudden increase in TB: the increased risk of infection due to overcrowding. Whether voluntarily or by obligation, people were living in cramped quarters, and their exposure to infectious cases may have extended beyond their households to other areas of crowding such as in crowded trains and other means of transport, in central kitchens, and distribution centers [13]. Dr. van Vliet, a public health clinician in Groningen, observed that because of the war, people mixed more outside their own families: the occupation created a sense of solidarity, leading to people who hardly knew each other before the war being united in their common hatred towards the Germans and becoming friends. The figures support this view: the number of extra-familial infections, where the source of infection had to be sought outside the family, markedly increased during the war [14].

A third explanation, which also was often suggested during WWII, was the role of psychological factors that may have affected immunity against TB. For decades, TB had been associated with "psychosocial stress situations" such as poverty, misfortune, misery and grief, particularly grief due to unhappy love. Music and literature is rich with examples on this theme. In her book, *Illness as Metaphor*, which deals with the myths surrounding diseases such as TB and cancer, Susan Sontag gives numerous examples on this theme from 19th–20th-century novels [15]. The novel *La Dame aux Camélias*, by Alexandre Dumas, formed the basis for Verdi's opera *La Traviata*, whose heroine, Violetta, dies of TB in a stupendous death scene. In Puccini's opera, *La Bohème*, the main female character, Mimi, suffers from TB and her death is accelerated due to love sickness. In James Joyces' famous story, "The death," a young man (Michael Furey), loses his will to live because of unrequited love and dies of TB. Dutch novels with similar themes include *Lament for Agnes*, by van Marnix Gijsen and *The woman eater*, by Theun de Vries.

Since its discovery by Robert Koch in 1882, it has been clear that TB is a contagious disease and that anyone can catch it. Yet, for many years, it was a mystery why only some people who were infected became ill and the majority did not. At the beginning of the 19th century, terms such as "pre-disposition" became rather fashionable, and psychological determinants gradually also began to receive medical attention. It was known that many patients experienced difficult life situations in the period prior to their illness: a divorce, loss of a loved one, poverty, debt, unemployment, etc. But it was unknown just how psychological factors could reduce host resistance to tubercle bacilli. In the meantime, research has shown that certain proteins (lymphokines) play an important role in immunological defenses, ensuring that the immune system reacts when certain antigens enter the body, serving to maintain a healthy balance. Stress disrupts this balance, resulting in a failure of the immune system [13]. More recently, Jaap Veen showed that among Vietnamese boat refugees on arrival in the Netherlands in the mid-1980s, a negative tuberculin skin test had changed to positive after a few months. He demonstrated that poor nutritional status at the time of entry was a confounding factor to the occurrence of temporary anergy and thought it plausible that stress (grief, anxiety, endured hardship) contributed to this poor nutritional state [16].

The WWII period from 1940 to 1945 offered a rich variety of stress situations: the worries associated with the daily struggle for survival, the fear of being arrested, the anxious hours spent in bomb shelters, the anger and hatred of the occupiers. A striking example was the rise in mortality in Rotterdam, after it was bombed in May 1940, followed in 1941 by 1,463 new cases of active TB being reported, including 352 people with open TB, versus only 132 cases in 1938 [13]. An interesting study by van Helsdingen showed the effects of a bombing near the Hoog-Laren sanatorium on the rate of disease. The bombing, which took place on 25–26 November 1944, caused 20% of the patients to experience a clear deterioration of their TB, with adverse manifestations in the temperature curve, blood picture, chest X-ray, and/or certain clinical symptoms [17].

In summary, both morbidity and mortality worsened during the war. To what extent increased mortally could be ascribed to increased morbidity or increased case-fatality is difficult to ascertain. The latter probably manifested more at the end of the war. Especially in the first years of the war, when the food situation was not so dire, stress played a major role. Obviously, in the last part of the war, in particular during the Dutch famine of 1944–1945, known as the Hongerwinter ("Winter of Hunger"), hunger, exhaustion, poor hygiene, and cramped living conditions in shelters took a far greater toll [18].

In addition, the crumbling health care system, including the slowly diminishing number of medical doctors, delays in care, shortages of medicines, and lack of hospital care, contributed to the increase in TB morbidity and mortality. Moreover, due to the circumstances, typical clinical symptoms such as weight loss became less specific, which sometimes made it difficult to establish the diagnosis [19].

Care and Control

Before the war, the most important TB treatment measures were focused on improving the immune response by: (i) eliminating those external factors that harm the immune system (irregular lifestyle, alcohol misuse, and sexual excess); (ii) using hygienic-dietary treatment (good food, fresh air, sunlight, and proper balance between rest and activity); (iii) at times using surgery (resection of extra-pulmonary lesions, artificial pneumothorax); (iv) personal protection (separating children from parents with TB); and last but not least, (v) rest. Rest included not only physical but also mental and intellectual rest. Mental rest was perhaps difficult to achieve, but bed rest and care was crucial. To prevent infection among family contacts, patients were sent away from their homes and, if possible, admitted to sanatoria or hospitals with strict time regimens, mainly of rest (Box 1) [20]. In the early 1940s, the Netherlands counted 4,970 beds in 36 sanatoria and 665 beds in 7 sanatoria for children. Those who could afford it went to the Dutch sanatorium in Davos [21]. However, not all patients could be admitted; for those who could not, special trained home advisors visited the pa-

tients' homes to provide health education, nutritional advice, hygiene measures such as the use of handkerchiefs, education about the infectiousness of the disease, psycho-social support and advice about reorganization of the house to prevent contact infection [22].

The large increase in the number of TB patients had a huge impact on the care and control system. Sanatoria and hospitals were soon overcrowded, not only due to the increased number of patients, but also to the reduction in the number of available beds; even before the war, some sanatoria were emptied to make room for the mobilization of the army. To compensate for the lack of sanatorium beds, rotating shelters were established throughout the country. Many of these could be seen along the road between the cities of Heerenveen and Groningen [23, 24] (Fig. 4).

The Dutch Central Association to combat Tuberculosis (NCV) established in 1903 (in 1953 it received its "Royal" (K) designation to become the KNCV [25] and in 2003 became the "KNCV Tuberculosis Foundation") used this situation for advocacy purposes. In 1943, they published the brochure *De Strijd van Meester Zonneschijn (the Struggle of Master Sunshine)*, focused on the growing number of patients who could not be admitted to sanatoria or hospitals and had to remain at home. It was a modern, fresh looking booklet, illustrated with photographs and drawings [26] (Fig. 5). The aim of the brochure was to educate patients to achieve cure without infecting their household contacts. It also stressed the importance of adhering to the strict rules of cure, and contained recipes and tips on how to use the meager rations available and still prepare a sensible meal.

<table>
<tr><td colspan="2">Box 1. A typical day in a sanatorium</td></tr>
<tr><td>6.30</td><td>Take temperature</td></tr>
<tr><td>7.00</td><td>Get up</td></tr>
<tr><td>8.15</td><td>Breakfast</td></tr>
<tr><td>8.45–12.00</td><td>Bedrest in the lounge (or) and prescribed walk</td></tr>
<tr><td>11.45</td><td>Take temperature</td></tr>
<tr><td>12.15</td><td>Lunch</td></tr>
<tr><td>1.00–2.30</td><td>Long rest and try to sleep</td></tr>
<tr><td>2.30</td><td>Take temperature</td></tr>
<tr><td>2.30–6.00</td><td>Bedrest in the lounge (or) and prescribed walk, with a 15 min tea break (3.45–4.00)</td></tr>
<tr><td>5.15–7.30</td><td>Evening meal; free time</td></tr>
<tr><td>7.30–8.30</td><td>Rest</td></tr>
<tr><td>8.00</td><td>Take temperature</td></tr>
<tr><td>8.45</td><td>To the dormitory</td></tr>
<tr><td>9.00</td><td>Bed time; lights out; complete rest</td></tr>
</table>

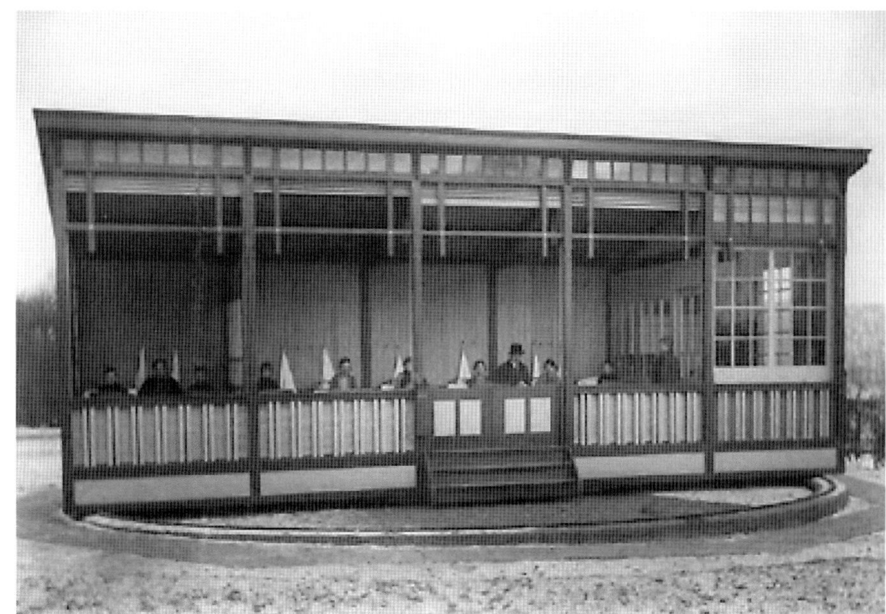

Fig. 4. A rotating tuberculosis shelter.

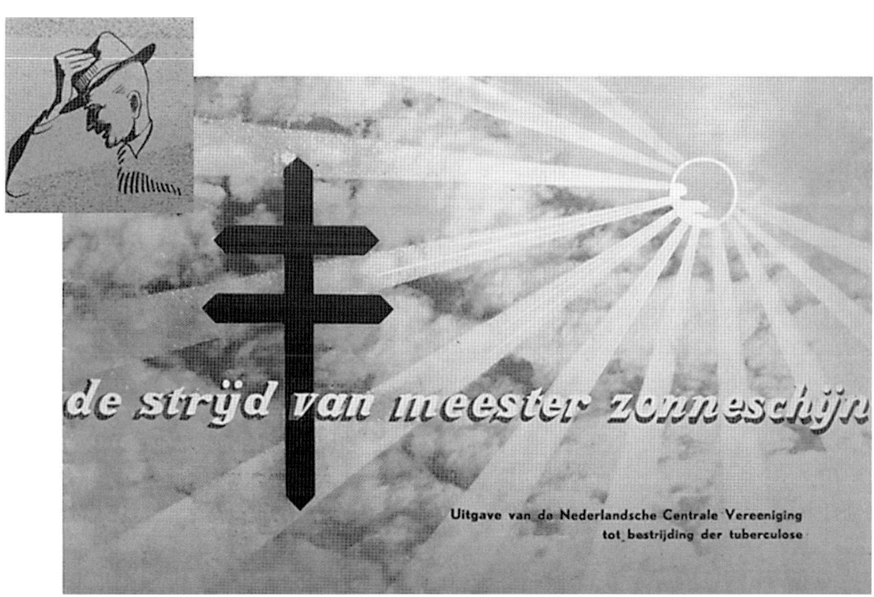

Fig. 5. The Struggle of Master Sunshine.

TB control was symbolized by the figure of Master Sunshine, an old man with a sunny mood, who visited various patients at home. In this way, different groups of patients with their specific problems were described: a housefather, whose TB was discovered during an inspection at work, but who did not adhere to the treatment rules at home; a three-year-old child, who continually jumped out of bed because the mother did not have time to take care of him; or a coughing teenage girl, whose bed was placed, on the advice of the nurse, in the living room from which the dusty carpets were removed. The brochure showed that in comparison with earlier NCV brochures there was a better understanding of the difficulties resulting from the treatment requirements. For example, issues around kissing which was still a taboo in the brochure of 1910, were now discussed in detail. Although it was limited to the affection between children and their parents (intimacies between husband and wife were not mentioned), this new approach was quite a big step forward. The above-mentioned girl of sixteen thanks her mother with a kiss. The mother hesitates:

"A kiss," the nurse told her, "Mother, don't kiss anymore, though Marietje is not a direct threat to her environment, you still must be careful. A kiss can be dangerous." And wouldn't she give a kiss? Marietje looked at her mother and understood. "No mother, no kiss but a Chinese kiss. You know, rubbing noses together." "Ah, child, do not be silly. You know what, you get a peach kiss." "A what?" "A peach kiss. Your cheek, child, is as rosy as a peach and you should press your cheek close to me. You are my sole Marietje, and a real kiss is something we keep for later, when you're better". [26]

Anti-TB Clinics

The system of anti-TB clinics played an important role in TB control, including early case finding, preventive measures and support of patient care [27]. They had to cope with large, sometimes excessive, numbers of patients. The number of first visits more than doubled from 60,377 in 1939 to 157,134 in 1943. This was caused by increased fear of TB among the public and general practitioners. In addition, many people hoped that by "having tuberculosis" they would be able to obtain extra food vouchers from the clinic or escape forced labor in Germany. Indeed, quite a few doctors interpreted the diagnosis of TB rather widely.

On average, 80 patients per day had to be examined, and soon a 6-week waiting time became common. In 1943, one of the doctors from district Noord Holland sighed in his annual report:

If one finishes busy days of investigation and sometimes doesn't find a single case with even suspected tuberculosis, one gets the disappointing impression of doing a monk's work. Office hours remain overcrowded by people who had not been referred anyway [...]. The real sufferers become victims, because for them there is insufficient time vailable. Also the clinic can perform less contact investigations than desirable. [28]

Nevertheless, during the early years of WWII, the consultation centers were able to continue their work. The Germans were afraid of TB, and the precautionary measures they took were sometimes so extreme as to be absurd: for example, all residents of camp Westerbork – the Dutch transit camp for the concentration camps in Eastern Europe – were screened with advanced equipment, and if sick put in a separate block for infectious diseases [29]. To illustrate another extreme, more than 20,000 prisoners from Buchenwald concentration camp and its sub-camps were employed in the arms industry. The prisoners were chronically malnourished and about 10% of them suffered from smear-positive TB [30].

TB control services, especially where the treatment of patients was concerned, continued to receive government sub-

sidies. These subsidies even increased, although this had little effect, as the payments regularly stagnated [28].

On the organizational level, however, the Nazi occupation intervened a great deal; Jews were no longer allowed to occupy positions on boards or in executive positions. Nursing and admissions of Jewish patients were forbidden; this became a clandestine process, using forged personal certificates. Sanatoria in the coastal regions had to be evacuated during the construction of the "Antlantikwall," and patients were accommodated as much as possible in the north and east of the country. The work of the NCV was seriously hampered; as for many other organizations and TB clinics, the Nazis ordered the dismissal of all Jewish employees and recruited a pro-German person to its board [31]. The Emma Flower Fund, a collection fund established by the Queens' mother Emma to raise money for TB patients, was banned, resulting in a significant loss of income.

The NCV initially took a rather hesitant attitude towards the occupying forces; they wanted to be able to continue to work as much as possible, and were prepared to make certain concessions. On January 22, 1942, the Germans set up the Dutch Culture Chamber, and one of their six guilds was the Press Guild. Anyone working in the press or in publishing had to report to the Press Guild within three weeks. When the NCV was also required to accommodate its magazine "Tegen de Tuberculose" (against TB) under the Press Guild, the Board of the NCV firmly rejected the demand, and in March 1942, "Tegen de Tuberculose" ceased the publication [31]. Scientific publications did not fall under this Guild, however, and the NCV was able to continue publishing their abstracts of international publications on TB.

Nevertheless, during all this misery, some control measures were introduced. In 1941, at the instigation of the Germans, the "Sickness Fund decision" was proclaimed, which included the decision that insurance funds were legally bound, in addition to paying for hospital care, to also (at least partially) pay the costs of sanatorium care. Initially these benefits were 1.50 guilders per day for a maximum of 1 year. Another important measure was the reduced risk of infection through contaminated milk. At the beginning of the war, much of the livestock, including cows infected with TB, was transported to Germany. As a result, measures were initiated to control bovine TB, and the pasteurization of milk in The Netherlands was made mandatory by decree in 1941.

Life in the sanatoria continued as it had before 1940, unless they were involved in combat operations or patients needed to be evacuated. The poet-writer Cees Buddingh, who was admitted to the "Zonnegloren" (Sun Glory) sanatorium, in Soest, during the war, wrote a poem, "Zonneglo-ren," about his experiences many years later, which provides good insight into the portrayed state of mind [32]:

It wasn't really uncomfortable.
I read and played a lot of chess.
Every other week Stientje came to visit me
And if you did well, you might
quickly get into the following bed.
You were not badly off: outside was war,
Eddy Hoornik sat in Dachau, lovers were
arrested or interned in Poland.
Also around me people sometimes died
from embolism or spitting blood, but
you knew: I didn't come here for that.

Last Year of WWII

In the last part of the war, particularly during the Dutch famine of 1944–1945, known as the Hongerwinter ("Winter of hunger"), hunger, exhaustion, poor hygiene, and crowded living conditions in shelters took their toll [18]. During the last three months of 1944, doctors in the anti-TB clinics noted a sharp reduction in patients' bodyweight. The number of patients increased, and the severity of the disease and the number of deaths rose (Table 1). Moreover, due to the circumstances, typical TB-related symptoms such as weight loss became less specific, which made it more difficult to make a diagnosis [19]. After October, trains were no longer running, and it became virtually impossible for patients to reach the clinics. For the same reasons, the work of home visitors and district nurses became appallingly difficult, although in some instances, they were able to distribute food (flour and milk powder) provided by the Red Cross in The Hague [8]. Due to fuel, electricity, and sometimes also water shortages, X-rays and blood and sputum examinations could no longer be performed. At the end of 1944, the activities of the anti-TB clinics came to a complete halt.

The TB certificates that protected people from deportation were not always sufficient. In German-sponsored raids, patients were also arrested and their blankets and clothes were no longer spared. But, as district Dr. Hulscher from Hilversum wrote:

By far the worst of all war torments was the poor and deteriorating nutrition, which despite the Central Kitchen was totally inadequate. Many non-sick members were constantly hungry, and many TB patients despite "extra-rations" just as much. In the last months of 1944, the food vouchers no longer included milk and butter. [28]

The situation had also become desperate in the sanatoria – those that had not been closed or destroyed. While, during a large part of the war, through the special distribution system, food and drug supplies had been relatively well maintained, in 1944, however, the drug supply system ceased to function and the patients could not return home either due to the lack of transport.

Finally, the crumbling health care system as a whole, including the diminishing number of practicing medical doctors, delays in care, shortages of medicines, and lack of hospital care contributed to the increase in morbidity and mortality due to TB. In 1945, 7,959 people died from TB, 5.6% of the total 141,000 reported deaths in The Netherlands. Many of these could probably have survived under normal conditions. However, hunger, exhaustion, and lack of health care ensured their deaths.

After WWII

After WWII, TB was widespread. In addition to the increased number of affected families, TB was also relatively frequent among the returning survivors of the concentration camps, prisoners of war camps and, a little later, among those who returned from the Japanese internment camps in Indonesia [33].

The number of new cases kept increasing for a while, with around 18,000 new cases per year. Particularly affected were young children (0–15 years), probably because many patients had to be treated at home due to shortages of sanatorium beds [34]. Nevertheless, TB mortality immediately started to decline, from 85.9/100,000 in 1945 to 28.9/100,000 in 1947, in a few years reaching even lower levels than in 1939 (Fig. 1) [35].

After May 1945, there were 7,000 beds available in sanatoria and hospitals – not enough for the 25,000 registered TB patients [13]. Priority for admission was given to those with active TB. Other measures to cope with the bed shortages included shorter hospitalization periods, the establishment of emergency sanatoria, and the so-called "Swedish barracks" (see below), as well as sending patients abroad.

The Swedish government donated 300 wooden barracks, each with a capacity of 20 beds (Fig. 6). However, due to all sorts of complicating factors in the organization, administration, and required adaptation of the barracks, it was years before sufficient beds were ready for use. Other donations came from a British NGO (medical equipment, microscopes and X-ray machines). In addition, the Marshall Plan included, apart from food, X-ray machines for screening purposes. A

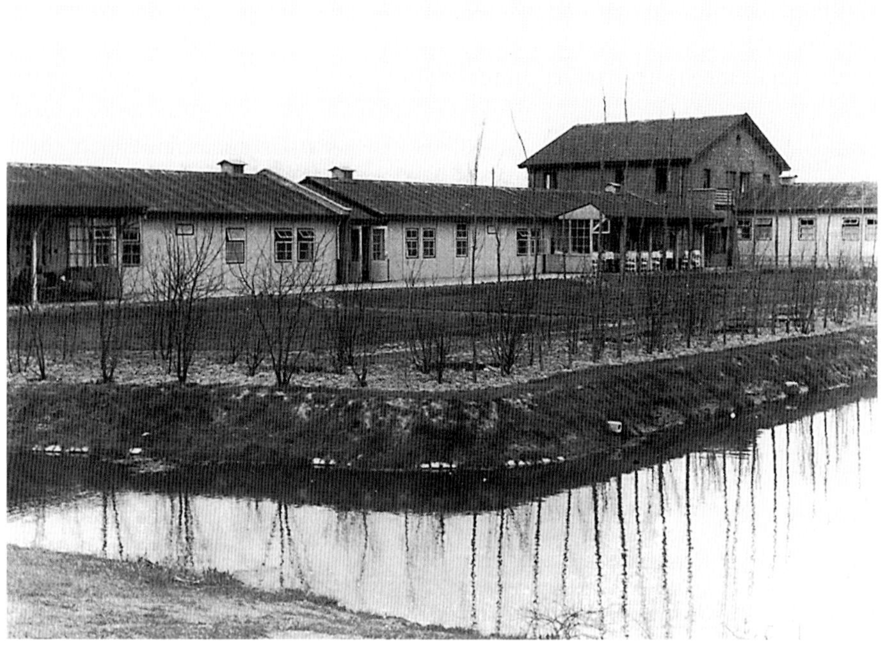

Fig. 6. Swedish barracks in Delft.

Swiss NGO donated funds to treat 681 patients in Swiss sanatoria (Davos and Leysin) and another 85 patients were treated in Danish sanatoria. With these measures, the number of beds in 1947 was almost doubled as compared to 1945 [8].

In 1947, TB control changed with the introduction of streptomycin as monotherapy. This was combined with PAS (para-aminosalicylic acid) after 1948. In 1952, isoniazid was added to this regimen. Initially, also to prevent resistance, medical treatment was considered as an addition to bedrest and surgery, but in the 1950s it became apparent that in many cases medical treatment alone was sufficient.

Pasteurization of milk, already introduced by the Germans during the war, became legally regulated along with other measures to control bovine TB. Initially only livestock with positive TB were culled; this later included animals with a positive tuberculin reaction. Farmers were compensated by Marshal Plan funding [33]. With all these new interventions, the lives of many TB patients were saved and TB gradually became a rare disease.

Conclusion

For the Netherlands, WWII began on May 10, 1940 and ended on May 6, 1945. Immediately after its start, TB morbidity and mortality worsened, reaching a peak at the end of the war. The increase in mortality could probably be ascribed to both increased morbidity and increased case-fatality. The latter worsened further during the Dutch famine of 1944–1945 known as the Winter of Hunger. In 1945, mortality had risen to 96.9/100,000, twice as high as in 1939. Several factors contributed to this exacerbation, including a deteriorating food situation, overcrowding, psychosocial stress, and at the end of the war also real hunger and the crumbling health care system.

Because the Nazi occupiers were afraid of TB, TB control services were left relatively unaffected; the network of anti-TB clinics could function, patients were admitted to sanatoria or hospitals and some new control measures were even introduced, including pasteurization of milk. On the organizational level, however, the Germans created serious problems: Jewish patients were forbidden to receive any form of health care and Jews were no longer allowed to occupy positions on boards or in executive positions. As such, the work of the NCV, as well as of anti-TB clinics and other related organizations, was seriously hampered.

It is remarkable that, despite the increased sources of infection, the risk of TB infection kept declining during the war. This may have been caused by the rapid and high mortality rate, offsetting the rate of spread of new infections and pasteurization of milk.

After WWII, the number of new cases kept increasing for about a year, with around 18,000 new cases per year. TB was relatively frequent among the returning survivors of the concentration camps, prisoners of war camps and, a little later, among returnees from the Japanese internment camps in Indonesia. The shortages of beds and problems with other TB control functions were (partly) resolved with help from the international donor community, including the Marshal Plan. TB mortality immediately started to decline, from 85.9/100,000 in 1945 to 28.9/100,000 in 1947, reaching even lower levels than in 1939.

In 1947, TB control changed dramatically with the introduction of streptomycin, in combination with PAS after 1948, and INH in 1952. With these and some other control measures, including the legally regulated pasteurization of milk, TB gradually became a rare disease in The Netherlands.

References

1　Wikipedia. "tweede wereld oorlog Nederland' https://nl.wikipedia.org/wiki/Holocaust_in_Nederland.

2　Styblo K: Epidemiology of Tuberculosis. Infectionskrankheiten und ihre Erreger. Band 4/VI. Jena, VEB Gustav Fisher Verlag, 1984.

3　Hueting E: 100 jaar Tuberculosebestrijding in The Hague. 2004, p 53.

4　van Geuns HA: De Tuberculose Bestrijding in Nederland. Ned. T. Geneesk, 1882, p 126.

5　Verslag van de staatscommissie van voorlichting over wetteijke maatregelen tot bestrijding van de tuberculose en over de beste wijze van Bestrijding. The Hague, July 3, 1918, p 29.

6　Honing JGA: Het vóórkomen van tuberculose in oorlogstijd en het vóórkomen na den oorlog. Tegen de Tuberculose 1946;42:7.

7　van den Berg H: Tuberculosis in Holland during the War. A paper read before the Tuberculosis Association, September 8 1945. Tubercle 1945: 181–185.

8　Gerbrandy HR: Over de opnemeing mogelijkheden voor tuberculose patienten in Nederland. Tegen de Tubercuolse 1947;43:13.

9　Styblo K: Recente ontwikkelingen in de tuberculose epidemiologie. The Hague, KNCV, 1982.

10　Ruys A CH: On tuberculosis in man due to the bovine type of the tubercle bacillus in The Netherlands. Tubercle 1939;XX (No. 12):556–560.

11　van der Hoeden J: Tubercelbacillen in Zuivelproducten Verlsag T.b.c. Studie Communication, 1940, p 14, 77.

12　Huitema H: Mycobacterial Infections and the Successful Eradication of Bovine Tuberculosis in Cattle in The Netherlands. The Hague, KNCV, 1992.

13　van Geuns HA: Tuberculose in Nederland voor en na de tweede wereldoorlog. Tegen de Tuberculose 1988;84:63.

14　van Vliet B: De Tuberculose; in Medische ervaringen in Nederland tijdens de bezetting. 1940–1945. Onder redactie van I. Boerema, 1947, p 435, 438.

15　Sontag S: Illness as Metaphor. New York, Farrar, Straus & Giroux, 1978.

16　Veen J: Aspects of temporary specific anergy to tuberculin in Vietnamese refugees. Groningen, Van Denderen BV, 1992.

17　Van Helsdingen RJ: De psychologie van de tuberculose; mogelijkheden voor psychotherapie. Amsterdam, Strengholt, 1951.

18　Roffel A: War in the Countryside: Re-examining Life in The Netherlands during World War II through the Memories of Dutch Immigrants to Ontario. Windsor, University of Windsor, 2014. http://scholar.uwindsor.ca/cgi/viewcontent.cgi?article=6120&context=etd.

19　van Lieburg M, Meinhardt MW: Geneeskunde en Gezondheidszorg in Nederland 1940-'45. Amsterdam, Editions Rodopi, 1991, p 183.

20　NCV: Leerboek de Tuberculosebestrijding. The Hague, NCV, 1944, pp 176–209.

21　de Goeij H: Korte geschiedenis van de organisatie van de tbc-bestrijding in Nederland. Tegen de Tuberculose 2014;110:8–17. https://www.kncvtbc.org/uploaded/2015/09/tdt_2014_nr_2_de_goeij_geschiedenis_organiatie_tbc_bestrijding_nederland1.pdf.

22　Hueting E: Sociaal-Verpleegkundigen en Tuberculosebestrijding. Een Beroep in Historisch Perspectief. Elzevier, 1998.

23　Vijfentwintig Jaar Sanatorium Verzekering, 1936–1961. Stichting Nederlandse Sanatorium-Verzekering, 1961.

24　de la Bruhèze AAA, Lintsen HW, Rip A, Schot JW: Techniek in Nederland in de twintigste eeuw. Deel 4. Huishoud Technologie, Medische Techniek, 2001.

25　KNCV. https://www.kncvtbc.org/wie-we-zijn/geschiedenis/.

26　Wilzen-Bruins EJ: De Strijd van Meester Zonneschijn. Illustraties door C. van der Baan. The Hague, NCV, 1943.

27　Sluier HJ: De Toekomst van het Consultatiebureau voor Tuberculosebestrijding. Ned T Geneeskunde, 1978, p 122.

28　Bloemsma AD: Gedenkschrijft: indrukken van 50 jaren tuberculosebestrijding in de provincie Noord Holland (behalve Amsterdam). Ter gelengenheid gouden jubuleum NCV May 4, 1985.

29　Mechanicus P: In Dépôt. Dagboek uit Westerbork, Amsterdam, 1987.

30　https://nl.wikipedia.org/wiki/Buchenwald.

31　Sickenga FN: Korte geschiedenis van de tuberculosebestrijding in Nederland 1900–1960. The Hague, KNCV, 1980, p 245.

32　Budding C: De eerste zestig. Amsterdam, De Bezige Bij, 1978, p 59.

33　Hueting E, Dessing A: Tuberculose. Negentig jaar Tuberculosebrestrijding in Nederland. Walberg pers, 1993, pp 87–92.

34　in't Zand PKA: Statistiek en Tuberculose. Tegen de Tuberculose 1947;53:12.

35　NCV. 45ste Jaarverslag van de NCV tot bestrijding van tuberculoses (1984). Tegen de Tuberculosis 1949;45:73.

Maarten R.A. van Cleeff
Rostocklaan 1
NL–1404AD Bussum (The Netherlands)
E-Mail mvancleeff@gmail.com

Murray JF, Loddenkemper R (eds): Tuberculosis and War. Lessons Learned from World War II.
Prog Respir Res. Basel, Karger, 2018, vol 43, pp 144–151 (DOI: 10.1159/000481482)

Tuberculosis in Belgium before, during, and after World War II

Maryse Wanlin[a, b]

[a]Belgian Lung and Tuberculosis Association (BELTA), and [b]Fonds des Affections Respiratoires (FARES), Brussels, Belgium

Abstract

World War II (WWII) began on September 1, 1939, when the Nazi German army invaded Poland and progressed relentlessly towards Warsaw. After silence from Germany, the United Kingdom, France, and several members of the British Empire declared war on September 3, 1939. Belgium's involvement in WWII began on May 10, 1940, when the Nazi army invaded Belgium on its way to France and Belgium was occupied by the Germans from May 28, 1940 until liberation by the allies. In 1850, the TB mortality rate was 376.7/100,000 and fell to 155.2/100,000 in 1900. As in most of Europe, TB mortality increased strikingly in WWI though less in WWII. But in 1941, TB mortality rose sharply to 98.3/100,000, remained high in 1942 to 95.3/100,000, and then fell progressively to 77.8/100,000 in 1945. Only in 1946 did the rate fall below that at the beginning of the war. The destruction and requisition of TB facilities worsened the plight of the rising number of active TB patients. The socioeconomic situation was desperate: 13% of men were prisoners of war; calories were restricted, malnutrition was prevalent. Nevertheless, TB treatment and prevention efforts, though compromised, were ongoing.

Belgium had a central situation among the Western European countries involved in World War II (WWII). During the 1940s, it had a surface area of 3,050 km^2, a little more than at the beginning of the century due to the annexation of part of one of the losers, Germany, after World War I (WWI) [1]. In 1930, 60.5% of the population was living in cities of more than 5,000 inhabitants, compared to 52.3% in 1900 [1]. The attraction to bigger cities was a trend that would continue into the future. At the beginning of WWII, the population of Belgium was estimated at 8,294,674, after excluding the 88,090 inhabitants of the Eastern cantons that had previously been annexed and were no longer under Belgian jurisdiction [1].

Belgium's involvement in WWII began on May 10, 1940, with the invasion of the Nazi German army, despite the fact that since the beginning of the conflict, in September 1939, Belgium had respected the principle of neutrality between its neighboring countries, France, England, and Germany [2, 3]. There was a chaotic exodus towards France of around 1.5 million people in the early days of the war [3]. After 18 days of fighting, King Leopold III signed the capitulation and became a prisoner of the Germans until the end of the war. The official Belgian government fled first to Paris and then escaped to exile in Bordeaux and subsequently London, until it returned to power in September 1944. From May 28, 1940, Belgium was taken over by the Nazis, and both Belgium and the North of France were occupied under the jurisdiction of the Wehrmacht [2].

Following D-day, most of Belgium was liberated during the advance of allied troops in September–October 1944, but the war continued as a new German offensive in the Ardennes took place in December 1944. However, the allies prevailed and the final German unconditional surrender was signed on May 8, 1945 [3].

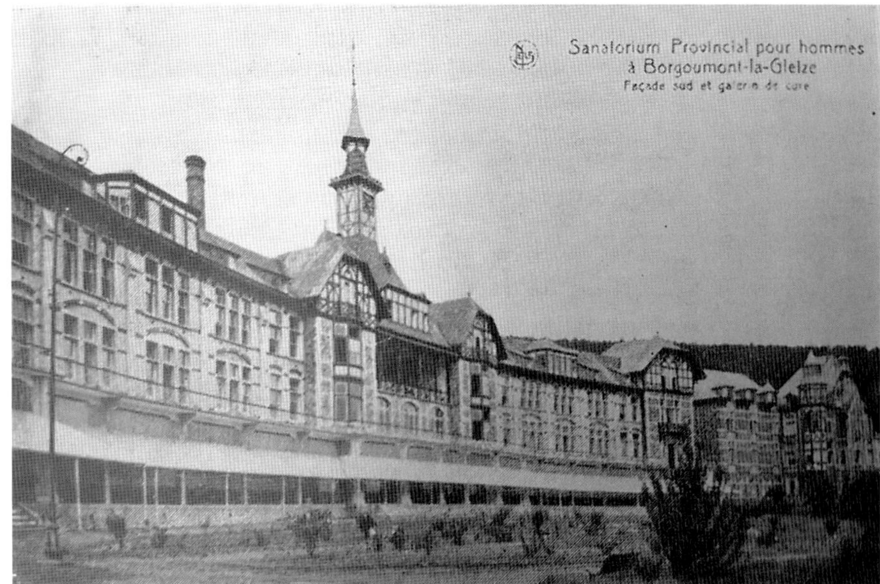

Fig. 1. The first sanatorium in Belgium [1], with permission.

An estimated 88,000 Belgians died during the conflict (1.05% of the total pre-war population), and one in 4 buildings was damaged in some way. The global loss suffered by Belgium was evaluated at 225–250 billion Belgian Francs, or 28–34% of the national wealth [3].

Tuberculosis Control in Belgium before WWII

Confronted with the ravages of tuberculosis (TB) in the 19th century, many health professionals, philanthropists, and other concerned people took private initiatives. In 1896, an order of nuns made beds available for TB patients in the first sanatorium, a former spa in Bokrijk [4], but it closed 12 years later in 1908 [5]. The first free medico-social TB clinic was established in Brussels by Dr Gustave Derscheid in 1897. In 1900, based on the idea of Albert Calmette in France, the first anti-TB dispensary was created in Liège by the visionary Dr Ernest Malvoz, who was also responsible for the construction in 1903 of the Borgoumont sanatorium (Fig. 1), for which he obtained the assistance of the provincial authorities. The same year, the first preventorium was opened on the North Sea coast [1]. The number of such institutions progressively increased, mostly after WWI, and in 1940 there were 103 dispensaries, 30 sanatoria (3,500 beds), 12 preventoria, and 4 open-air institutions for the protection of children [4].

The beginning of the 20th century is marked by the creation of 3 non-profit anti-TB organizations:

– the "Ligue Nationale contre la Tuberculose" in 1900, which took over the coordination of the dispensaries;

– the "Association Nationale Belge contre la Tuberculose" in 1923, which grew out of a number of organizations founded after 1902 that were involved in the construction and management of sanatoria;

– the "Oeuvre de Préservation de l'Enfance contre la Tuberculose" (1911), which managed the preventoria and foster care for children.

In addition to these organizations, health insurance agencies played a major role for their own beneficiaries [1, 4, 6].

Given the lack of coordination of TB activities, in 1929 the government created a unique public utility foundation, the "Oeuvre Nationale Belge de Défense contre la Tuberculose," into which all 3 previous organizations were integrated and which became the reference for all other TB initiatives. In 1919, before deciding on this fundamental reform, the Minister of Health requested the Superior Council of Public Hygiene to develop a plan for TB control as a basis for future legislation and as leverage for obtaining the budget to put these legal measures into place and make improvements in TB control. This plan confirmed the validity of the strategic approach applied until then and was based on the following pillars [1, 4, 6]:

1. Early diagnosis of infectious TB patients in dispensaries or through targeted mass screening.

2. Socioprophylaxis for patients and their families by social nurses performing home visits: education, social surveys, contact investigations, and welfare.

3. Isolation of infectious patients in sanatoria, hospitals or at home, if possible.

Table 1. Mortality rates in Belgium from 1900 to 1948

Years	Overall mortality (/100,000)	TB mortality (/100,000)			Contribution of TB to overall mortality, %
		pulmonary TB	non-pulmonary TB	all forms	
1900	1,928	136.2	20.0	156.2	8.1
1910	1,520	97.2	25.3	122.5	8.1
1920	1,384	88.7	26.5	116.0	8.4
1930	1,328	68.3	23.0	91.3	6.9
1940	1,612	54.1	14.9	69.0	4.3
1941	1,467	77.7	20.6	98.3	6.7
1942	1,473	74.3	21.0	95.3	6.5
1943	1,345	65.8	16.1	81.9	6.1
1944	1,574	66.2	15.5	81.7	5.2
1945	1,472	61.2	16.6	77.8	5.3
1946	1,340	52.1	13.7	65.8	4.9
1947	1,312	50.9	12.5	63.4	4.8
1948	1,239	43.9	10.9	54.8	4.4

Adapted from [1], with permission.

4. Transfer of infected children/adolescents to preventoria and non-infected children to open-air institutions or foster families in the countryside.

5. Treatment of active TB cases in sanatoria and hospitals, and follow-up and rehabilitation in active life after cure.

6. Targeted BCG use, especially for children living in contact with an infectious case.

7. Media campaigns to inform the population.

From initial private initiatives, TB control became progressively more organized and more structured with the assistance of the State, provincial and local authorities. In addition to regular allocations to the official institutions, a TB fund of 100 million Belgian Francs was allocated by law in 1930 for the construction and improvement of anti-TB institutions (dispensaries, sanatoria, and preventoria) [1].

Epidemiology of TB

Mortality

With the exception of WWI and WWII, the overall mortality rate decreased in Belgium as living conditions improved [1, 7]. During the period from 1900 to 1948, mortality dropped from 1,928 to 1,239/100,000 (Table 1).

TB was a real plague in the 19th century in Belgium with a TB mortality rate of 376.7/100,000 around 1850 [1, 6]. The situation improved, and in 1900, 1 death in 12 was caused by TB [8], corresponding to a TB mortality rate of 156.2/100,000; 50 years later it had fallen to 54.8/100,000 [1].

Evolution was favorable, in spite of an increase during the 2 World Wars, which was particularly steep in WWI [9]. Social hygiene, early diagnosis, and isolation of infectious patients gradually improved the TB situation [7, 8, 10]. From 1900 to 1948, the mortality rate for pulmonary TB decreased by 65%, while the overall mortality rate diminished by only 32%. The decrease in mortality due to other forms of TB was approximately 30% [1].

Jeurissen [11] reported that the mortality rate due to TB in Belgium decreased more quickly in the younger population and that among the deaths due to respiratory TB the proportion of persons over the age of 50 years increased progressively: 23% in 1935, 26% in 1940, 34% in 1945, and 43% in 1950. In comparison with other countries, the TB mortality in Belgium was more favorable at the beginning of the 20th century than in 1935, when the country was overtaken mainly by The Netherlands, the United States, Denmark, Germany, and Scotland [1, 6].

TB mortality decreased from 74.8/100,000 in 1935 to 68.2/100,000 in 1939. When the war broke out, there was no immediate impact on TB mortality, which remained at 69.0/100,000 in 1940. But it rose sharply to 98.3/100,000 in 1941, and remained high in 1942 (95.3/100,000). During the subsequent war years, it fell progressively to reach 77.8/100,000 in 1945. Once the war ended, TB mortality dropped to 65.8/100,000 in 1946, well below the rate at the beginning of the war [1, 6] (Table 1).

According to Daniels [9], there were 3 main groups of countries in Europe: one in which there was little or no wartime rise in TB mortality (e.g., Denmark), a second group in which there was a rise in the early years of the war and then a continuous fall (e.g., Belgium, England and Wales, Ireland, and France), and a third group in which there was a rise in the latter part of the war (e.g., Hungary and Austria).

In Belgium, the chaos of the first 2 years of the war is sufficient to explain the TB mortality peak in 1941, with the destruction and occupation of the sanatoria, discharge of patients to their homes, breakdown in food distribution, overcrowding, and lack of hygiene. However, the central TB organization was rapidly re-established, and by 1942 there were almost as many sanatorium beds available as before the war. Double rations were provided by dispensaries not only for patients with acute TB but also for those who had had active lesions in the last 5 years. All of the above can explain the rapid improvement after 1941 [9].

One particularly interesting aspect of the wartime rise in TB mortality was the more pronounced increase in men. This phenomenon was especially striking in Belgium. In 1941, at the peak of TB mortality, the increase over the 1938 rate was 49% in males and 36% in females. The subsequent decline was much slower in males: in 1944, the rate among females had returned to the pre-war level, and was 20% below this by 1947; the rate among males in 1944, however, was still 32% above the pre-war level and did not reach it till 1947. There was much less difference between the sexes for non-pulmonary TB [9]. This unequal trend in the decrease in TB mortality by sex was also highlighted by Tuyns and Fontaine [12].

Based on results from 1945, another specificity of TB mortality in men is that it continued to climb until the age of 60, while it remained almost stationary in women [1, 8]. The excess TB mortality in males was also observed in young children and in adults [1]. In the middle of the 19th century, this excess did not exist in Belgium; on the contrary, TB mortality was much higher among females than among males [1].

There has been much conjecture regarding the nature of the wartime rise. The additional deaths could be explained by patients who under normal conditions would have lived a little longer (premature death), or patients who would normally have overcome their disease and survived. In both events, the main factor responsible would be the deterioration in living conditions and nutrition, aggravating the prognosis of established disease [4, 6, 9]. These deaths could also have occurred among individuals who were being infected for the first time in greater numbers than normal due to increased exposure. There is no doubt that in most countries the increase was due to a combination of all 3 factors [9].

Morbidity

All statistics should be interpreted with caution, particularly morbidity [6, 7], which was not an epidemiological standard at that time [8]. In conditions of war, these are of practically no value for comparative purposes, either for comparison between successive years in the same country or between different countries [9]. In 1945, Gengou [6] wrote that the Belgian TB rate was not established correctly due to the lack of systematic and uniform notification by practitioners in dispensaries, even though TB was classified by the law of June 7, 1941 as an infectious disease that was legally notifiable [1, 4, 6]. Dispensaries may also not have diagnosed all the TB cases [6]. This situation changed during the war, however. Attendance at dispensaries rose significantly, in particular because TB patients were receiving food benefits [1, 6]. In addition, TB screening was organized in schools and factories with mobile X-ray units [1, 6]. The higher proportion of the population undergoing X-ray screening and the precise data collection by the dispensaries provided a better overview of the TB epidemic during this troubled period. Between 1940 and 1945, the number of TB patients registered by dispensaries increased from 79,000 to 156,299 [1] (Table 2).

Was this due to the better detection, or did it represent a real increase in TB? Some facts can attest to the veracity of the increase, particularly the greater proportion of new cases reported by the dispensaries in 1940 (44%) in comparison with 1939 (18%). However, due to the lack of good prewar statistics the exact rise cannot be precisely demonstrated [6].

What is questionable is the discrepancy between the trend in TB mortality and morbidity from 1943, with the former falling and the latter increasing [6, 9]. One explanation given by Gengou [6] is that during the first 2 years of WWII, attendance at dispensaries was lower, and as a consequence the proportion of TB patients who could benefit from the double food ration to reinforce their resistance to the disease was lower than in subsequent years. Daniels [9] reported that the Belgian authorities themselves evoked the possibility of over diagnosis by dispensaries confronted with hungry patients they could not refuse to help during the German occupation.

According to reports from medical doctors in the Belgian sanatoria, the lower resistance to TB as a consequence of the war could have been responsible for a change in the presentation of the disease, with more serious and evolving forms, mostly before 1942 and during 1944 [6].

Table 2. Workload of the TB dispensaries in Belgium from 1901 to 1948

Years	Dispensaries, *n*	Persons examined, *n*	TB patients registered, *n*	Medical doctors, *n*	Nurses, *n*
1901	1	1,250			
1930	97	67,598		199	140
1939	103	82,769	31,069	186	158
1940	105	101,993	43,900	188	156
1941	118	216,658	79,000	201	203
1942	126	290,548	111,752	222	247
1943	129	285,694	131,380	230	264
1944	129	273,496	131,049	228	259
1945	130	246,963	156,299	226	240
1946	130	277,548	146,904	233	250
1947	134	247,276	154,389	236	253
1948	129	300,579	123,443	230	239

Adapted from [1], with permission.

TB Control during and in the Aftermath of WWII: Situation and Special Measures

When the Germans invaded Belgium, the country was not ready to deal with the consequences of the war on the TB epidemic. Although there had been a considerable increase in the numbers of dispensaries and sanatoria since the beginning of the century, there were insufficient facilities, mainly in terms of sanatoria, preventoria, and institutions for isolating infectious patients [1, 6]. Based on an estimation of 2 beds per TB death, Belgium should have had about 14,000 beds, but only 6,098 beds were available in 1939 [6]. Education of the population on prophylactic measures was also deficient, as was BCG vaccination coverage [6].

During WWII in Belgium, the availability of facilities for TB management deteriorated, with both the destruction and requisition of institutions. At the beginning of the conflict, an estimated 4,400 TB beds were lacking in sanatoria and patients had to wait for months before entering [1, 6]. The objective of the health authorities was to increase institutional capacity to manage the growing numbers of TB patients. In 1942, the government voted to allocate 50 million Belgian Francs for the construction or renovation of dispensaries, sanatoria, and preventoria; this fund was managed by the Oeuvre Nationale Belge de Défense contre la Tuberculose. This allowed the number of dispensaries to be increased from 105 in 1940 to 129 in 1948 [1] (Table 2). However, even with these new or transitional constructions, the number of beds remained insufficient, and around 1,500 beds were still lacking in 1948 [6], mostly for men [13]. One alternative was to send patients to Switzerland, where buildings were rented or bought by Belgian organizations to care, in priority, for soldiers, prisoners of war, and children with TB [1].

In 1943, another decision taken by Belgian authorities was to allocate funds under certain conditions to hospitals, with the objective of creating specific wards to receive chronic bedridden TB patients not eligible for sanatorium care, TB persons requiring urgent hospitalization for medical/social reasons, and those who were waiting to enter a sanatorium [6]. Another objective was to create sorting centers where patients with presumptive TB could be referred to when the diagnosis required special methods and hospitalization [6].

If providing for beds for TB patients was a priority during and after the war [14], early TB diagnosis was another priority. Efforts were made to maintain dispensaries in all regions of the country, but emphasis was also placed on systematic screening of collectivities by X-ray mobile units [1, 6]. Belgium was one of the first countries to follow this approach in the 1930s [1]. During the war, more than 300,000 individuals were screened at the request of schools, factories, and administrations [6]. In 1943, the Department of Justice also requested systematic annual screening in institutions hosting child and adult patients with mental illness [1].

Just before the war, in response to the lack of nurses, Derscheid, the practitioner who had created the first free medico-social TB clinic in Belgium, established a new certificate for a "sanatorium auxiliary." In this way, trained women with TB who were receiving treatment in a sanatorium could work under the supervision of graduate nurses and take on duties that did not require nursing skills [1]. In the dispensaries, which were pivotal structures for TB control in Belgium, there was also a chronic staff shortage to take on the considerable workload even though staffing levels were raised from 156 nurses and 188 doctors in 1940 to 264 nurses and 230 doctors by 1943 [1] (Table 2).

The socioeconomic situation was desperate during the war, and the population suffered mostly at the beginning due to the total disorganization of everyday life, particularly for the refugees who had fled during the exodus, most of whom returned to Belgium in mid-October 1940 [3]. In addition, at the beginning of October 1940, 225,000 men, 13% of the active male population, were being held as prisoners of war in Nazi Germany. This situation had a massive impact on work and the organization of family life. Women thus played a key role in occupied Belgium in an extremely difficult context of general shortages, limited family resources, support to prisoners, and psychological stress [3]. At the end of 1942, the introduction of forced labor in Germany further exacerbated the shortage of active men [3].

One of the first actions of the new military administration during the occupation was to establish food rationing [3]. While during peacetime, the average daily diet was estimated at 2,480 calories, it was only 1,400–1,900 calories with rationing, and even less when there were shortages [6]. A diet lacking in animal protein, fat and calcium was the rule [6]. Apart from those who resorted to the black market or who had their own gardens, the search for food was difficult and hunger progressively appeared, particularly in the cities. Food shortages were further aggravated by the requisitions by the German army and exportation towards Germany [3]. Importation of food supplements from neighboring countries was necessary for the population's survival [3]. For the most underprivileged, including some TB patients, a system of mutual assistance was created in October 1940 under the name of "secours d'hiver" (winter aid) [4] ; from 1940 to 1944, around 1.3 million people, of whom 750,000 were children, received help to survive [2, 3]. From July 1940, a double food ration was granted to TB patients, provided they were enrolled in a dispensary which was responsible for delivering a specific certificate confirming that the patient suffers from TB [6].

Social and material aid for TB patients and their families was already being organized before the war by TB organizations, and continued during the conflict. The role of health insurance services and their TB funds based on mutual assistance was also very important [6]. Although registration was not mandatory, around 50% of the population had health insurance [1, 6]. As pointed by Daniels [14], there was great progress in social medicine in Europe during and after the war, and the concept of the community's duty to protect itself as a whole as well as each individual who may suffer misfortune, was adopted in many countries. In Belgium, a new compulsory health insurance scheme was established with the law of December 28, 1944 [1].

After the worsening of the TB situation at the beginning of the war, TB notification became mandatory by law in June 1941 for epidemiological and prophylaxis purposes [1, 4, 6]. This was very controversial, as private practitioners were worried about privacy and breaches of professional secrecy; accordingly obligatory notification was not properly applied during the conflict and its aftermath, except by TB institutions [6].

TB vaccination in Belgium is far from having had the development observed in some neighboring countries. Although there was a certain interest at the end of the 1920s, the skepticism and indifference on the part of practitioners led to only targeted use of BCG [1, 6]. During WWII, one of the main applications was the protection of young children with a negative tuberculin reaction, who were in contact with an infectious TB patient. Belgium never applied systematic BCG vaccination at birth. From 1935 to 1943, around 55,000 doses of BCG were produced by 4 laboratories [6]. In 1947, the steering committee of the "Ligue Nationale contre la Tuberculose" decided to create a BCG technical working group to revise the Belgian position. The final report recommended establishing a central office to centralize BCG activities which was implemented in 1948. Its objective was not only to organize BCG vaccination in targeted communities, but also to raise awareness in concerned institutions and inform the population through flyers and conferences [1].

Propaganda for good hygiene was organized in Belgium from the start of its TB control activities [1], with messages and means of communication being adapted over the years (Fig. 2). Films were used in the field of TB prevention to reach as much of the population as possible; 2 of these date from 1938 and 1948, respectively. A special commission was created after the war to extend the education and information program [1].

Conclusion

Similar to what had occurred during WWI, Belgium paid a high price for TB in WWII, with an increase in mortality and morbidity; however, these years of conflict were also an opportunity to stimulate energy, good will, and political commitment to improve TB control [1].

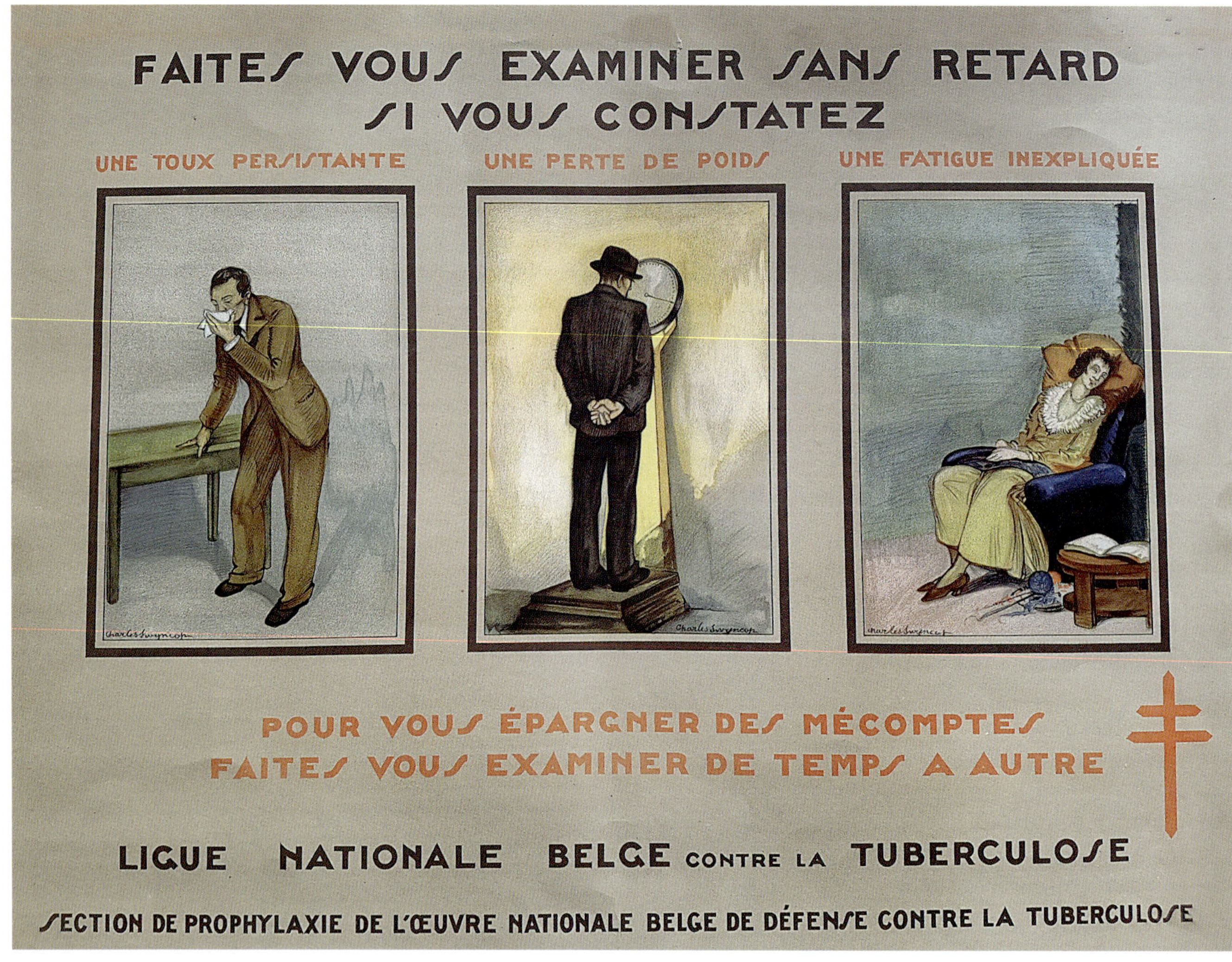

Fig. 2. TB poster edited in Belgium. Private collection of the Belgian Lung and TB Association, with permission.

According to Daniels [9], the TB disaster was not as pronounced during WWII as in previous wars, most notably WWI. This was particularly the case in countries like Belgium, where public health services had expanded significantly between the 2 wars. These services were initially able to absorb the impact of the war, but as living conditions worsened, the TB situation deteriorated as well. It was possible to reverse this trend by providing a strong response as soon as the situation allowed. This effort was maintained once the war was over.

References

1 Œuvre Nationale Belge de Défense contre la Tuberculose. 50 années de lutte contre la tuberculose en Belgique, 1897–1947. Brussels: Œuvre Nationale Belge de Défense contre la Tuberculose, 1950.

2 De Launay J: La Belgique à l'heure allemande. Brussels, Editions J. M. Collet, 1981.

3 De Launay J, Offergeld J: La vie quotidienne des Belges sous l'occupation 1940–1945. Brussels, Editions Paul Legrain, 1982.

4 Praet G: La lutte antituberculeuse en Belgique. Brussels, Editions La Flambée, 1943.

5 Vanhees B, Marut A, Zoons J: Het sanatorium van Bokrijk. Van Kneipp-inrichting tot TBC-behandeling. Retroscoop. http://www.retroscoop.com/maatschappij.php?artikel=103 Accessed August 2017.

6 Gengou O: L'endémie tuberculeuse et sa prophylaxie. Brussels, Ligue Nationale Belge contre la Tuberculose, 1945.

7 Millet M: Cinquante ans de lutte antituberculeuse en Belgique. Acta Tuberc Pneumol Belg 1975;66:27–35.

8 Gyselen A: Tuberculosis in Belgium: past, present and future. Acta Clinica Belgica 1994;49:125–131.

9 Daniels M: Tuberculosis in Europe during and after the Second World War-I. BMJ 1949;2:1065–1072.

10 Millet M: Remarques sur l'état actuel de l'endémie tuberculeuse. Brochure: 1–14. Extrait de la revue l'Enfant de l'Oeuvre Nationale de l'Enfance, 1964;no. 1 (This last publication is available in the archives of the Belgian Royal Library).

11 Jeurissen A: La fréquence et la gravité de la tuberculose respiratoire selon le sexe et l'année de naissance du malade. Acta Tuberc Pneumol Belg 1963; 54:345–431.

12 Tuyns A, Fontaine Y: La mortalité par tuberculose en Belgique. Acta Tuberc Belg 1958;49:331–343.

13 Tuyns A, Landrain J: Etude statistique sur l'endémie tuberculeuse en Belgique (1948). Brussels, Acta Medica Belgica, 1952.

14 Daniels M: Tuberculosis in Europe during and after the Second World War-II. BMJ 1949;2:1135–1140.

Dr. Maryse Wanlin
Belgian Lung and Tuberculosis Association (BELTA)
rue de la Concorde, 56
BE–1050 Brussels (Belgium)
E-Mail maryse.wanlin@fares.be

Murray JF, Loddenkemper R (eds): Tuberculosis and War. Lessons Learned from World War II.
Prog Respir Res. Basel, Karger, 2018, vol 43, pp 152–164 (DOI: 10.1159/000481483)

Tuberculosis in Southern European Countries and the Balkans before, during, and after World War II

Giorgia Sulis[a] · Lia D'Ambrosio[b, c] · Rosella Centis[b] · Raquel Duarte[d] ·
José-María García-García[e] · Giovanni Battista Migliori[b]

[a]University Department of Infectious and Tropical Diseases, WHO Collaborating Centre for TB/HIV and TB Elimination – University of Brescia, Brescia, and [b]WHO Collaborating Centre for TB and Lung Diseases, Maugeri Care and Research Institute, Tradate, Italy; [c]Public Health Consulting Group, Lugano, Switzerland; [d]National Reference Centre for MDR-TB, Hospital Centre Vila Nova de Gaia, Department of Pneumology, Public Health Science and Medical Education Department, Faculty of Medicine, University of Porto, Porto, Portugal; [e]Tuberculosis Research Programme, Spanish Respiratory Society (SEPAR), Barcelona, Spain

Abstract

As observed throughout, virtually all of Europe, the burden of tuberculosis (TB) in Southern Europe and the Balkan region was significantly influenced by World War I (WWI) and World War II (WWII) during the first half of the 20th century. The already precarious socioeconomic and living conditions of these countries were dramatically worsened by both wars, which fostered the spread of epidemic TB infection and disease for decades. TB was generally recognized as a major public health concern, and the introduction of sanatoria after the turn of the century, though slow and unevenly distributed throughout the national territory, led to considerable improvements in TB care. The first social protection measures aimed at providing support to affected patients and limiting the catastrophic impact of the disease on individuals and the community, were adopted in that period and opened the way for future strategic interventions. Based on the limited data that are available through scientific literature, national/regional surveys and other relevant reports, we provide an overview on the epidemiological situation and TB disease control efforts in Greece, Italy, Spain, Portugal, Bulgaria, Romania, and former Yugoslavia from WWI throughout the second post-WWII period.

© 2018 S. Karger AG, Basel

The aim of this chapter is to describe the efforts to control tuberculosis (TB) during, between, and after the 2 World Wars (WWI and WWII) in Southern European countries (Greece, Italy, Portugal, and Spain) and in the Balkan region (Bulgaria, Romania, and former Yugoslav countries). Figure 1 shows which of these countries were German allies in 1943, occupied by Germany or neutral (Fig. 1).

Published articles, books, and national or regional reports were searched to retrieve relevant information on the epidemiological situation and organization of the health system in each country. TB experts from all the selected organizations were interviewed to increase the sensitivity of the inquiry. Unfortunately, only a fragmented picture of the fight against TB in the period could be obtained from available documents. However, important information on epidemiology – incidence, prevalence, and mortality and their trends through the war times, and including the development of health services (sanatoria, dispensaries, etc.), response of the national anti-TB associations and organization of health schemes, plus the precursors of the currently recommended universal health coverage and social protection measures – were described to the extent possible. Images useful to introduce the reader to the spirit of the fight against TB infection and disease at the time were also included.

Italy

Epidemiological Trends

Like other European countries, TB represented an important public health problem in Italy during the first half of the 20th century. Available data show that the mortality rate from all forms of TB fell by as much as 70% over a 50-

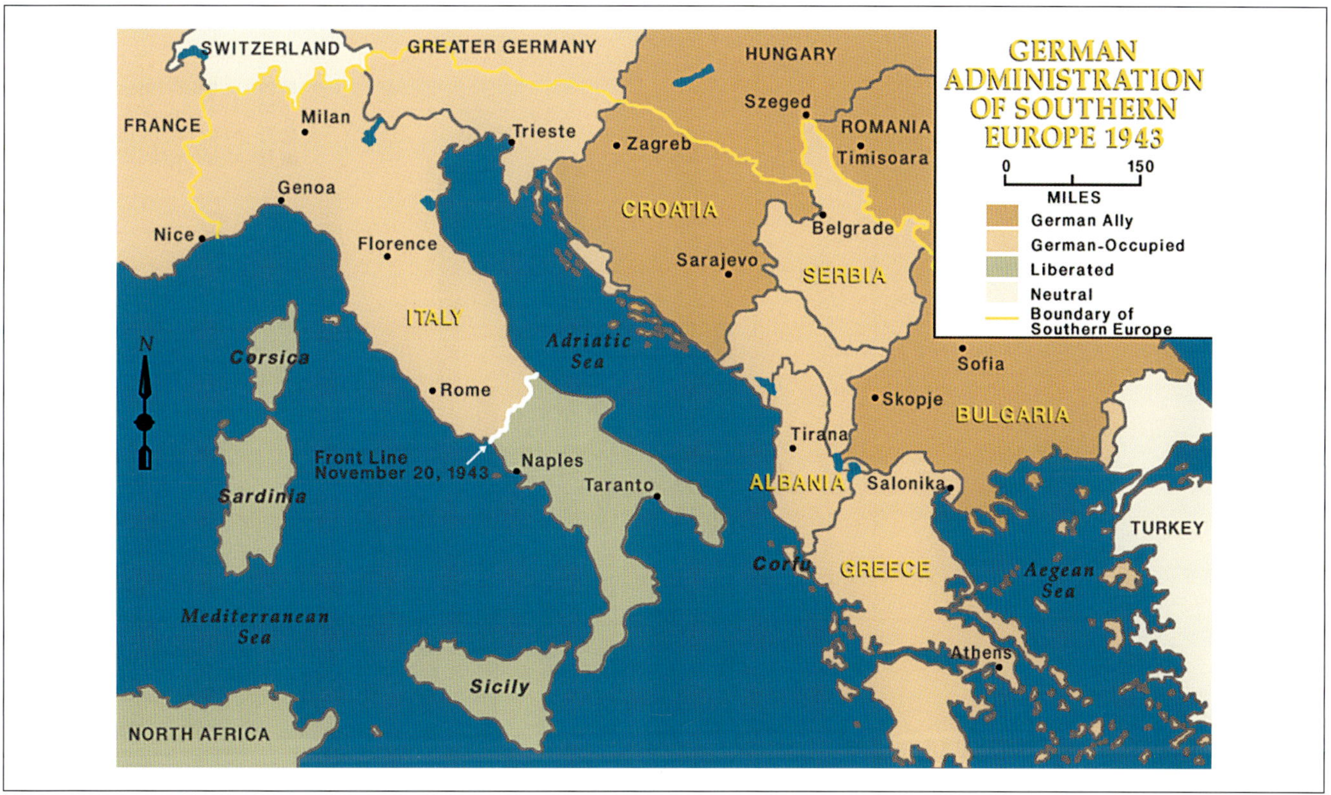

Fig. 1. German administration of Southern Europe and the Balkans in 1943 showing which of these countries were at that time German allies, occupied by Germany or neutral. US Holocaust Memorial Museum, with permission.

year time span, declining from a national average of 177/100,000 in 1898–1899 to 55/100,000 in 1948–1949 [1]. In 1898–1899, most TB deaths were reported in Northern Italy, with Liguria and Lombardy accounting for the highest rates (226 and 214/100,000, respectively), but epidemiological trends evolved at a different pace in different regions such that in 1948–1949 TB was responsible for a higher number of deaths in Trentino-Alto Adige (89/100,000) and Sardinia (72/100,000; Fig. 2). Despite the overall decline, the proportion of pulmonary cases rose over time compared to that of extra-pulmonary forms of TB: the ratio between them changed from 1.4 to 3.2 during the period, corresponding to an increase of 230% [1]. Interestingly, the proportion of patients who died from extra-pulmonary TB constantly exceeded that of pulmonary cases in all areas with a prevalent rural economy – such as most of the South – compared to more industrialized settings, which are predominantly concentrated in the North of the country.

Besides the direct consequences of war, the rising phenomenon of rural-to-urban migration across Italy significantly contributed to the heterogeneity of TB epidemiology between and within regions since the turn of century [2]. In fact, urban centers with a population of over 100,000 inhabitants accounted for the greatest TB burden, reflecting the effects of poorer housing conditions, overcrowding, and air pollution secondary to industrialization: mortality rates due to TB in these contexts exceeded the national average by 12% at the end of the 19th century and by 36% in the middle of the 1900s (202 and 86/100,000, respectively), which is in line with the 3-fold increase in the urban population in the whole country [1].

The rapid deterioration of general living conditions accompanied by the partial dismantlement of health care services that occurred during war led to a sharp increase in TB mortality in the country in both 1914–1918 and 1942–1944, particularly in the Northern and Central regions that were more heavily affected by the conflicts [3]. Of note, while the overall TB death rate reached a peak of 210/100,000 at the end of WWI and then decreased to about 140/100,000 population in the period 1920–1925, it then plummeted to around 75/100,000 in 1938 (Fig. 3). However, during WWII it rose again up to 100/100,000 in 1942–1944 and almost returned to the pre-war levels by 1946 [3–5].

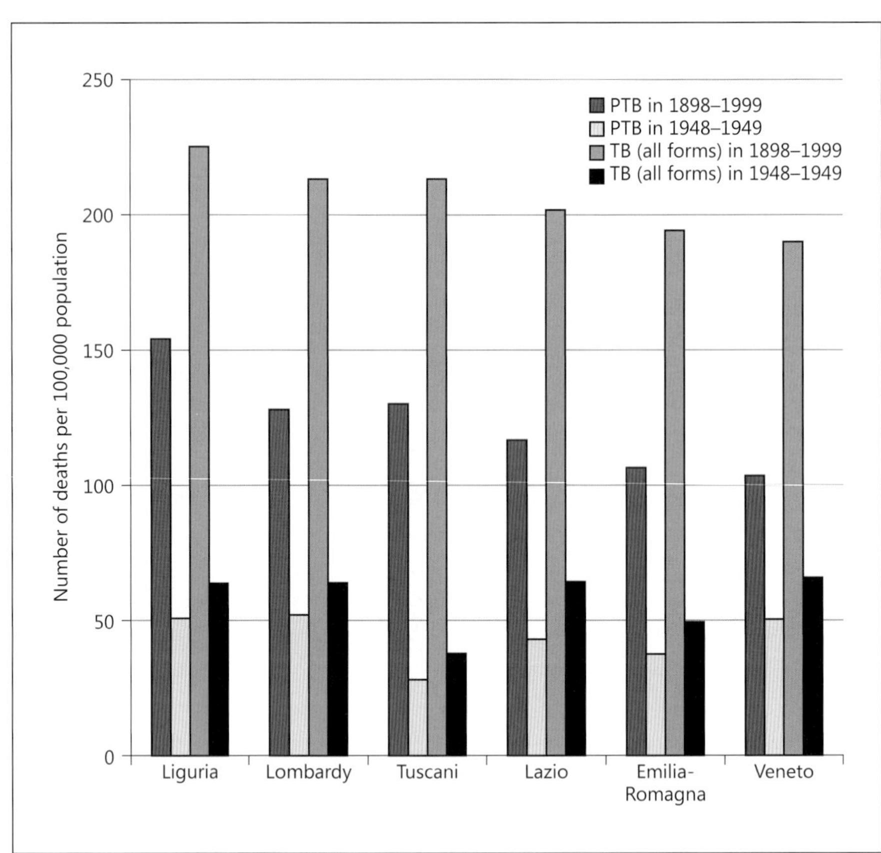

Fig. 2. Number of deaths from pulmonary tuberculosis (PTB) and from all forms of TB in 6 Italian regions with the highest burden of disease in 1898–1999 and 1948–1949, data from [5].

It is worth noting that among the major infectious diseases, TB was by far the highest cause of mortality: according to available data, it accounted for 63% of all deaths due to infections in 1938–1940, 33,928 out of a total of 53,812, which included influenza, typhus, diphtheria, pertussis, syphilis, measles, malaria, scarlet fever, and smallpox, with a considerable growing trend in comparison with half a century before, 64,500/190,086 deaths caused by TB in 1887–1889, corresponding to 34% of the total [6].

Evolution of Anti-TB Response Around World War II
Under the influence of the significant scientific advancements that occurred in the field of microbiology during the last few decades of the 19th century, culminating in 1882 with the discovery of *Mycobacterium tuberculosis* by Robert Koch, a number of local associations were established in many Italian cities to promote the fight against TB, together with the growing awareness that this subtle yet incredibly dreadful disease could not be addressed through the quarantine-based measures that were usually adopted to cope with common epidemics such as those of typhus or diphtheria. However, until the 1920s the bulk of anti-TB efforts

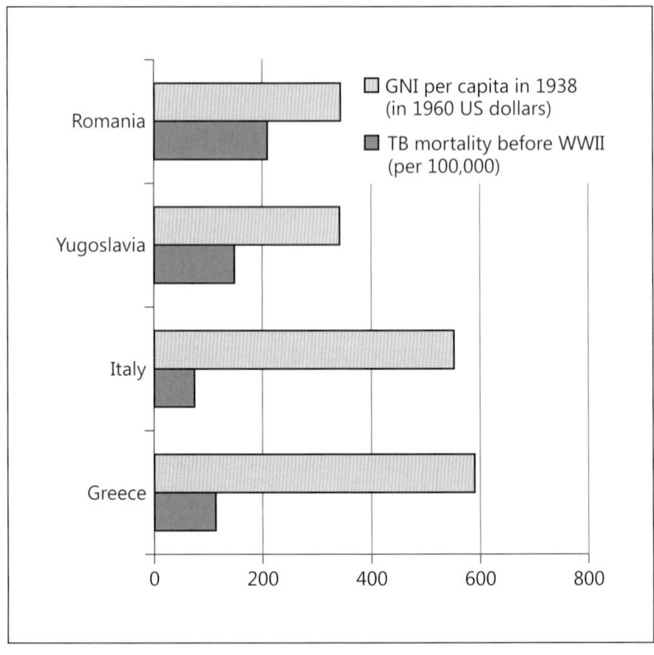

Fig. 3. Estimated TB mortality (per 100,000 population) and gross national income (GNI) per capita (in USD 1,960) in 4 European countries before the outbreak of World War II, data from [4, 5, 17, 18].

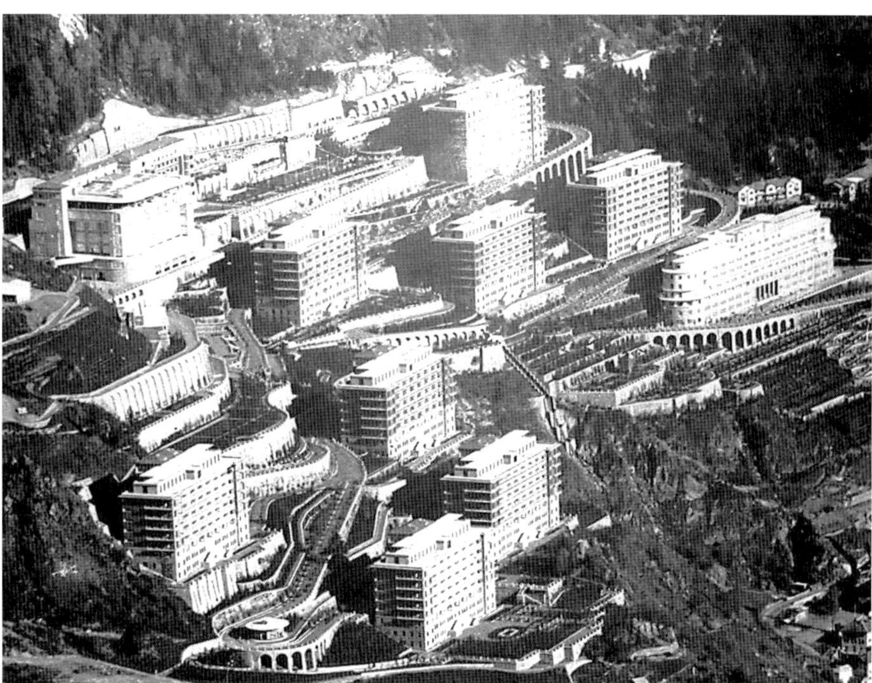

Fig. 4. Historical picture of Sondalo TB Sanatorium, Italy, courtesy of Prof. Giovanni Battista Migliori.

arose from the community through the use of private funds, while governmental institutions seemed not to recognize the importance of TB in the overall health situation of the country. Sanatoria, as well as TB dispensaries, appeared in Italy at the beginning of the 20th century but they were mostly isolated developments rather than part of a nationwide design [5]. The very first Italian sanatorium was built in 1903 near Sondalo, in the Alps of Northern Italy at 1,240 m above sea level, though it achieved worldwide fame between 1932 and 1940, when a new complex of buildings was erected farther below (at an altitude of approximately 1,000 m) to become the largest sanatorium throughout Europe with its 3,500 beds and a total area of 350,000 m^2 (Fig. 4) [6, 7]. In accordance with the pioneering German and Swiss experiences, the therapeutic approach to TB in these institutions was mainly based on a combination of residence at high altitude, rest, overfeeding, and adoption of strict hygienic precautions, all aimed at restoring the physical fitness of patients who were often weak and debilitated because of their precarious living and working conditions.

Since 1919, anti-TB services began to be institutionalized and a royal legislative decree of 1927 (R.D.L. 27 October 1927 n. 2055) established that specific public offices devoted to TB care and prevention at provincial level had to be developed in compliance with well-regulated tasks and objectives. The nationalization of TB-related intervention was accompanied by the introduction of a compulsory insurance

program provided by the National Institute of Social Providence to all affected patients or their families [8]. The general improvements in the management of TB together with the provision of financial benefits significantly contributed to the steep decline in TB mortality throughout the 1920 and 1930s.

Thanks to such interventions, the capacity of national-level sanatoria nearly tripled between 1923 and 1930, when 32,000 beds were available for TB-affected individuals. This trend continued during the following years and, despite the difficulties encountered during WWII, 3 years after the end of the conflict as many as 90,000 hospital beds were reserved for TB. Nearly one third of them were in urban centers with a population of over 100,000 people, corresponding to a ratio of 3 TB beds per 1,000 inhabitants, compared to the national average of 2 per 1,000 [1]. Yet, in the biggest cities, such as Milan, dispensaries were considerably more developed and numerically prevalent than sanatoria, and they were mostly involved in preventative and supportive interventions rather than therapeutic ones [6].

Unlike other European countries, Bacille Calmette-Guérin (BCG) vaccination was never introduced as a compulsory measure in Italy. Although prevention had been widely mentioned throughout the 1920 and 1930s as a pivotal aspect of TB control, no specific reference to BCG has ever been made in national policies. Public and expert opinion on the advantages and disadvantages of this intervention remained a matter of debate for several years, such that the first legislative decree to explicitly give directions on its use was issued as late as 1970 [9, 10].

The development of a widely distributed network of TB care centers with a homogeneous distribution throughout the national territory favored the growth of scientific and academic activities in the speciality of TB, with the aim of better understanding the physiopathological mechanisms of the disease, improving its clinical and surgical management, and optimizing public health measures to prevent further transmission. The first Medical Specialty Schools of Pneumology and Tisiology were inaugurated a few years before the outbreak of WWII in Rome (1935) and Naples (1939), thus reflecting the new commitment of governmental institutions against TB. The Italian Federation against Social Lung Diseases and TB, that was founded in 1922 and joined the International Union against Tuberculosis (The Union) 1 year later, convened national conferences almost annually since 1923 and, after an inevitable 5-year suspension during the war, organized a new edition soon after the conflict ended [11]. Note that after the closure of the Paris Office of the International Union against Tuberculosis by the Germans in 1940, a new Union (Vereinigung) was founded in November 1941, with its headquarters in Berlin. Fifteen states, all belonging to the Axis Alliance, became members. Raffaele Paolucci from Italy was elected as President (for details, see Chapter 5). In spite of the limited participation to these activities because of the logistic difficulties in attending the meetings as a consequence of the desperate situation that had befallen the country, and notably the Northern regions, in the immediate post-conflict period. The group of experts who managed to gather in Rome in June 1945 underlined the need to urgently promote bold policies to address the threat of TB which had spread exponentially over the previous years. Nevertheless, even in the middle of WWII TB research never stopped and as soon as peace was restored, important findings were promptly discussed and distributed between 1947 and 1950 concerning the biological basis of susceptibility to infection, the factors associated with disease progression, and the benefits of streptomycin for the treatment of active TB [12–16].

Romania and Bulgaria

The evolution and trends of infectious diseases in most Eastern European countries are unfortunately poorly known, because most of the relevant documents were lost during WWII and the Soviet occupation. According to the 1881 estimates, TB mortality among Romanian males and females was around 464 and 338/100, respectively, with a peak in infants up to 12 months of age and in adults aged over 40 years. Statistics from Bucharest reveal that the rate of TB-attributable deaths constantly decreased over time, declining from 362 to 209/100,000 between 1900 and 1940, with 85% of cases having pulmonary involvement (Fig. 3) [4, 5, 17, 18]. In line with what happened elsewhere, the burden of TB was typically greater in densely populated urban settings: in fact, mortality rates were higher in the capital city than in other towns and considerably lower in rural areas. We can reasonably assume that a similar situation could be observed in Bulgaria, although specific data are lacking.

In accordance with the archives of the Bulgarian Society of Lung Diseases, the first sanatorium of the country (with a capacity of only 50 beds) was opened in 1905 and a few others developed in the following years. The first dispensary was established in Sofia in 1910 to provide diagnostic and therapeutic services including radiographic examination. Preventative measures began to be put in place after the end of the WWI, and BCG vaccination made its appearance in Bulgaria in 1928, though no mass vaccination campaigns were conducted until many years later. By 1944, 22 dispensaries and 2,900 hospital beds were available in the entire country, but their number rapidly rose to 95 dispensaries and 5389 beds in 1952, though still far from the needed number.

TB continued to represent a major scourge in both Romania and Bulgaria, which were among the least economically developed European countries in the interwar period (Fig. 3), with a very slow and troubled growth after the end of WWII. By contrast, in western countries the modern transformation of social progress and longevity was reaching ever higher levels with considerable improvements in life expectancy and population health status: the southern and eastern peripheries of the continent could not keep the pace and disparities remained huge [19].

Greece

Epidemiological Trends
In spite of its glorious past history, by the first few decades of the 20th century, Greek economy was among the weakest in Europe, being largely based on agriculture and highly dependent on importation of goods from abroad. The modernization process had evolved quite slowly after obtaining independence from the Ottoman Empire in 1829, thus lead-

ing to little progress in a mostly undeveloped country [20]. Since the 1920s, the industrial sector began to emerge in circumscribed areas and was accompanied by a massive population movement from the countryside, such that by 1928 over 45% of all Greeks lived in urban or semi-urban areas. Nevertheless, the general living conditions remained dreadful and it is estimated that more than 30% of the population suffered from undernutrition before the outbreak of WWII [17]. The effects of the conflict on an already devastated country were massive, and the overall mortality rapidly grew by at least 5-fold during that period. The German, Italian, and Bulgarian occupations, the blockage of imports and the long-lasting hyperinflation put a severe strain on Greece, and things got much worse after 1944, when the 6-year civil war began [20]. In such a dramatic scenario, health conditions became extremely compromised.

However, as clearly described by a medical officer from UNRRA (United Nations Relief and Rehabilitation Administration), who explored Greece in the immediate post-war period to assess the TB situation in the country, no sharp increases in the incidence and mortality of the disease seem to have occurred [17]. In fact, since TB services were almost absent throughout the national territory, patients converged to the capital for TB diagnosis and treatment, thus favoring a sort of segregation of persons with active disease into some locations, which probably limited the spread of the disease in the rest of the country. However, since diagnostic tools such as radiology and diagnostic laboratory equipment were essentially unavailable, TB confirmation could not be obtained for most cases, thus making it very difficult to draw a reliable epidemiological picture over time. The TB mortality rate in Greece was estimated at 116/100,000 in 1938, corresponding to some 8,230 deaths in the whole country, though this figure is likely to underestimate the real burden of the problem, because notification was not compulsory (Fig. 3) [17, 18]. In accordance with what was known, available data show an important discrepancy between urban and rural areas, with an average ratio between them of 5 to 2. Substantial differences were also observed among the diverse regions, with Central Greece afflicted by the heaviest burden, while Crete and the Aegean Islands had the lowest rates (Fig. 5). This geographic distribution probably reflects the more favorable climatic conditions of certain areas as well as their limited population density.

Evolution of Anti-TB Response Around World War II
Before WWII, a considerable number of TB-affected individuals became concentrated in the Attic region, around Athens, where the majority of anti-TB services of the entire country were located, with 4,527 beds reserved for TB [17]. Because several structures were severely damaged during WWII, fewer than usual beds were actually available at the beginning of 1945, but returned to the pre-war levels within a year or so, which was unfortunately considerably far from the real needs (Fig. 3).

In 1945, the distribution of dispensaries throughout the national territory was also rather uneven, with 23 of them located in Athens and a total of 26 countrywide, whereas extended areas such as Macedonia, Thrace, Thessaly, Epirus, and the Islands had none (Fig. 5) [17]. The Sotiria Sanatorium (near Athens) and the Asvestochorion Sanatorium (at Salonica) stood out as the most famous institutions, the former being among the largest in the world with its nearly 2,000 potentially available beds, and the latter with a capacity of about 600 beds. However, these structures had very little in common with their equivalents in most Western European countries, where rigorous therapeutic schedules were followed to ensure patients the best possible hygienic and nutritional conditions. In sharp contrast with this approach, Greek sanatoria were overcrowded places run by untrained personnel, with almost no rules for resident patients. Such a precarious situation should not be surprising if we think that the national health expenditure, which had always been negligible, accounted for only 6% of the total governmental budget in 1940–41 and that less than 8% of this inadequate amount was allocated for TB [17].

Thanks to voluntary organizations (the Red Cross above all), a few "preventoria" were opened in Greece after 1943, with the aim of isolating infected patients (especially children) who did not have symptoms of active disease but were considered at high risk of progression. Unfortunately, these institutions had short lifespans due to the huge financial shortage of the country, which did not allow sustainability of their costs. Besides this attempt, the most important preventative intervention that was put in place was definitely the vaccination campaign with BCG in early childhood, started in 1925 by the Red Cross [21]. Until the end of WWII, the only vaccination site was in Athens, but by 1948 a nationwide campaign on tuberculin-negative individuals up to 18 years of age was actively promoted since 1948 and a full coverage was reached within 1951. By that year, 22.7% of the eligible population had a positive tuberculin skin test, and the other 77.3% received BCG and were kept in isolation for 6–8 weeks afterwards as per national protocols [21].

In early 1945, a new tailored program to fight TB in Greece started to be implemented by the Ministry of Hygiene under the guidance of UNRRA. Special attention was

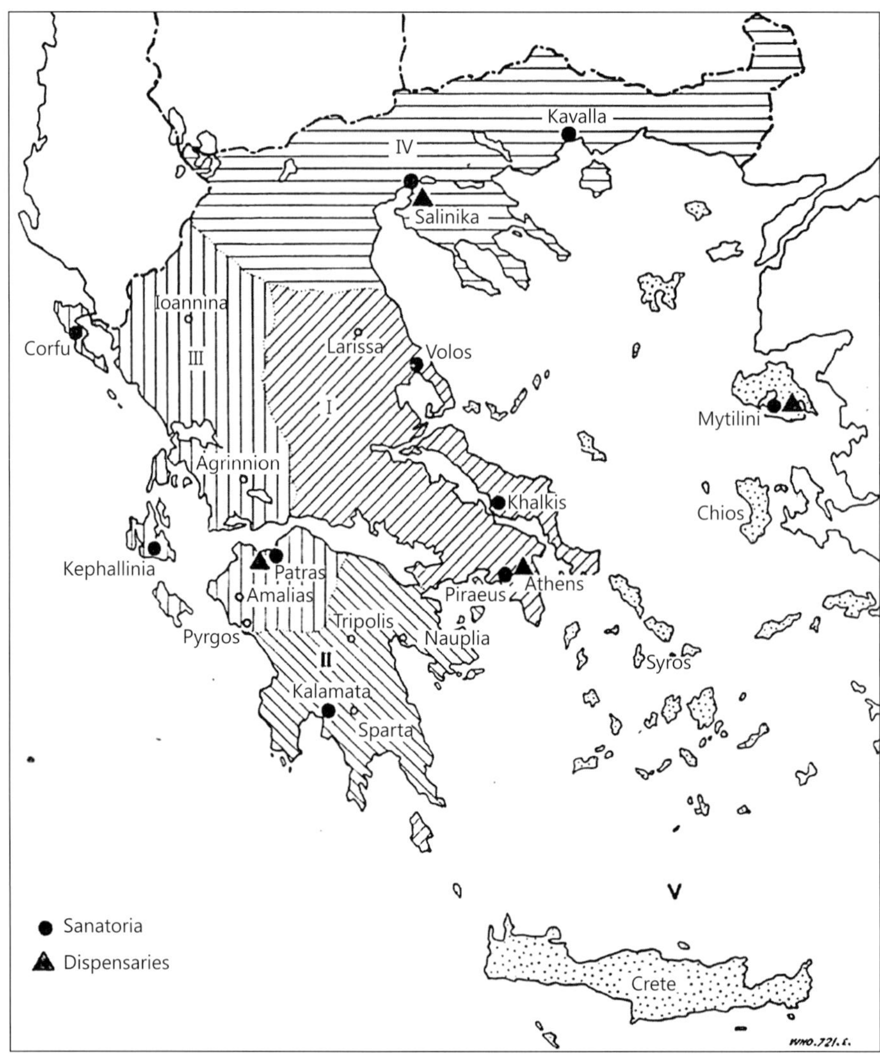

Fig. 5. Distribution of anti-tuberculosis institutions (sanatoria and dispensaries) in Greece at the beginning of 1945 [17], with permission.

reserved to training, because most health professionals operating in the country had very little knowledge of TB and its management principles. Mass radiology, which was also performed for the first time in Athens, permitted the calculation of some rough estimates of TB prevalence – approximately, 3% of the urban population – but large-scale implementation of this technique remained impractical, due to high cost, lack of skilled personnel, and poor acceptability among the local population [17].

Although plans had been made for the reconstruction and expansion of the TB services network throughout Greece, implementation took a long time, and the results were poorer than expected, as other priorities were set by the government and insufficient funds were actually allocated for TB. Of course, the continuation of the Civil War until 1951 worsened the already precarious circumstances.

Yugoslavia

Very little information is available concerning the TB situation in former Yugoslav countries around WWII; moreover, available documents mostly cover only circumscribed locations, thus providing a fragmented picture that cannot be generalized at the national level. In spite of the Kingdom's attempt to create a centralized state, socioeconomic gaps among different regions created sharp differences. It should not be surprising that most of our current knowledge about TB epidemiology and the organization of TB care services actually comes from the wealthiest parts of the country (Serbia and Slovenia above all).

Since documents were intentionally destroyed after the foundation of the Socialist Federal Republic of Yugoslavia, no reliable statistics are available to document the burden of

Sulis et al.

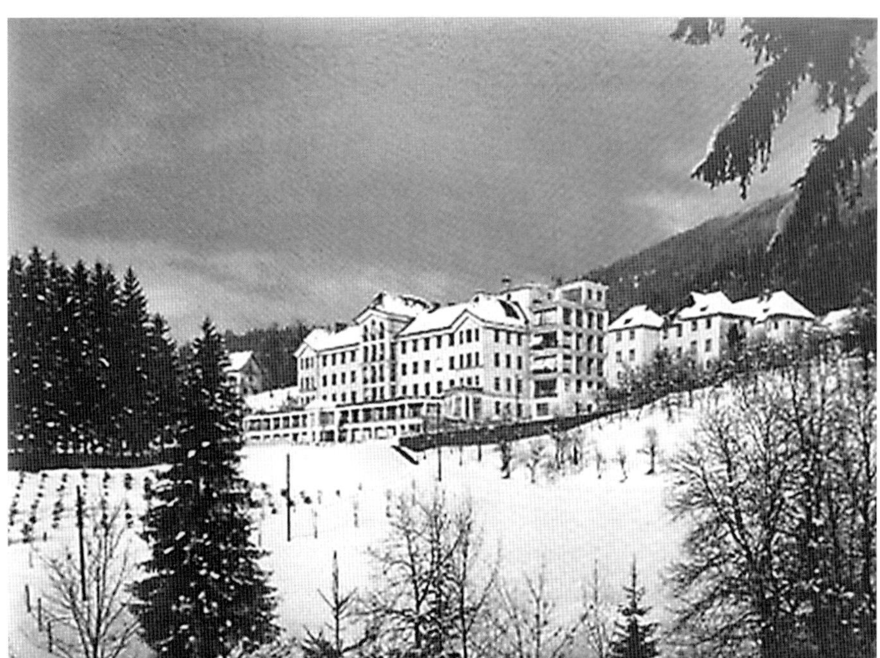

Fig. 6. Historical picture of Golnik TB Sanatorium, Slovenia [22], with permission.

TB in the area during the first half of the 20th century. It was estimated that the TB death rate exceeded 150/100,000 in the 1920s and very few changes seem to have occurred over the next 2 decades (Fig. 3) [4, 5, 17, 18]. In 1947, national TB mortality almost touched 200/100,000, though lower rates were registered in some areas such as Slovenia, where less than 110/100,000 were due to TB, but still reflected the deplorable effects of WWII [22].

In the interwar period, the sanatorium system thrived, with as many as 27 new centers built in Serbia, mostly around the city of Novi Sad, in Vojvodina, between 1920 and 1939 in addition to the 14 already in existence, modeled after their equivalents in Western Europe. Yet, all such improvements remained unevenly distributed throughout the country. Curiously, only 2 of the above-mentioned new institutions (one private and one public) were devoted to the management of active pulmonary TB cases, while the majority were mainly focused on surgical treatment of extrapulmonary TB forms and other diseases [23]. The medical staff operating in Serbian sanatoria were highly trained professionals with extensive experience abroad, and tried to introduce the most modern technologies and therapeutic approaches that were already being used in other countries. However, most of these institutions were privately run and had a very limited bed capacity, both of which hindered people's ability to access care.

By contrast, in the mid-1930s only 3 sanatoria were operative in Slovenia (Topolšica, Golnik, and Vurberg, respectively, which were founded in 1919, 1921, and 1923), and 5 were established in Croatia (Klenovnik, Brestovac, Strmac, Novi Marof, and Kraljevica). Golnik sanatorium was among the largest centers of the entire country, with its 240 beds in 1940 that survived WWII and nearly doubled the capacity in 1950; thereafter there was an exponential increase in the number of annual hospital admissions [19]. As in other parts of the Yugoslav state, very few people could afford these elite health care facilities: free access to treatment was only reserved to disabled veterans, civil servants, and orphans (Fig. 6).

On the other side, dispensaries constantly remained a rarity in the pre-war period and preventive interventions aimed at containing TB transmission were only sporadically and inefficiently implemented in most well-off provinces.

During the 1930s, Yugoslavia was stuck between the fascist powers on the west and the Soviet Union on the east, all struggling to impose their supremacy on the Balkan peninsula, which favored political instability and the exacerbation of ethnic conflicts within the country with detrimental consequences on social and health conditions. The German invasion in 1941 and the subsequent Nazi domination up to 1945 brought the Kingdom of Yugoslavia to its knees, including the almost complete dismantlement of the already weak health system [24].

It was only after 1945, following the end of WWII and the birth of the Socialist Federal Republic of Yugoslavia, that a national health system based on public funding was first introduced, which led to substantial improvement in the management of TB [22, 24].

Portugal

In the early 19th century, the TB epidemic in Portugal became a true state matter. After the French invasions and the Civil War that followed, the country entered a quiet political period, and attention was drawn to various problems needing a solution, one of them being TB: considered by the government and public opinion a relevant public health issue.

In 1899, Queen Amelia initially created a Charity Institution called "Assistência Nacional aos Tuberculosos" (National Support for Tuberculosis, ANT), which was defined with special status and promulgated by King Charles I. In 1895, with the intention of discussing this scourge, the first Portuguese Congress on TB was held in Coimbra, the same year that Roentgen discovered X-rays. The total number of TB deaths in Portugal, at that time, was around 20,000 per year. In the same year, famous Portuguese physiologists (among them Dr. de Sousa Martins) strongly promoted the "sanatorium-based anti-TB treatment in altitude climate," with the consequence that cities like Guarda (altitude 1,600 m) were invaded by large numbers of people suffering from TB, seeking cure for their disease [25]. Dr. de Sousa Martins, with distinguished colleagues, strenuously promoted the campaign aimed at obtaining sufficient funds to build large sanatoria – such as the one in Serra de Estrela – large health facilities that were able to host and systematically treat many people affected by TB (Fig. 7).

A following decree issued in July 1911 officially approved the status of the "National Assistance to Tuberculosis," establishing a permanent committee for prophylaxis of TB, presided by the Minister of the Interior and having as vice-president the professor of hygiene of the Faculty of Medicine, Lisbon. The national assistance to TB was still kept as a private initiative, based in Lisbon and acting both in the country and in the adjacent islands and colonies (Fig. 8).

The first Portuguese sanatorium was built in Funchal, Madeira, in 1862 as per initiative of the former Empress of Brazil, the widow of D. Pedro IV, in memory of her daughter, Princess Maria Amelia, who died from TB 3 years earlier when she was only 22 years old. Due to the ideal climate of the island, this sanatorium was acclaimed by patients from all over Europe, especially from the United Kingdom. Thirty-seven years later, in 1899, Queen Amelia developed

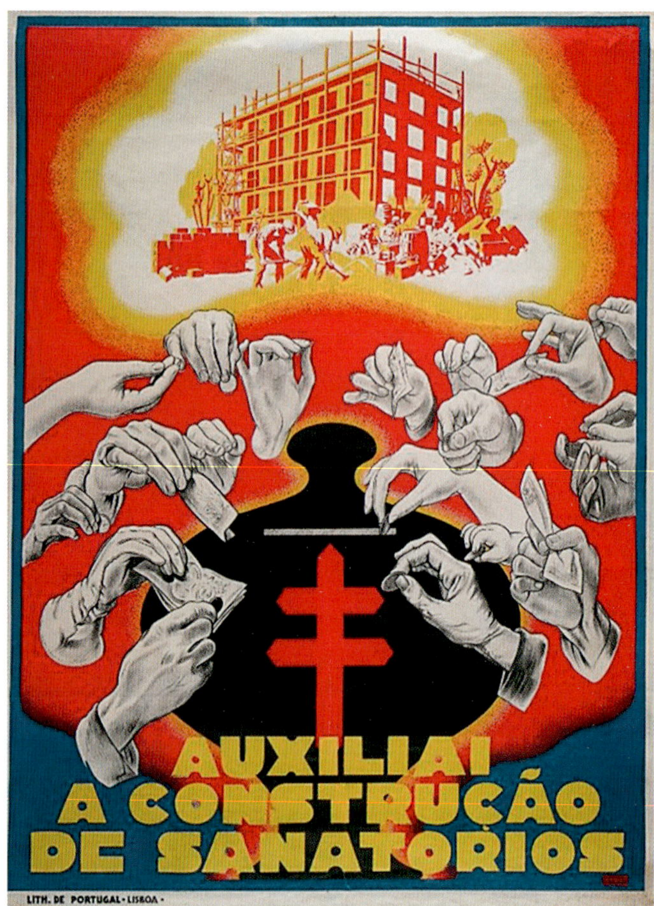

Fig. 7. Poster promoting the campaign to build TB sanatoria in Portugal, 1928. Restos de Coleção, with permission. http://restosdecoleccao.blogspot.pt/search?q = tuberculose.

a network of outpatient clinics, hospitals, sanatoria, and preventoria: where the children of patients with TB could be lodged in order to prevent transmission of the disease [26].

By the end of 1926, TB was responsible for 9% of all deaths in Portugal and had a mortality rate of 150/100,000 inhabitants [27]. Portugal had, at the time, 5 sanatoria (388 beds) and 7 dispensaries for outpatient management [28]. In 1927, the government decided that all public workers paying taxes were entitled to hospitalization for TB free of charge, without impact on their salary; this decision anticipated what today's World Health Organization recommends as universal health coverage and social protection.

A movement started in 1928 to increase the number of hospitals and dispensaries [25]. Three years later, a plan was implemented to set up a network of dispensaries all over the country with sufficient capacity to treat patients on an outpatient basis and equipped with laboratory and radiological

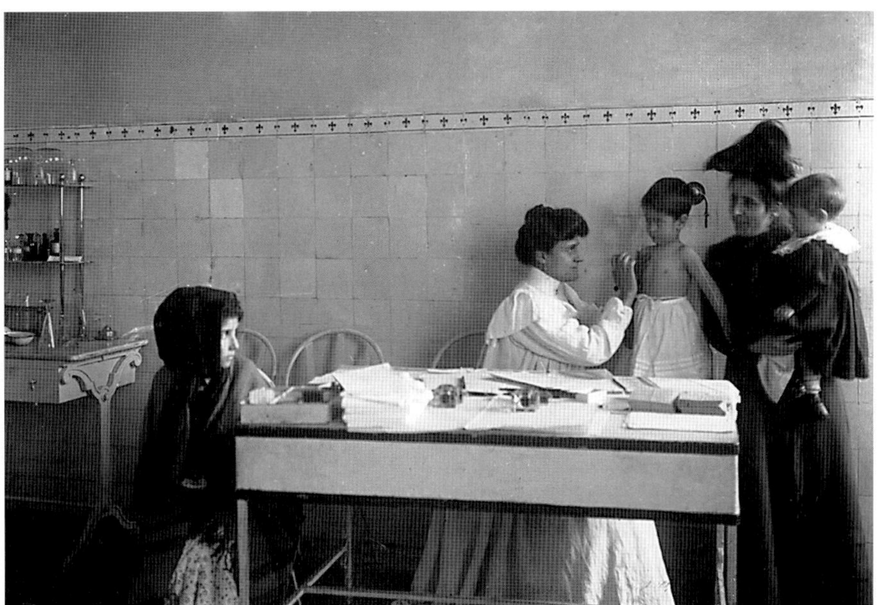

Fig. 8. Prophylaxis of tuberculosis under the "National Assistance to Tuberculosis" program in Portugal. Restos de Coleção, with permission. http://restosdecoleccao.blogspot.pt/2011/04/instituto-de-assistencia-nacional-aos.html.

services as well as with modern pneumothorax devices. The dispensaries had the mission to prevent, diagnose, and treat cases of active TB. At that time, sanatoria received only patients who could benefit from ongoing hospitalization. In 1939, Portugal had 7 sanatoria (900 beds), 3 sanatoria near the sea (600 beds) plus 5 new sanatoria being built (600 beds) and 63 dispensaries [28].

Portugal remained neutral during WWII and compared to other European countries, experienced a "quiet war," which contributed to the survival and health of a large number of refugees [29]. But in the meantime, huge problems arose internally: the Spanish Civil War (1936–1939), soon followed by WWII, brought food shortages to Portugal, spread of disease, rationing of goods, and triggered inflation. The general population became poorer and poorer, with deterioration of social and health conditions [29, 30]. After the war, several strikes were organized and soon after a political crisis followed.

In 1939, TB was responsible for 10% of all deaths in the country, corresponding to about 150/100,000 inhabitants, which increased to 12% in 1950 and then started to decline [27]. The first surveillance data that were reported in 1958 showed a TB incidence rate of 215/100,000 population. Accordingly, TB was still responsible for 5% of deaths [27]. Later after the revolution, in 1975, Portugal received a massive influx of more than 500,000 citizens from former African colonies, mostly with a high TB burden and poor socioeconomic conditions, thus leading to an increased TB incidence [26].

Spain

At the beginning of the 20th century, there were an estimated 30,000–50,000 TB deaths in Spain out of 500,000 TB patients in a population of 20 million people. Thus, the disease was responsible for 20–25% of all the deaths in the country [31].

In Spain, the "sanatorium era" in the fight of TB began at the end of the 19th century. The first sanatoria were inaugurated in 1887 in Porta Coeli (Valencia, 14 beds) and in Busot (Alicante); then in 1911 another sanatorium was built in Terrassa (Barcellona), another in 1913 in Humera (Madrid), and more were inaugurated between 1918 and 1948 (in Madrid, Barcelona, Oviedo, and Zaragoza), when 10,000 beds in 56 TB sanatoria became available nationwide [31–33].

In 1901, TB was considered an important public health problem at the national level when mandatory notification was officially introduced. In 1903, the "Asociación Antituberculosa Española" was founded with the aim of organizing and implementing the country-wide fight against TB. At the same time, the Association promoted the construction of sanatoria for isolating and treating TB patients and dispensaries for diagnosing and preventing TB infection. In 1907, under King Alfonso XIII, whose father Alfonso XII had died from TB, the "Real Patronato Central de Dispensarios e Instituciones Antituberculosas" was created to raise funds for fighting against TB, and a festival tradition, "La fiesta de la flor" or "Flower Day Festival" was inaugurated

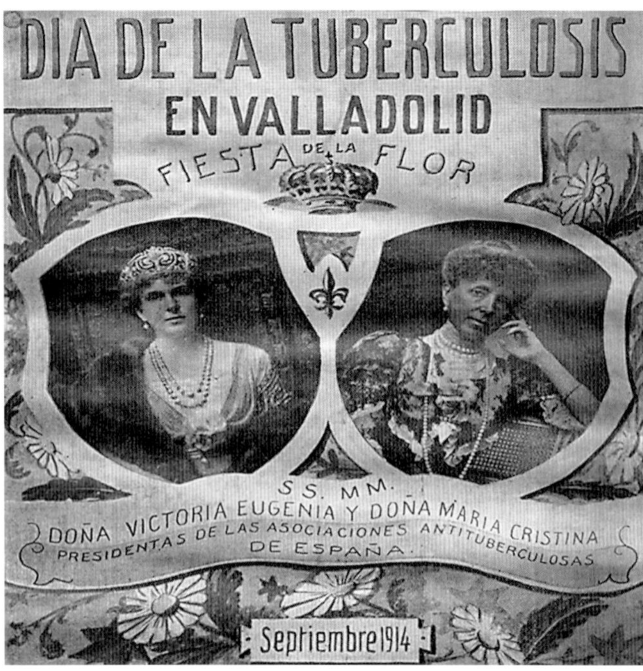

Fig. 9. Poster of the TB day (Fiesta de la Flor) in Valladolid, Spain, September 2014. La Real Academia Nacional de Medicina, with permission. http://www.bancodeimagenesmedicina.com/banco-de-imagenes/categorias/publicaciones/actos/dia-de-la-tuberculosis-valladolid-1914–5193.html.

[31] (Fig. 9). After the inauguration of the first TB dispensary in 1901 in Madrid, a progressive expansion of these health units continued until 1944, when 76 dispensaries were serving the Spanish population [31].

Spain did not participate directly in either WWI or WWII, but both conflicts had a significant impact on TB incidence and mortality in Spain during that period [34, 35] (Fig. 10).

TB mortality rate rose steadily until 1918 and in 1919–1920 stabilized at a higher level as compared to the pre-war period (1913). TB incidence rose accordingly during the same time span, from 153/100,000 population in 1913 to 172/100,000 in 1917 and 180/100,000 in 1920. The incidence rate was considerably higher in the capital city, 301/100,000 in 1913 and rose to 392/100,000 by 1920 [34].

In 1924, during the period of General Primo de Rivera, the "Real Patronato de la Lucha Antituberculosa" was created as a private initiative, but was later cancelled in 1931 at the beginning of the Republican government, when the idea of having a specific budget for the construction of dispensaries and sanatoria and for recruiting TB specialists (phthisiologists) was launched. In that period Spain developed a study on TB mortality among different regions of the country, which was mainly aimed at raising awareness on the implementation of an effective anti-TB campaign in the country (1931–1935) [36, 37].

During and after the Spanish civil war (1936–1939), the country faced a significant increase in TB mortality with rates ranging from 101/100,000, before the war, to 129/100,000 in 1945 and 90/100,000 in 1950 [27]; such numbers clearly reflect the key role of TB in social and political issues at that time [36, 37].

Similar to what happened in Italy under fascism, the anti-TB campaign was among the main goals of Gen. Franco's "regime" starting from the beginning of the civil war. The "Patronato Nacional Antituberculoso" was created in 1936, but due to lack of resources was perceived as an obvious propaganda instrument. After the war, a plan of "Seguro Obligatorio" (mandatory health insurance) similar to the Italian one was initially developed, but soon it turned out to be impossible to implement due to the political differences among the different factions within the "regime" [37]. Thus, the "Patronato" remained more a political than a scientific or public health instrument, receiving little support from TB specialists. During this period, although a large number of TB specialists remained in their sanatoria, a major proportion of doctors from other specialities were exiled for political reasons. In 1941 the "Seguro Obligatorio de enfermedad" (mandatory health insurance) was approved and insurance against TB was rejected. Despite the political difficulties, the TB budget for 1941–1944 was increased and some sanatoria were built and in 1954 the "Patronato" had 14,000 beds to manage TB cases in the country.

In summary, both WWI and WWII significantly influenced the epidemiological trends of TB in Spain despite the official neutrality of the country during the conflicts.

Conclusion

In contrast to many countries that had both qualified personnel and sufficient financial resources, recovery from the colossal death and destruction of WWII in Southern European countries and those in the Balkan region was extremely slow and to some extent still lags behind the level of progress in wealthy countries. Modernization efforts to upgrade the decade-long TB epidemic have been stifled by long-standing severe poverty. Among other major obstacles in Greece was the 6-year long civil war. In Italy, significant increases in urban-to-rural migration patterns worsened the TB mortality. Portugal remained neutral dur-

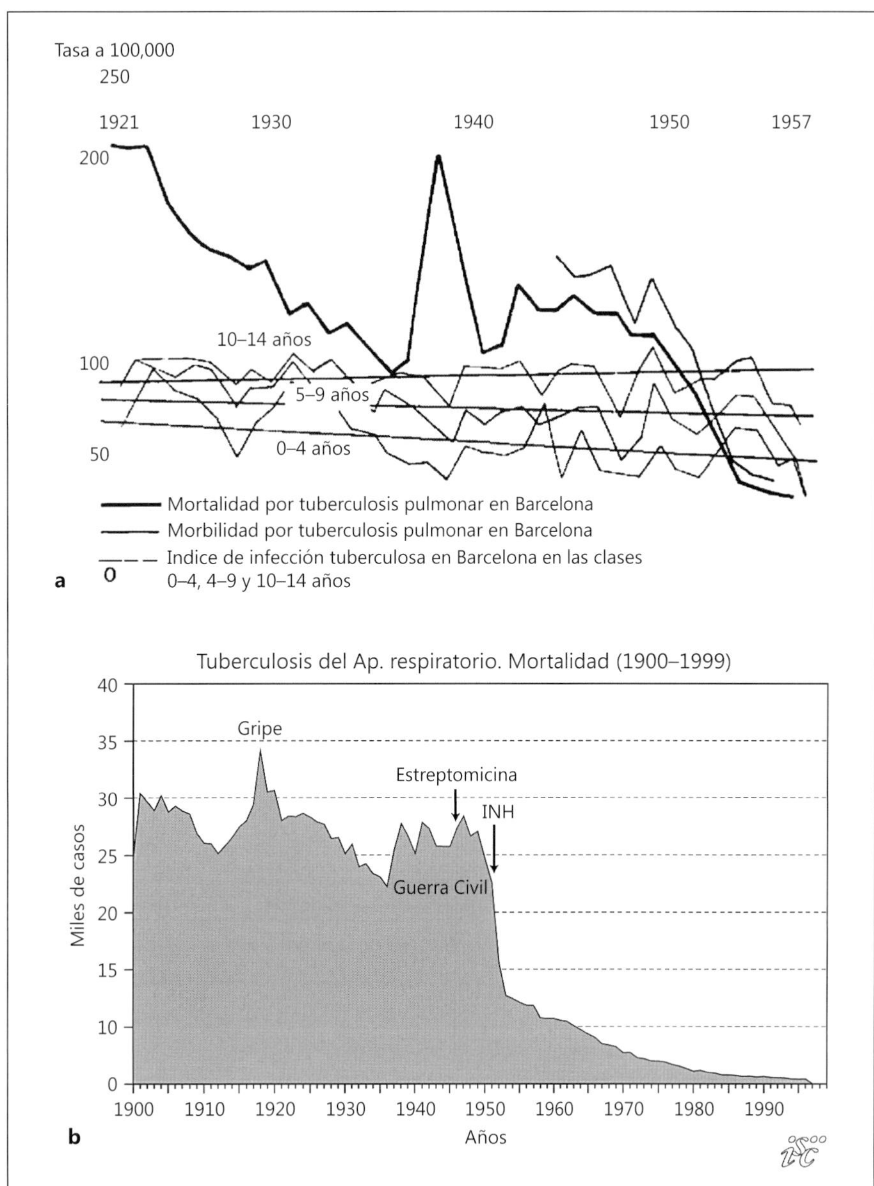

Fig. 10. Epidemiology of tuberculosis in Barcelona (**a**) and in the whole country (**b**) with clear evidence of increased incidence and/or mortality at the time of the two world wars. **a** [35]. With permission. Copyright 1987 SEPAR. All rights reserved. **b** With permission of Instituto de Salud Carlos III-Ministerio de Sanidad y Consumo, Madrid. "Análisis de la sanidad en españa a lo largo del siglo XX" Trabajo de investigación aprobado por el Fondo de Investigaciones Sanitarias del Instituto de Salud "Carlos III" (99/0208) (Proyecto no SBPY 1059/99) page 224.

ing WWII, but deficiencies during the civil war in Spain created food shortages as well in Portugal, leading to rationing and caused inflation; both countries suffered increased TB mortality. Both Romania and Bulgaria were among the poorest European countries during WWI, WWII and the interwar period and active TB remained high throughout and afterward. Finally, Yugoslavia sanatoria thrived between 1930 and 1939, but during and after WWII, political divisions and recurrent warfare greatly impaired progress in TB control.

References

1 L'Eltore G, Rustichelli V: [Evolution of tuberculosis in Italy in the last fifty years in relation to the development of receptive capacity of the anti-tuberculosis organizations]. Lotta Tuberc 1951;21: 25–43.

2 Malanima P: Urbanisation and the Italian economy during the last millennium. Eur Rev Econ Hist 2005;9:97–122.

3 Capri U: The fight against tuberculosis in Italy in the war. Tubercle 1946;27:60–62.

4 Daniels M: Tuberculosis in Europe during and after the second world war. Br Med J 1949;2: 1065–1072.

5 Sabbatani S: [The fight against tuberculosis and developments in public health from 1890 to 1930 in Italy]. Infez Med 2005;13:123–132.

6 Cosmacini G, De Filippis M, Sanseverino P: La peste bianca: Milano e la lotta antitubercolare (1882–1945). Franco Angeli, 2004.

7 Inzirillo F, Giorgetta C, Ravalli E, Tiberi S, Pona CD, Robustellini M: Protecting ourselves from tuberculosis. Describing a historic poster printed in Italy on 1937. Lung India 2014;31:425–427.

8 Renga S: Social Security Law in Italy. The Netherlands, Kluwer Law International BV, 2010.

9 Balice A: [Specific anti-tubercular prevention in Italy]. Ann Sanita Pubblica 1964;25:557–562.

10 L'Eltore G: [Vaccination against tuberculosis]. Lotta Tuberc 1951;21:436–438.

11 De Palma M: La tuberolosi in Italia dal 1882 al 1950: Scritti, Congressi, Sanatori: GPAnet, 2003.

12 Daddi G, Panà C: Recettività e resistenza nella tubercolosi polmonare: Vallecchi, 1947.

13 Daddi G, Savarino S: Sull'attività antitubercolinica dei filtrati di miceti; nota preventiva. Acta Neurol 1947;22:229.

14 Daddi G, Pana C: Reperti anatomici di un caso di tubercolosi miliare generalizzata trattato con streptomicina. Ann Ist Carlo Forlanini 1948;11: 317–323.

15 Omodei-Zorini A, Daddi G, Nuti B: La streptomicina nella cura degli empiemi tubercolari. Ann Ist Carlo Forlanini 1948;11:260–262.

16 Costanini G, Daddi G, et al: Aspetti clinici ed anatomo-patologici della tubercolosi nel periodo bellico e post-bellico. Arch Tisiol 1948;3:XXX-VIII–XLII.

17 McDougall JB: Tuberculosis in greece: an experiment in the relief and rehabilitation of a country. Bull World Health Organ 1948;1:103–196.

18 Bairoch P: Europe's gross national product: 1800–1975. J Eur Econ Hist 1976;5:273–340.

19 Berend IT: An Economic History of Twentieth-Century Europe: Economic Regimes from Laissez-Faire to Globalization. Cambridge University Press, 2016.

20 Freris AF: The Greek Economy in the Twentieth Century. Routledge, St. Martin's Press, 1986.

21 Charocopos SA: B.C.G. vaccination in Greece. Indian J Pediatr 1954;21:158–160.

22 Zupanic SZ: Slovenias Golnik Sanatorium and TB in Central Europe. Lang ББК: Р194. 94–3, Р54, 0; 2011.

23 Dobanovački D, Breberina M, Vujošević B, Pećanac M, Žakula N, Trajković V: Sanatoria in the first half of the XX century in the Province of Vojvodina. Arch Oncol 2013;21:34–43.

24 Kunitz SJ: The making and breaking of Yugoslavia and its impact on health. Am J Public Health 2004; 94:1894–1904.

25 António Fernando Castanheira Pinto Santos. Combate à Tuberculose uma abordagem demográfico-epidemiológica o Hospital de Repouso de Lisboa (1882–1975). Dissertação orientada pelo Professor Doutor João Cosme. Universidade de Lisboa, Faculdade de Letras, Departamento de História. 2010. repositorio.ul.pt/bitstream/10451/3857/1/ulfl096136_tm.pdf.

26 Antunes ML, Fonseca-Antunes A: The tuberculosis situation in Portugal: a historical perspective to 1994. Euro Surveill 1996;1:19–21.
Daddi G, Pana C: Reperti anatomici di un caso di tubercolosi miliare generalizzata trattato con streptomicina. Ann Ist Carlo Forlanini 1948;11: 317–23.

27 Cancela de Abreu L: Algumas considerações sobre o problema da tuberculose em Portugal. Jornal do Médico 1966;LIX(1207):657–690.

28 Carvalho Augusto da Silva: A Lucta Contra a Tuberculose e a Obra da Assistência Nacional aos Tuberculosos, 1899–1928: Typographia Adolpho de Mendonça, Lda., Lisboa, 1928.

29 Leite JC: Neutrality by agreement: portugal and the British alliance in World War II. Am Univ Int Law Rev 1998;14:185–199.

30 *Portugal e a Segunda Guerra Mundial* in Artigos de apoio Infopédia [em linha]. Porto: Porto Editora, 2003–2017. [consult. 2017-03-29 15:49: 26]. https://www.infopedia.pt/$portugal-e-a-segunda-guerra-mundial (last access: March 29, 2017).

31 José Antonio Maradona: Tuberculosis. Historia de su conocimiento. Ediciones de la Universidad de Oviedo. Oviedo, 2009.

32 Jesús Sauret Valet: La tuberculosis a través de la historia. Rayma Servicio Editorial, Madrid, 1990.

33 Ruiloba Quecedo C: Arquitectura sanitaria: sanatorios antituberculosos. Escuela Nacional de Sanidad. Instituto Carlos III. Madrid, 2014.

34 Drolet GJ: World War I and tuberculosis. A statistical summary and review. Am J Public Health Nations Health 1945;35:689–697.

35 De March P: La evolución de la tuberculosis en España. Situación actual. Dificultades y errores epidemiológicos. Arch Bronconeumol 1987;23: 181–191.

36 Jorge Melero Mesa: Historia social de la tuberculosis en España (1889–1936). Granada, Tesis Doctoral, 1989.

37 Jorge Melero Mesa: Enfermedad y previsión social en España durante el primer franquismo (1936–1951). El frustrado seguro obligatorio contra la tuberculosis. Acta Hispanica ad Medicinae Scientiarumque Historiam Illustrandam 1994;14:199–225.

Giovanni Battista Migliori
World Health Organization Collaborating Centre for Tuberculosis and Lung Diseases
Maugeri, Care and Research Institute
Via Roncaccio 16
IT–21049 Tradate (Italy)
E-Mail giovannibattista.migliori@icsmaugeri.it

Murray JF, Loddenkemper R (eds): Tuberculosis and War. Lessons Learned from World War II.
Prog Respir Res. Basel, Karger, 2018, vol 43, pp 165–170 (DOI: 10.1159/000481484)

Tuberculosis in Hungary before, during, and after World War II

Gábor Kovács · István Gaudi · Ildikó Horváth

National Koranyi Institute for Pulmonology, Budapest, Hungary

Abstract

Tuberculosis (TB) mortality in Hungary in 1900 was 381/100,000. Between the 2 World Wars (WWI and WWII), TB mortality fluctuated until 1924, but then declined impressively and relatively steadily until 1939 (136/100,000). During the interwar period, decreases in TB mortality were achieved through consistently implemented measures, such as isolating patients with active TB, screening patient's environments, and adopting social measures. The battle against TB included TB sanatoriums, inpatient wards, and the network of TB outpatient clinics. Worsening TB mortality erupted during WWII (1939–1945) in regions re-annexed from neighboring countries to Hungary in 1938 and 1940. Hungary joined the Nazi war effort in 1941, after which the treatment of TB patients deteriorated rapidly. It became increasingly difficult to provide satisfactory amounts and quality of food, which was important for patients. Researching patients' environmental contact screening could no longer be carried out with the required efficiency. It became increasingly difficult to transport laboratory samples and to perform activities in diagnostic laboratories due to the mobilization of physicians for military services. When Hungary turned into a theatre of war during 1944–1945, sanatorium buildings and TB outpatient clinics suffered substantial damage. After 1946, post-WWII TB services were gradually restored. © 2018 S. Karger AG, Basel

Until 1918, the historical Kingdom of Hungary constituted a co-equal part of the Habsburg Empire (Austria-Hungary). The territory of the country was 280,000 km^2 and it had a population of 18.3 million. Following World Wars I (WWI), as a result of the Treaties of Paris, the Habsburg Empire disintegrated, causing historical Hungary to lose two-thirds of its territory and half of its population. The beneficiaries of these changes included Romania, Czechoslovakia, Yugoslavia and, to a lesser extent, Austria. After 1920, the territory of Hungary was reduced to 93,000 km^2, while its population decreased to 9 million. In 1938 and 1940, the First and Second Vienna Awards modestly reversed the former territorial reductions that had been extremely disadvantageous to Hungary. As a result of the Awards, about 67,000 km^2 of its former territories and 4.3 million citizens, overwhelmingly of Hungarian ethnicity, were returned to the motherland. Following World War II (WWII), however, the victorious Allied powers reinstated the pre-1938 status quo with regard to Hungary's national borders.

WWII consisted of a series of diverse and complex political actions and military operations both within Europe and on other continents. In Europe, military action began as early as September 1939, but Hungary did not consider itself as a belligerent party and did not actually enter into war on Germany's side until June 1941. One must be familiar with the massive and relatively frequent political changes to understand the demographic and epidemiological trends that manifested themselves in the number of TB cases and in public health measures taken to combat TB in Hungary during the first half of the 20th century.

Table 1. TB mortality in Hungary, 1896–1955, data compiled from [3, 4, 6]

Year	Per 100,000 persons	Year	Per 100,000 persons	Year	Per 100,000 persons	Year	Per 100,000 persons
1896	384.0	1911	358.0	1926	243.0	1941	142.0
1897	369.0	1912	340.0	1927	240.0	1942	157.0
1898	362.0	1913	314.0	1928	225.0	1943	143.0
1899	380.0	1914	294.0	1929	219.0	1944	144.0
1900	381.0	1915	328.0	1930	198.0	1945	148.0
1901	363.0	1916	318.0	1931	199.0	1946	134.0
1902	376.0	1917	324.0	1932	193.0	1947	118.0
1903	380.0	1918	355.0	1933	169.0	1948	109.0
1904	387.0	1919	351.0	1934	157.0	1949	96.0
1905	434.0	1920	315.0	1935	158.0	1950	79.0
1906	378.0	1921	275.0	1936	151.0	1951	77.0
1907	379.0	1922	308.0	1937	148.0	1952	61.0
1908	362.0	1923	308.0	1938	140.0	1953	44.0
1909	353.0	1924	324.0	1939	136.0	1954	36.0
1910	337.0	1925	256.0	1940	140.0	1955	34.0

TB before WWII

In 1900, 77,000 inhabitants died from TB in the territory of historical Hungary. Projected to a hundred thousand citizens, it defines a mortality rate of 381/100,000. Based on contemporary observations, the number of people suffering from active TB is estimated at 7 times the number of actual TB deaths. According to this prediction, there were about 500,000 active TB patients in 1900, one of the highest rates in Europe. By comparison between 1896 and 1900, the annual mean TB mortality was 190/100,000 in England, 180/100,000 in Italy, and 194/100,000 in the German Empire. The moderate improvement after the first decade of the 20th century was halted by WWI and the mortality curve continued to fluctuate until 1924 [1]. As Table 1 and Figure 1 show, the mortality rate declined firmly and relatively steadily until WWII (1939–1945). During the first year of the war, TB mortality in Hungary had dropped to 136/100,000 [2, 3]. By contrast, during WWII and until 1946 – as a direct consequence of the war – TB mortality rates increased [4, 5]. Thereafter, in 1946 as a combined result of measures taken during the peace period, new anti-TB drugs and the general introduction of BCG vaccination (in 1948), TB mortality rates subsequently decreased [2, 5, 6].

When assessing various sections of the mortality curve, it must be seen that during the consolidated peace period between WWI and WWII, that is, between 1925 and 1939, mortality declined almost as steeply as immediately following WWII and until 1946 (Fig. 1). It was achieved without medication, through consistently implemented measures, by isolating patients with active TB, screening patients' environments, the consistent application of contemporary therapies, and the adoption of social measures, for which health politicians and public health, epidemiology and pulmonary disease specialists deserve our highest appreciation [1, 2, 7].

Important institutions in the battle against TB included sanatoria, hospital inpatient wards, TB clinics, and residences for TB patients established to isolate patients with active disease. In 1920, the country had 2,500 hospital beds and 25 TB clinics [2]. While the number of beds increased to 4,047 then 5,742 by 1932 and 1938, respectively, according to contemporary recommendations, the number of available beds should have corresponded to the mortality rate, which would have been 12,000 beds at the time. Interestingly, that number was finally achieved in 1955, well after WWII, by which year, however, mortality had declined significantly [5, 7]. The missing hospital beds were partly made up for by relying on substantially cheaper beds in TB patients' own homes, which, however, enabled the isolation of patients. There was also a steady increase in the number of TB clinics. In 1932, 1938, 1940, and 1941, immediately before Hungary's entry into war, there were 73, 83, 103, and 141, respectively, TB clinics throughout the country [2].

TB clinics became the focus of the battle against the disease. They were responsible for diagnosing the disease while at the same time they also managed further activities. Their working practices were determined by the recognition that TB was both an infectious disease and a social disease. The government scheduled the organization of TB clinics in all districts and, in smaller municipalities, in 1908 extended the operation of the established "Green Cross Health Protection Service," which enabled district nurses to trace down, screen and, where appropriate, forward contacts to clinics [8, 9]. During that period, the equipment of TB clinics was standardized and provided by the government.

TB During World War II

As illustrated by the TB mortality curve (Fig. 1), the decline of mortality reversed in 1940, even though Hungary did not go to war before 1941. What was the reason for the worsening of results 2 years earlier? It was due to the higher TB mortality rates in regions re-annexed to Hungary following the First and Second Vienna Awards. Whereas in 1938, the

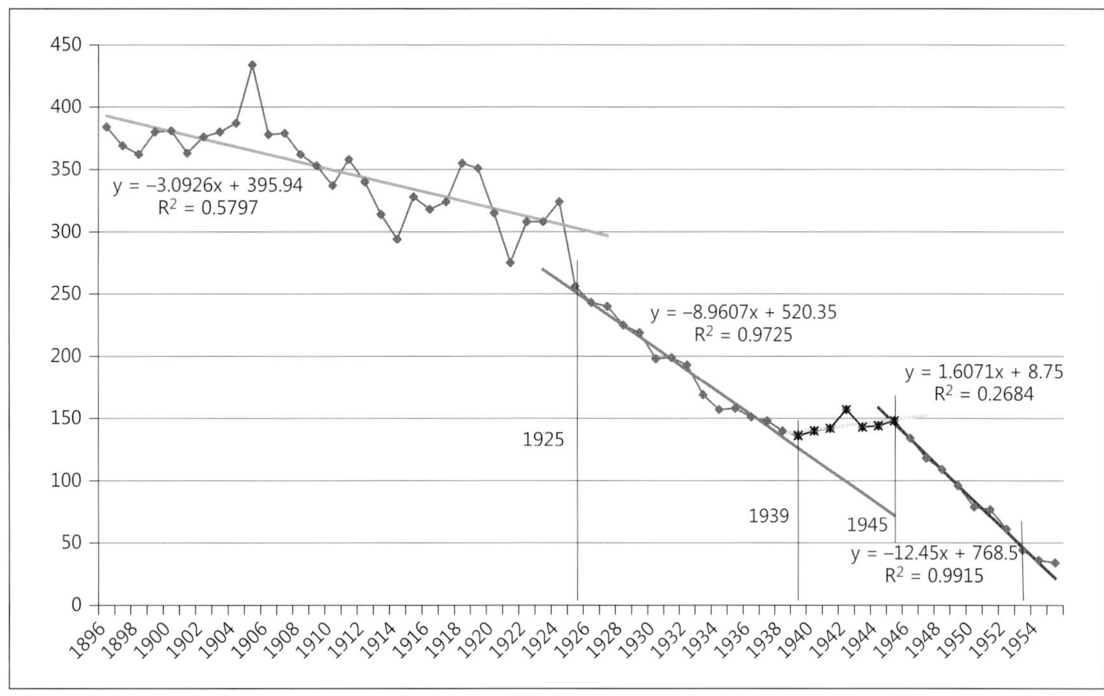

Fig. 1. TB mortality and different periods in trends in Hungary, 1896–1955, data compiled from [3, 4, 6].

TB mortality rate was 139/100,000 in Hungary, it was 180/100,000 in the former Czechoslovakian territories in the north, 188/100,000 in Northern Transylvania formerly belonging to Romania, and 170/100,000 in the South in former Yugoslavian territories [3]. The situation was aggravated by the scarcity of appropriate infrastructure in the re-annexed regions. In Northern Transylvania, 450 hospital beds were allocated for about 60,000 patients, whereas 15,000 TB patients had to share a mere 9 hospital beds in the South, in former Yugoslavia [10].

In 1941, the country became a belligerent party when Parliament declared that Hungary was going to war on Germany's side. Subsequently, the conditions of the treatment of TB patients deteriorated rapidly. Following the introduction of rationing, it became increasingly difficult to guarantee both a satisfactory amount and quality of food, which is vital for patients suffering from TB. Requisitioning rendered transportation and researching patients' environment more difficult and contact tracing could no longer be carried out with the required efficiency. It became more difficult to transport laboratory samples and to perform diagnostic laboratory activities in general. Screening programs became incidental. Medical staff became insufficient due to the declining number of physicians who were incorporated into military services and as a result of restrictive measures affecting

Jewish doctors – who from 1939 onwards became enlisted men and were held politically unreliable – initially were forced to work in Hungary, but later during the war were forced to serve in the armed forces on the battlefront and suffered significant human casualties [11]. In 1944 and 1945, the final years of WWII, Hungary turned into an active theatre of war, sustaining substantial damages to homes and other buildings owing to regular air bombardment. Even greater damage was caused by battlefront fighting, street conflicts, and destruction in towns. Most hospitals, sanatoriums, and TB clinics fell victim to the ravages of war. While the number of TB clinics had increased to 141 by 1941, as a result of bombardment and local warfare, the number of operating clinics dropped to 34 by 1945. Moreover, the number of hospital beds declined from 6,000 to 500.

At the same time, it was very interesting to observe that clinics continued to operate under increasingly difficult conditions. In 1943, 367,000 people, about 2.7% of the population visited a clinic, while 388,000 participated in pulmonary screening. In 1944, 422,000 visited a clinic and 201,000 participated in screening, and even in 1945, amidst the wartime activities, 477,000 people visited a clinic, while 154,000 participated in screening. The only major setback occurred in the number of tuberculin tests, probably as a result of the limited availability of skin test reagents. As opposed to 62,000 tests in 1943, only 16,000 and 23,000 tests, respectively, were carried out in 1944 and 1945 [12]. The number of pneumothorax therapies also declined as a result of local warfare; in 1943, 93,000 pneumothoraces were performed in Hungary, whereas their number decreased to 66,000 in 1944 and a mere 43,000 in 1945. In 1946, however, the number of interventions had increased to 76,000 [12]. The change in the number of sputum tests indicates the limited accessibility of laboratories. While in 1943, 52,000 tests were performed, their numbers dropped to 30,000 and 15,000, respectively, in 1944 and 1945, which was clearly insufficient. In 1946, the number of sputum tests had already increased to 30,000 [12].

Taking into account the wartime damages of TB clinics, it can be ascertained that the buildings of 6 clinics were completely destroyed while 74 buildings suffered substantial damages. X-ray equipment was either lost or seriously damaged in 57 pulmonary clinics: including 49 pneumothorax devices, 61 microscopes, 54 coat aprons, and 61 lead mittens. By early 1945, only 34 clinics remained operable. It was from that deplorable condition that anti-TB networks had to be restored, their staff re-organized, and the lost infrastructure rebuilt following the end of war. By the end of 1945, the number of clinics had increased to 110, whereas as many as 126 clinics were operating by late 1946.

The priorities of the SAS (Hurry, Give, Help [Siess, Adj, Segíts in Hungarian]) movement included the rapid restoration of the anti-TB infrastructure, and the fact that it donated 42 complete X-ray machines greatly contributed to progress. The success of restoration and renovation is clearly illustrated by the mortality figures. From 1946 onward, mortality begins to decline, at a consistent and ever increasing rate in Hungary. The TB-related mortality rate was 136/100,000 in 1939 and 148/100,000 in 1945. By 1946, mortality had decreased to 134/100,000; in other words, we had returned to the 1939 mortality level and there were more reductions ahead [4, 5]. Studying the chart, one is inevitably forced to reflect on how the rate of mortality could have changed in Hungary if the ravages of WWII had been avoided. Had the steady improvement of the post-WWI years continued, the significantly lower values achieved in the 1950s would have been attained 5 or 6 years earlier. It could have helped to avoid 1,000–1,500 TB-related deaths per year and saved around another 10,000 young lives. In the sea of world conflicts, this was only a small slice compared to the tens of millions of war victims. For Hungarians, however, their loss appears just as painful and pointless.

TB as a Continuum

Although TB is an infectious disease, it is also obvious that patients' social circumstances play a significant role in the dynamics of a person becoming infected by *Mycobacterium tuberculosis* and whether or not the disease develops, which depends on the body's immunologic resistance, state of nutrition, and associated factors. Following the identification of *M. tuberculosis* in 1882, governments started to introduce both a series of public-level preventive measures and legislation required by the circumstances to prevent and control the disease.

In Hungary, the first piece of legislation addressing infectious diseases in a wider sense, was Chapter XIII of the Public Health Act of 1876, which addressed epidemics [13, 14]. The 1908 amendment of that law (Act 1908/XXXVIII) provided for specific measures concerning TB [15]. First of all, it defined TB as an endemic disease and identified the struggle to control it as a duty of both society and the government. The law included provisions of the official medical services, the welfare/sanitary service and, particularly in rural areas without district doctors, establishing the Green Cross Health Protection network of district nurses. It provided that the costs incurred in connection with the prevention of infectious diseases were to be shared between the national patient care fund and local municipalities on a fifty-fifty basis. Infectious diseases had to be reported to the municipal authorities. The law provided for the setting up of provisional quarantines in epidemic situations, the possibility of seconding physicians, the provision of required funds, and the forced isolation of infectious patients if their contacts were at significant risk of being infected and if the patient did not adhere to provisions for preventing the spread of infection. One of the most important outcomes of the 1908 law was the establishment of the so-called "National and Central Committee for anti-TB Struggle," whose president was vested with the powers of a government commissioner. These definite provisions, which properly addressed the requirements of the age, along with the improving infrastructure, enabled the precipitous decline in TB mortality in Hungary between WWI and WWII. As a result of new scientific achievements and the evolution of society, however, it became unavoidable to draft a new, adequate, and modern legislation to provide for all aspects of the disease in proper depth, from administrative and organizational issues to the conditions of therapies to social aspects. The more comprehensive new health policy goals could not be achieved until the administrative system was properly modernized through legislation.

After lengthy preparation and professional consultations, the Hungarian Parliament finally passed Act VI of 1940 on the prevention of TB and venereal diseases. Parliament amended certain provisions of public health laws ("Lex Tuberculosis") and implemented other regulations of the law (Regulation No. 888/1940 of the Minister of Interior) [16, 17]. For posterity, this is another indication of how much Hungarian politicians of the age still hoped that Hungary might steer clear of WWII. By 1940, Poland had been divided, war was raging all across Europe, France had become a theatre of war and England was being heavily bombed by German aircrafts. The fight against TB was hardly a top priority in those countries. In Hungary, on the contrary, Parliament took time during those months for a debate concerning the most important issues of controlling the disease and the financing of those efforts. At the time, it was certainly a very progressive law, even by international standards.

The first chapter of the law addresses general issues of TB control. Article 1 of the law provides that promoting TB control is a public service mission carried out by the government in cooperation with towns and municipal governments, insurance institutions, and the associations and institutions established for that purpose. Article 2 provides for the reporting and registration obligations, the rules of which were laid down in a decree issued by the Minister of Interior. The reporting obligation applied to patients once they had become aware of their disease as well as to physicians, including private, hospital or military conscription doctors if they had diagnosed a virulent or possibly virulent case of TB. The attending physician, the coroner, and patients themselves were responsible for reporting the recovery, death or change of address of a notified patient, respectively. Article 3 provided for confidentiality with a view of protecting patients through the confidentiality obligation imposed on civil servants and physicians. They were, however, relieved of their confidentiality obligation if patients were uncooperative and refused to obey the doctor's instructions to prevent the spread of infection and disease. Confidentiality was not compulsory vis-à-vis persons living in the same household with patients who were informed of the consequences, including death, of their condition.

Article 4 provided for compulsory medical examination prior to the admission of children into nursery schools, children's homes or day care centers and compulsory examination at 6, 10, and 15 years of age. Based on the provision concerning the compulsory treatment of children, the age limit for medical treatment was increased from 7 to 18 years. Workers employed by children's institutions had to undergo regular screening tests, while people suffering from TB were not allowed to work in such institutions. Domestic servants (housekeepers, live-in maids, nannies, family tutors, female companions, readers, and nurses) had to be regularly examined for TB. If a servant's license was issued to such persons, they had to be examined beforehand, and the result of the examination recorded in the servant's log. Where the suspicion of TB arose, the mayor or an official appointed by the mayor had the power to instruct the medical examination of the persons or groups concerned. The detailed rules for ordering the examination were laid down in a decree issued by the Minister of Interior. At the same time, the law permitted persons found to be ill to seek an independent review. Articles 5 and 6 provided for the quarantining of patients where their virulence posed a risk to their environment. The quarantine had to be maintained until the full recovery of the patient or until the disease had lost its virulence. The quarantine could be ordered by force if the patient failed to adhere to the instructions. For persons employed by the government, the law provided for a year of sick-leave with full pay, which could be extended with another year with 40% of the patient's former pay where appropriate. Article 7 provided for the disinfection, following the patient's change of address, hospitalization or death, of premises regularly used by the patient.

Further provisions were devoted to the organizational conditions of battling TB. The responsibility for the organization and consistent guidance of anti-TB measures and the monitoring and supervision of institutions set up to prevent the disease was assigned to the National Institute of Public Health. The law identified the institutions of TB prevention: they included TB clinics, health protection services, TB sanatoriums, public hospitals, university clinics, and the hospitals and homes for TB patients, maintained by insurance companies. At TB clinics, examinations were carried out free of charge. A network of TB clinics was to be set up for preventive purposes. The underlying idea was that a TB clinic should be set up in each district. The law restricted the right to establish institutions for prevention and medical treatment. Private individuals were deprived of this right. It raised the concern that, with time, problems might arise concerning institutions founded by private individuals if the charitable nature of an institution wears off and is replaced by entrepreneurial spirit. The important and forward-looking provisions of the law included its intention to provide for the costs of operation. Both municipal governments and insurance companies were required to bear costs at equal proportions. Insurance companies were required to share the costs of maintaining TB clinics in proportion with their insured population. In its day, the law essentially enabled the health authorities and experts to increase the efficiency of their strenuous efforts with a view of controlling TB, hand in hand with municipal governments and insurance companies. It was not the legislators' fault that, not long after the law had been proclaimed, Hungarian health policy was already facing completely different challenges. As Hungary got directly involved in WWII, the noble idea of controlling TB soon fell into the background. Nearly continuous warfare, day-to-day survival and physical subsistence continued to define the everyday life of the country and its population in the years that followed.

Conclusion

The creed of the struggle against TB was articulated perhaps with the highest precision and at the same time, most poetically by Béla Johan, a crucial figure in Hungarian public health policy between the 2 wars:

Tuberculosis is one of the most exciting and most instructive issues in medicine. Tuberculosis is never about the problem of a single person, a single patient. The lesson taught by tuberculosis is that, in the practice of good physicians, the ideas of therapy and prevention must be united and must complement each other. The roots of battling tuberculosis reach down into the soil of epidemiology and social sciences. The arsenal of physicians specialising in tuberculosis contains equal parts of medical science, medical art and philanthropy [18].

The Latin motto "inter arma silent musae" probably rang true during WWII. The muse of medical art also kept silent for long years. Following the war, however, with renewed energy and backed to a considerable extent by scientists and governments, it finally enabled TB to be driven back. That, however, would be another story.

References

1 Pólya J: The Roman of the Medicine (Hun: Az orvostudomány regénye) Edit: Béta Irodalmi R.T. Budapest, 1941, pp 335–337.
2 Kapronczay K: Hungarian epidemics since the early 19th century. (Hun: A magyarországi járványok a XIX. század elejétől kezdődően) http://tankonyvek.tudomanytortenet.hu/a_kozegeszsegugy_tortenete.
3 Hungarian Statistical Yearbook, New Series L. 1942. Budapest, Hungarian Royal Statistical Office, 1944.
4 Hungarian Statistical Yearbook, New Series. LI., LII., LIII., LIV.; 1943, 1944, 1945, 1946. Hungarian Central Statistical Office, Budapest,1948.
5 Zádor A: The TB mortality (Hun: A tbc mortalitásáról), http://demografia.hu/kiadvanyokonline/index.php/demografia/article/viewFile/1570.
6 Hungarian Statistical Yearbook 1949–1955. Budapest, Central Statistical Office, 1957.
7 Kováts F: Fighting against TB in Hungary (Hun: A gümőkór elleni küzdelem Magyarországon) docplayer.hu(19233364-A-gumokor-elleni-kuzdelem-magyarorszagon-irta-prof-kovats-ferenc.

8 Scholtz K: Népegészségügy 1926;7 No.1. p 53.
9 Johan B: The recovering Hungarian village (Hun: Gyógyul a magyar falu) 1939, Budapest, M.Kir. Orv.Közeg.Int. ISBN:0299001442517;pp 229–243.
10 Hungarian Statistical Reports, CXIV. Budapest, Hungarian Royal Statistical Office, 1941.
11 Kapronczay K: The Hungarian medicine between the two world war (Hun: A magyar medicina a két világháború között). Magyar Tudomány, www.matud.iif.hu/2016/05/13.htd.
12 Nyárády I: Statistical data on the battle against TB. (Hun: A tbc elleni küzdelem statisztikai adatai) Compiled by the Centre for TB Statistics, (1951, manuscript).
13 The 14th Law of 1876 Year about the Public Health. http://www.1000ev.hu/index.php?a=3¶m=5727.
14 Papp D: Epidemic and Public Health in Hungary: The 14th Law of 1876 Year and it's effects. (Hun: Járványos és közegészségügy Magyarországon: az 1876 évi XIV. törvénycikk és hatásai) Joghistória XVIII. 2016;2:7–12.

15 The 38th Law of 1908 Year: The Modifying of the 14th Law of 1876 (Part II, Chapter I) about the Public Health (Hun: A közegészségügy rendezéséről szóló 1876. évi XIV. törvénycikk II. rész I. fejezetének módosításáról szóló 1908. évi XXXVIII. törvénycikk) http://www.1000ev.hu/index.php?a=3¶m=7038.
16 Székely M: Hungary's "Lex Tuberculosis" and "lex veneris." Népegészségügy 1940;2:78–86.
17 The 6th Law of 1940 Year: The Protection of TB and Venereal Diseases and the Certain Commissions of the Public Health Acts (Hun: A gümőkór és a nemibetegségek elleni védekezésről, valamint a közegészségügyi törvények egyes rendelkezéseiről szóló 1940. évi VI. törvénycikk) http://www.1000ev.hu/index.php?a=3¶m=8120.
18 Johan B: The tuberculosis question and the battle against tuberculosis in Hungary. (Hun: A tuberkulózis kérdés és a tuberkulózis elleni küzdelem hazánkban). Orvosi Hetilap1939;4:101–107.

Gábor Kovács
National Korányi Institute for Pulmonology
Pihenő út 1
HU–1121 Budapest (Hungary)
E-Mail kovac@koranyi.hu

Murray JF, Loddenkemper R (eds): Tuberculosis and War. Lessons Learned from World War II.
Prog Respir Res. Basel, Karger, 2018, vol 43, pp 171–178 (DOI: 10.1159/000481485)

Tuberculosis in the Soviet Union before and during World War II

Marina V. Shulgina[a] · Irina A. Vasilyeva[b]

[a]I.I. Mechnikov North-West State Medical University, Saint-Petersburg, and [b]The National Medical Research Centre of Phthisiopulmonology and Infectious Diseases of the Russian Ministry of Health, Moscow, Russia

Abstract

World War II (WWII) started for the majority of the Soviet people on June 22, 1941. It was a socioeconomic and demographic catastrophe for the country, and its aftershocks are still being felt. According to the latest research, losses among civilians totaled 28,378,000, and the total number of people killed or dead of hunger, cold, overwork, and epidemics amounted to 37.3–42.0 million, including military losses. Tuberculosis (TB) did not play a major role because the number of TB deaths was greatly outweighed by the enormous number of overall deaths. Research in TB epidemiology in the USSR after 1931 was complicated by the fact that conventional statistical data on TB morbidity and mortality had not been published and had been substituted with rates of case finding among individuals (workers, collective farmers, soldiers) screened for TB, and rates of patients with different forms of TB. We, therefore, reviewed data on the socioeconomic situation during the war in regions of the Soviet Union that were not directly involved in the war – mainly the Urals and Siberia, the TB control program in the civilian and military sectors, and the peculiarities of TB caused by conditions of stress and starvation during the war.

© 2018 S. Karger AG, Basel

World War II (WWII) started for the majority of the Soviet Republic on June 22, 1941. It was a socioeconomic and demographic catastrophe for the country, and its aftershocks are still being felt. By 1941, the Soviet Union was a union of 16 republics, which are now all independent states: some of which have joined another union, the European Union, whereas others have different levels of partnership and cooperation with neighboring former Soviet republics. In WWII, however, they performed as one nation and one state, sharing the burdens of war and the glories of victory.

The estimated number of total human losses by the Soviet Union in WWII, as published at the end of the 20th century, was 26.6 million, including 8.9 million due to military losses [1]. According to the latest research, however, losses among civilians amounted to 28,378,000, and the total number of people killed or who died of hunger, cold, overwork, and epidemics amounted to 37.3–42.0 million, including military losses [2]. This is almost a quarter of all citizens of the Soviet Union registered in the census of 1939. It is difficult for the human mind to comprehend the true weight of these figures.

TB did not play a principal role in the disaster. The number of deaths due to TB was greatly outweighed by the enormous number of total deaths that occurred during WWII. However, a review of the data on TB epidemiology and TB control in the USSR demonstrates catastrophic consequences of war. At the same time, the particularities of the epidemic and the clinical course of the disease, as well as the structure and effectiveness of TB control programs implemented in the Soviet Union in the variable conditions of those times, might be useful for planning TB programs today.

Our research into the past was significantly limited by the lack of epidemiological indicators for TB in those times. After 1931, no statistical data on TB morbidity and mortality were published: these were substituted by rates of case finding among individuals (workers, collective farmers, soldiers) screened for TB, and rates of patients with different forms of TB [3, 4]. There were governmental regulations for TB control, including TB case finding procedures, treatment, and rehabilitation of TB patients. We also found a number of recent publications describing the socioeconomic situation and the state and functioning of medical services in civilian settlements in different regions of the Soviet Union in the period from 1941 to 1945.

Much of the data highlight the link between TB and famine. Malnutrition was a severe complication of civilian life in both occupied and unoccupied territories, and one of the causes of the huge human losses among civilians [5]. There are also published observations by Leningrad practicing TB specialists on the clinical picture of TB under the extreme conditions of starvation during the 1941–1944 siege of Leningrad [6, 7].

TB Before 1941
Anti-TB activities in the Soviet Union were based on 2 main principles that were common to the socialist health care system in general:
– a state-supported health care system, and
– a trend towards integration of medical treatment and
    prevention.

The latter led to a new concept of dispensary activities, targeted at both diseased and healthy people, involving the whole population of the supervised region or facility. A new type of multifunctional TB dispensaries (TB departments) were introduced that became responsible for all TB control activities in the supervised region – organization and performance of screening for TB, diagnosis and treatment of the disease, rehabilitation of patients in the sanatoria, introduction of measurements of improvements in working and living conditions, and epidemiological surveillance of TB [3, 4].

After 1929, the "Great Break" program – which involved the accelerated industrialization and collectivization of farming – started to be implemented in the Soviet Union resulting in massive migration and deterioration of socioeconomic conditions for hundreds of thousands of people. TB statistics inevitably demonstrated an increase in TB morbidity and mortality, as well as increases in the rates of other diseases. Nevertheless, the Government blamed the poor health statistics on inappropriate organi-

zation of the public health services and started its reform [8].

As of 1931, TB program activities were concentrated on industrial workers at working sites such as new building projects, factories and plants, and collective farms. TB dispensaries were responsible for the implementation of TB control programs, named "The struggle against TB" in a supervised region, industrial or rural formation. TB dispensaries cooperated closely with the Communist party and Soviet authorities and trade unions [3, 4]. In 1940, there were 1,687 dispensaries, including 554 self-maintained TB centers and 1,133 TB ambulances functioning as part of the general medical facilities. There were over 28,800 beds for TB patients in hospitals and sanatoria in urban settlements and 1,700 in rural areas [8].

According to Governmental Decree No 1176 of December 10, 1934, early diagnosis of TB was to be assured by systemic medical screening of the supervised population for TB by X-ray examination. From 1935, all acid-fast bacilli (AFB)-positive patients accommodated in workers' or students' hostels were compulsorily isolated in inpatient TB hospitals. Urgent surgery for TB was also considered [3, 4]. The Governmental decrees obliged urban administrations and other authorities "to consider the necessity of providing extra square meters" for AFB-positive TB patients in dwellings allocated to their families [3, 8].

Implementation of the Governmental decrees was not comprehensive. However, systematic X-ray for TB screening was introduced as of 1934 in several population groups, for child-care and food industry workers, and for the military. In 1937, BCG vaccination was introduced and 3 years later (1940), fluoroscopic examination of the chest was started as a pilot project in one of the military units and proved highly effective for pulmonary TB case finding [8].

Although TB dispensaries were organized in the large industrial centers, their network did not include all settlements of the huge country. Rural and sparsely populated regions were inadequately covered by the program, reflecting their generally poor representation within the general health care network [9, 10]. For example, Siberian cities and towns were poorly covered, not only by general medical facilities but also by specialized medical services, including TB dispensaries (Table 1) [10]. Siberia was and still is a territory with low population density, but most of the regional centers were densely populated industrial cities at the beginning of 1941 [9].

Reformation of the health care system and consequent improvement in the population's health status resulted in a decrease in the number of latent TB cases among conscripts by 1940. Annual TB screening by X-ray examination was successfully implemented in the army, and all TB cases identified were demobilized and treated, mostly in civilian TB hospitals [11, 12]. We failed to find any data on TB case finding during the pre-mobilization medical examinations before the beginning of the war.

Although data were not published in the open press, monitoring of epidemiological data was ongoing in governmental structures, and the data were leaked. According to official reports, the average mortality index had halved by 1940 compared to 1913, from 270/100,000 in 1913 to 130/100,000 in 1940 [11, 12]. According to further data published by Averbukh [8], this increased by 85% in 1941 compared to 1930. Averbukh's assumption was that it was prohibited to publish statistical data on the TB epidemic after 1931 due to the dramatic increase in mortality indices. According to data obtained from personal communications with a retired official of All-Union Ministry of health, in 1940 the TB mortality had increased in 45 cities of the USSR included in TB monitoring to 287/100,000, as shown in Figure 1 [8].

TB During WWII

The beginning of WWII significantly affected the TB programs. The whole health care system collapsed in the first months of the war. This was true both for the army and the civilian medical services.

TB in the Army

The Soviet Army medical services had analyzed the negative experiences of losses due to TB in Russian history and during WWI. In peacetime, TB mortality in the army in 1913 amounted to 607/100,000, while the TB incidence was 1,300/100,000 [11]. By 1940, military medical services had developed a multistep system of TB case finding and a method for evacuating those with active disease. This was based on regular medical screening of those with suspected TB by medical specialists in the military medical units at all levels: soldiers who were healthy, wounded or with non-TB diseases were examined for clinical TB symptoms in the army hospitals and on the front, while those behind the lines underwent clinical examination and X-ray screening. Two methods of X-ray screening were used: total screening and examination of those with suspected TB. Total X-ray screening was done for troops who had been withdrawn from active operations to reform or during quiet periods. Total screening provided more focal forms, whereas examination

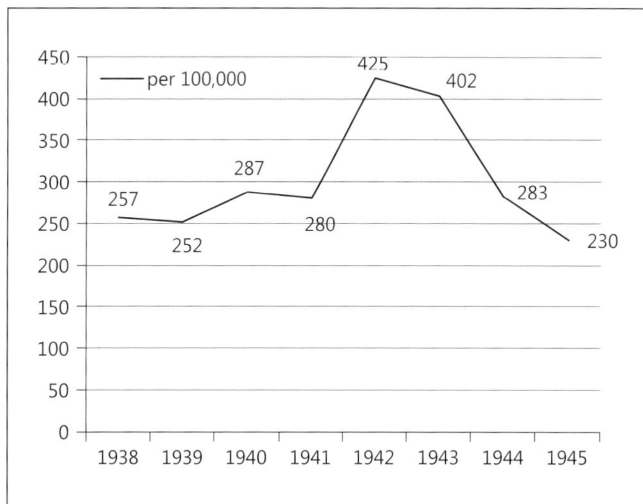

Fig. 1. Average tuberculosis mortality in 45 major USSR cities, compiled from [8].

Table 1. Number of TB hospitals in Siberian regions in 1941

Name of the region (as in 1941)*	Population, mln (Census 1939) [9]	No of TB hospitals	No of beds
The Altay Territory	2.5	3	65
Novosibirsk region	4.1	6	365
Omsk region	2.4	3	95
Irkutsk region	1.304	–	–
The Krasnoyarsk Territory	2.0	1	50
Chitinskaya region	1.2	–	–

* Administrative borders of the regions changed after 1941.

of TB suspects – more infiltrative and disseminated forms. By the end of the war mass fluorography screening had been introduced [12].

In 1943, AFB-smear microscopy was organized in some medical and sanitary battalions (medical facilities located close to the active operations on the front). The anti-TB program had started to function as an effective unit in 1942–1943. The average rate of active TB among soldiers in 1941–1945 was 1% (compared with 1.3% in peacetime in 1913) [11, 12].

Based on the results of their medical examinations, all TB patients and those with suspected TB were divided into 3 groups with different treatment and evacuation strategies. The first group of patients, with "active TB," primarily smear-positive, were immediately isolated in special wards of designated hospitals located behind the lines for anti-TB

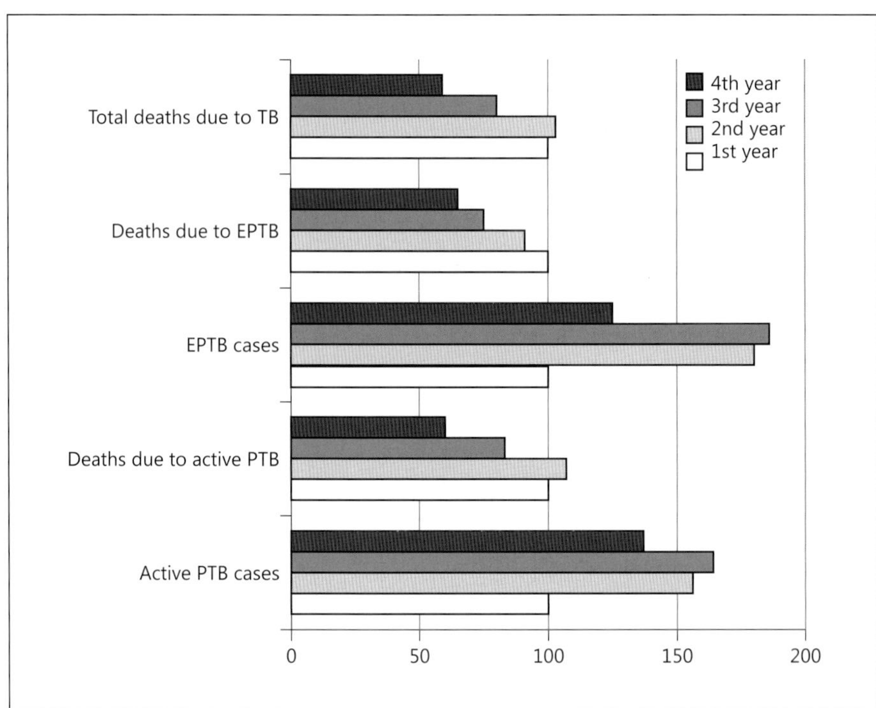

Fig. 2. Dynamics of the relative numbers of tuberculosis cases and deaths registered during the 1941–1945 war in the military medical services (%). 100% = number registered during the first year of the war: June 1941–May 1942. Following years: 2nd year: June 1942–May 1943; 3rd year: June 1943–May 1944; 4th year: June 1944–May 1945, diagrams compiled from [12].

treatment. These represented 28% of all TB patients [12]. The second group included AFB-smear-negative patients who nevertheless needed medical supervision and additional examinations, for which they were evacuated to the army hospital. Depending on the results of the additional examinations and supervision, they were either returned to active military units or hospitalized in special wards behind the lines. According to the published data, these represented 18% of all TB patients [12]. The third group, and the largest, was a group of patients with residual lesions of previous TB (cured TB). These comprised 54% of all registered TB cases and were left for intensive medical supervision in their subunits, with frequent medical examinations [12].

TB diagnosis was a problem in certain medical units, especially during the first months of WWII. TB was misdiagnosed as bronchopneumonia (30% of TB cases), malaria (18%), bronchitis, influenza or enteric fever. Over diagnosis of TB was also frequent: active TB was not confirmed in 49–67% of cases. The highest rates of incorrect diagnoses were in the medical units in active operations on the front, without X-ray examinations, where only 33% of diagnoses were correct. The highest rates of correct diagnoses were in referral hospitals with infectious disease wards and services.

The final diagnoses were made in army and front-line hospitals and in hospitals behind the lines. The number of cases of active and inactive pulmonary and extra-pulmonary TB registered in referral military hospitals increased in 1942–1943 compared to the first year of the war, while deaths decreased for all groups, as shown in Figure 2. The increase in numbers of TB cases diagnosed in the military units could be a result of the increasing numbers of people from liberated territories joining the armies. Indirectly, it may reflect TB morbidity in the occupied territories. The number of TB cases had decreased by the end of the war in 1945, and the number of deaths due to TB started to decrease in 1944 [12].

The diagnosis of TB in many front-line military medical units was not efficient, resulting in delayed isolation of infectious TB cases.

Although the total rate of correctly diagnosed TB patients was 99%, with only 1% of cases diagnosed post-mortem [12], the post-mortem rate cannot be considered as an unbiased proof of excellent diagnostic methods in the army during the war, as autopsy practices could not be comprehensive: many, many soldiers were killed in battle or died of their wounds in medical units close to the sites of battles, and were buried without autopsy.

TB cases in the military units occurred mainly in soldiers with a previous history of TB (75% of all TB patients) and/or who had been in contact with a case of TB before joining the army (47%). Age less than 25 years, being wounded, and staying in an occupied territory or in prisoner of war camps were risk factors for TB. No correlation was observed with duration in the army: most TB patients stayed in the army for 6–18 months and were mobilized in 1941 in the period of mass mobilization. Military TB specialists have estimated that 24% of cases were infected and developed TB disease in the army [12].

TB in the Civilian Sector

The Soviet health care system was in complete disarray after the beginning of WWII. Medical personnel were mobilized and hospitals were destroyed. By the end of the war, there were 616 TB dispensaries in urban areas and only 11 in rural areas, compared to 1687 before the war. Most of the dispensaries were located in derelict premises, 50% of which had neither X-ray machines nor laboratories. In Odessa (in today's Republic of Ukraine), the estimated damages to the TB facility infrastructure in 1944 amounted to 78% of their original state in 1940, while the number of staff had decreased by 20% [8].

The invasion of the Soviet territories by the Wehrmacht troops in 1941 led to the mass migration of civilians to the east of the country. Most of the industrial facilities from the industrially developed West of the country began to be evacuated immediately to the Volga region, the Urals, Western Siberia, Kazakhstan, and other Soviet republics. Whole factories were disassembled, embarked to railway platforms, transported to the sites allocated by the USSR commission for evacuation, installed at the new sites and resumed the production of the armaments, ammunition, medicines, and so on, needed by the army. Animal herds and vehicular and railway transport facilities were moved away from vulnerable regions; large areas of infrastructure were destroyed. People left their native settlements. Part of this migration was organized by the Governmental committees: workers and engineers of the evacuated plants and organizations, their families, families of the army officers, regional leaders of the communist parties, scientists, museum staff, professors and students, and many others. Many fled on their own. According to official data, over 2,500 factories and over 17 million people were evacuated. The number of people who moved to the East on their own accord is unknown [13].

During the evacuation, people were transported mainly by rail. The evacuation started in July 1941; the journey to their places of destination thousands of kilometers away took several months, and the majority arrived in the Urals, Siberia, and Kazakhstan in late November 1941–February 1942, in the depths of the Russian winter. The evacuation was one of the most successful operations of WWII. Most

researchers today agree that it was crucial for retaining industrial productivity to support the war activities of the Soviet Army and its eventual victory. It also saved the lives of those who succeeded in moving away from the occupied regions and would otherwise have been executed due to their ethnicity, political views or other reasons [13].

Although the evacuation was considered successful, this does not exclude the fact that there were many losses. With 17 million migrants, even a presumed 1% of losses amounts to 170,000 human lives. People traveled in overcrowded carriages, with limited access to water, food, and heat. Infectious disease outbreaks were common: dysentery, measles, and scarlet fever are mentioned in documents from the time [13–15]. The number of people who died during transportation or just after their arrival at their destination is unknown. Emergency measures were developed and introduced to facilitate transportation several months after the beginning of the evacuation, but their implementation started after the peak of migration was over [13, 14].

The conditions of housing provided for refugees varied from one region to the other. For example, in Uzbekistan and Tajikistan, the flow of newcomers seems not to have affected the quality of life of the local people and appeared relatively comfortable compared to other regions of the USSR. However, the situation in Siberia, the Urals, and Kazakhstan was catastrophic. The population in many settlements was increased by 25–30%, and the local infrastructure, including the health care services, was not sufficient even for the existing population. In rural settlements, the living conditions for refugees were much worse than in urban areas, and the conditions for the local people deteriorated significantly [10, 13–16]. There was no housing for the refugees. People were settled in earth-houses, barracks, garrets, and in industrial sites. The average living space in Barnaul (Altay territory) was 2 m^2 per person, which no doubt fuelled TB transmission [16]. Refugees often received no administrative support, requiring clothes and utensils, while the local people, who were already experiencing acute shortages before the war, had to share limited resources with newcomers.

The greatest disaster in the majority of the non-occupied territories of Russia was malnutrition. The full mobilization of able-bodied males from the rural areas and requisition of food resources for the army minimized the rations available for those who were left. The evacuation of so many people from the west to the east of the country further aggravated an already critical situation. The population of the rural regions decreased by 20% on average between 1939 and 1945 in the Urals and Siberia [17, 18].

Hunger was a severe complication of the epidemiological situation in the Soviet Union during the "Great Patriotic War," the 1941–1945 conflict between the Soviets and Nazi Germany in WWII. The most well-known and horrific tragedy was the Siege of Leningrad, when hundreds of thousands of civilians were blocked in the city without food, heating or water, under daily bombardment, for 871 days. Many thousands died of alimentary dystrophy and infections. In one of the analyses of the health of the population during the siege, the living conditions were termed "semi-starvation" [6]. This does not adequately describe all the clinical and social effects of these conditions that led to so many deaths: it was deadly hunger [6, 7].

Due to the critical living and health conditions in the unoccupied territories, and the inadequate health care system, TB incidence and death rates increased in major Soviet cities (see Fig. 1). In 1942, TB mortality had increased to 425/100,000 population [8].

TB in the Occupied Territories
No statistical data are available on TB in the Nazi-occupied territories. According to statements of the military medical services, TB rates were high among people from the liberated territories who joined the army. Remaining in an occupied territory was considered a TB risk factor [12]. High TB morbidity could be expected in these regions, given the destruction of the infrastructure, the well-known policies of the Nazi administration in repressing the Slavic population, and requisition of food for Germany's needs. The rate of TB cases among war prisoners revealed by fluorography mass screening by the end of the war was 2.5 times higher than in militaries in the army [12]. In 1946, the population of the liberated regions had decreased by 17–30% compared to 1939 [17, 18].

TB Program in 1941–1945.
The Soviet government was conscious of the threat of TB and tried to prevent the destruction of its TB services. In August 1941, a critical period in Russia's war operations, the USSR People's Commissariat of Health issued an instructive letter on maintaining and improving the TB services. In this letter, the necessity of notification and of providing medical services for evacuated TB patients was stipulated. To replace TB specialists who had been mobilized, physicians of other specialties were to be involved in TB management [8]. In 1942, the People's Commissariat of Health order was issued making BCG vaccination of newborns obligatory. Orders and instructions of the People's Commissariat of Health concerned the management of osteo-articular TB and TB in children, sanitary inspections of the disinfection of sites with AFB-positive TB patients plus isolation of these patients [7, 8].

In 1943, the Government issued a decree "On anti-TB activities," initiating the organization of new TB hospitals and mini sanatoria in factories, kindergartens, and country boarding schools located outside the industrial centers [7, 8]. In Siberia, the number of TB dispensaries and hospital beds increased in most of the regions. However, these were still insufficient for the increased numbers of TB patients, and were negligible in rural areas [10].

TB patients working in ammunitions factories were provided with extra rations to increase their dietary intake. From an initial 70,000 people receiving ration coupons, this was later increased to 206,000 [8].

The increased TB prevalence in children and adolescents was recognized as an urgent problem. New child-care facilities, sanatoria, and schools specializing in TB were opened, with a total of 83,000 beds. To deal with the major problems of malnutrition, dining halls for children and adolescents with TB were organized [8]. Health inspections included regular medical examinations of factory workers in intensive contact with children, adolescents, and others [7, 8].

The USSR People's Commissariat of Health orders and instructions were also adapted to the army medical system [12].

Although the edicts issued in 1941–1942 were inappropriate in the context of the time, under war conditions and the extreme socioeconomic difficulties, they started to be put in place after 1943. By the end of the war, TB mortality had started to decrease with social stabilization (see Fig. 1). Similar improvements in the TB situation were reported by the military medical corps (see Fig. 2) [7, 8, 12]. By 1945, the TB mortality index was similar to that in 1940, at 230/100,000, in 45 cities of the USSR. Although the indicators in 1940 and 1945 are ambiguous, the conclusion that the TB situation had improved is supported by memoirs of many TB specialists who were there during those difficult times [8].

Peculiarities of the Clinical Course of TB in Conditions of War
In a retrospective study of medical histories, no difference was observed in the rates of the various forms of TB in different cities of the USSR, for both pulmonary and extrapulmonary TB [7]. However, some peculiarities in the disease's clinical course and manifestations were described.

TB dispensary data omitted acute cases of primary TB in both the civilian and military services. The disease was probably diagnosed as another acute infectious disease or a manifestation of alimentary dystrophy [7, 12, 19]. Differently in the general health care facilities, an increase in primary acute TB among adults was observed [7, 19]. Post-mortem examinations reported increased rates of exudative forms and caseous pneumonia, and a decrease in non-exudative fibrosis forms [7]. Severe miliary TB was rare. In 1942, an increase in the number of cases of tuberculous lymphadenitis was reported by clinicians (5.6% in 1942 compared to 3.8% in 1939–1940 in Moscow), and as a result of post-mortem examinations (up to 32–40%) in several cities among civilians and war casualties [7, 19]. This was interpreted as a result of immune system failure during primary infection with hematogenic spread and activation of latent infection. Rates of TB lymphadenitis in children remained low [7]. Low rates of serositis among civilian population were registered, with 2–4% exudative pleurisy among all TB cases registered [7]. However, high rates of serous pleurisy, both in the background of other forms of TB and as a single registered symptom, were reported in Leningrad in the context of severe famine and siege, and among the military (up to 27%) [7, 19]. Military TB specialists reported focal TB in 56%, disseminated TB in 15%, and infiltrative TB in 23% of all TB cases registered [19]. In patients with cachexia, manifestations of pulmonary TB were suppressed, and no bacilli were found in the sputum [7].

The clinical course of infiltrative TB was frequently complicated with dissemination, fibrocavernous TB was complicated by acute lymphadenitis and serous pleurisy, and caseous pneumonia by laryngeal TB and serous pleurisy [19].

Observations during the Siege of Leningrad revealed a paradoxical effect: chronic patients with fibrocavernous pulmonary TB proved to have higher tolerance "to malnutrition and deteriorated living conditions" [7].

Conclusion

Although the indices of the TB epidemic are dubious, the general trends are supported by numerous memoirs of people who lived through in those times. They also reflect dynamics of the war and the socioeconomic situation in the USSR in 1941–1945. The catastrophic events of 1941 and the tectonic economic and demographic shifts of 1941–1942 inevitably resulted in outbreaks of TB. The course of the disease in both the civilian and military sectors demonstrated features conditioned by severe depletion of the immune system manifesting as severe disease and dissemination. Governmental edicts and decrees concerning TB issued from the very beginning of the war could be implemented only when some stabilization of the situation was achieved in the areas of conflict and behind the lines and proved to be effective by the end of the war, bringing down TB morbidity and mortality rates.

References

1 Krivosheev GF: Great Patriotic war in Krivosheev G (ed): Russia and the USSR in wars of the 20th century. Losses of the military forces. Statistical research. Moscow, OLMA-Press, 2001, Chapter V. http://lib.ru/MEMUARY/1939–1945/KRIWOSHEEW/poteri.txt#w05.htm–_Toc536603347.

2 Great Patriotic War: Anniversary Statistics Collection. Stat. Coll, Rosstat, Moscow, 2015 (in Russian).

3 Skachkova EI, Nechaeva OB, Punga VV: Organization of anti-TBcare in Russia. Social Aspects of Public Health 2008;2:6–15, http://vestnik.mednet.ru/content/view/66/30/lang,ru/ (in Russian).

4 Yablonskii PK, Vizel AA, Galkin VB, Shulgina MV: Tuberculosis in Russia. Its history and its status today. Am J Respir Crit Care 2015;191:372–376.

5 Zima VF: Soviet rear human losses of famine and diseases in 1941–1945 in Population of Russia and the USSR: new sources and research methods. Ekaterinburg 1993;41–42 (in Russian).

6 Brozek J, Wells S, Keys A: Medical aspects of semistravation in Leningrad (siege 1941–1942). Am Rev Sov Med 1946;4:70–86.

7 Rabukhin AE: War and Tuberculosis. Am Rev Sov Med 1946;3:198–204.

8 Averbukh LG: Tuberculosis: Stages of Fight, Findings and Losses. Optimum publishing house, Odessa, 2005 (in Russian).

9 Historic encyclopedia of Siberia, Historic heritage of Siberia, Novosibirsk, 2009, vv 1–3. http://irkipedia.ru/content/omskaya_oblast_istoricheskaya_enciklopediya_sibiri_2009 (in Russian).

10 Davydova YA: Structure and dynamics of medical – sanitary facilities network in Siberian cities during the Great Patriotic War in 1941–1945. Vestnik of Moscow Region University 2013;3:14, www.evestnik-mgou.ru (in Russian).

11 Ravich-Sherbo VA: Problems with TB in the USSR before the Great Patriotic War in Smirnov E, Girgilav S, Orbeli L (eds): Experience of the soviet medicine in the Great Patriotic War 1941–1945, v.25. Pulmonary TB (peculiarities of genesis, clinical course, prevention and treatment during the war), Moscow, Medgiz, 1955, pp 26–31 (in Russian).

12 Talanov SI, Ivanov IN: Organization of anti-TB struggle in active army in Smirnov E, Girgilav S, Orbeli L (eds): Experience of the soviet medicine in the Great Patriotic War 1941–1945, v.25. Pulmonary TB (peculiarities of genesis, clinical course, prevention and treatment during the war), Moscow, Medgiz 1955;37–67 (in Russian).

13 Kumanev GA: Evacuation of the USSR population: achievements and losses in: USSR human losses in the period of the II World War, Saint-Petersburg, 1995;137–145 (in Russian).

14 Usol'tsev NL: Assurance of Sanitary and Epidemic Welfare of the South Ural during the Great Patriotic War, Magistra Vitae E-Journal in History and Archelogy Sciences, 2016;1:128–137. http://magistravitaejournal.ru/ru/archive/6-aprel-2016.html (in Russian).

15 Zhanggutin BO: Evacuation of the Soviet Population to Kazakhstan (1941–1942), 2010. https://cyberleninka.ru/article/v/evakuatsiya-sovetskogo-naseleniya-v-kazahstan-1941-1942-gg (in Russian).

16 Shevlyakov AS, Cheremnyh OA: Every-day Life of People in Western Siberia during the Great Patriotic War: On Housing and Household, Rusin Journal Library, 2015;2:7–21 (in Russian).

17 Isupov V, Korobeinikova N, Semenov M: Population of the West Siberia during the II World War, Demographic Reviews, 2016;3:143–168 (in Russian).

18 Zima VF: Mortality of Rural Population in the Soviet Rear (Archive Summaries 1941–1945) in: USSR Human Losses in the Period of the II World War, Saint-Petersburg, 1995;160–165 (in Russian).

19 Ravich-Sherbo VA (ed): Peculiarities of the Primary forms of Pulmonary TB in Military Units during the Great Patriotic War in Smirnov E, Girgilav S, Orbeli L (eds): Experience of the soviet medicine in the Great Patriotic War 1941–1945, v.25. Pulmonary TB (peculiarities of genesis, clinical course, prevention and treatment during the war), Moscow, Medgiz, 1955;68–146 (in Russian).

Marina V. Shulgina
I.I. Mechnikov North-West State Medical University
1/28, Santiago-de-Cuba str.
RU–194291 Saint-Petersburg (Russia)
E-Mail m_shulgina@mail.ru

Murray JF, Loddenkemper R (eds): Tuberculosis and War. Lessons Learned from World War II.
Prog Respir Res. Basel, Karger, 2018, vol 43, pp 179–187 (DOI: 10.1159/000481486)

Tuberculosis in the United States before, during, and after World War II

Philip C. Hopewell

Curry International Tuberculosis Center, Division of Pulmonary and Critical Care Medicine, San Francisco General Hospital, University of California, San Francisco, CA, USA

Abstract

With war looming, both civilian and military tuberculosis experts, aware of the impact of WW I on tuberculosis mortality, began to make plans to prevent a similar occurrence in yet another war. In 1940, the country was in a better position to confront the public health challenges of the war. As reflected by the mortality rate, there was less than half as much tuberculosis as there had been at the conclusion of the previous war. Resources for case detection and care were available. Radiography was commonly used for screening and case detection. Care facilities for patients with tuberculosis were more widely available. An enlarged public health infrastructure was established with tuberculosis control agencies in many county and state jurisdictions, and a federal agency initiated in 1942. Although anti-tuberculosis drug development was an active area of research during the war years, utilization of the drugs did not occur until after the war. In the United States, the decline in tuberculosis death rates continued through the war years. Mortality fell from 45.8/100,000 in 1940 to 40/100,000 in 1945, a 15% decline However, between 1940 and 1945 the case rate increased from 76/100,000 to 89/100,000 a 17% increase, likely a consequence of the war.

On September 3, 1939, 2 days after Germany invaded Poland, France and England declared war on Germany, a near final step in setting the stage for World War II and making the entry of the United States into the war largely inevitable. In late 1939 and 1940, with war looming, public health authorities and clinicians, both civilian and military involved in tuberculosis care and control in the United States, being well aware of the impact of World War I on tuberculosis mortality in the civilian and military (including former military) populations of the country, began to make plans to prevent a similar occurrence in what was sure to be a protracted conflict [1, 2]. Sir Authur McNaltey, Chief Medical Officer of the British Ministry of Health called tuberculosis, – "one of the camp followers of war," and this was very clearly borne out by World War I [3]. The effects of World War I on tuberculosis in the United States were felt not only during the war but also later and, thus, influenced the situation when World War II began. However, by the time it became clear that the United States would be drawn into the global conflagration, in spite of just emerging from the economic devastation of the Great Depression, the country was in a much better position to confront the public health challenges, including tuberculosis, brought about by the war. Thus, the overall impact was, perhaps, less than anticipated, but, nevertheless, appreciable.

Although this chapter is focused on the impact of the Second World War on tuberculosis in the United States, the events occurring in the war years, 1941–45, cannot be assessed in isolation from events that occurred and circumstances that prevailed prior and after the war as well as during war time.

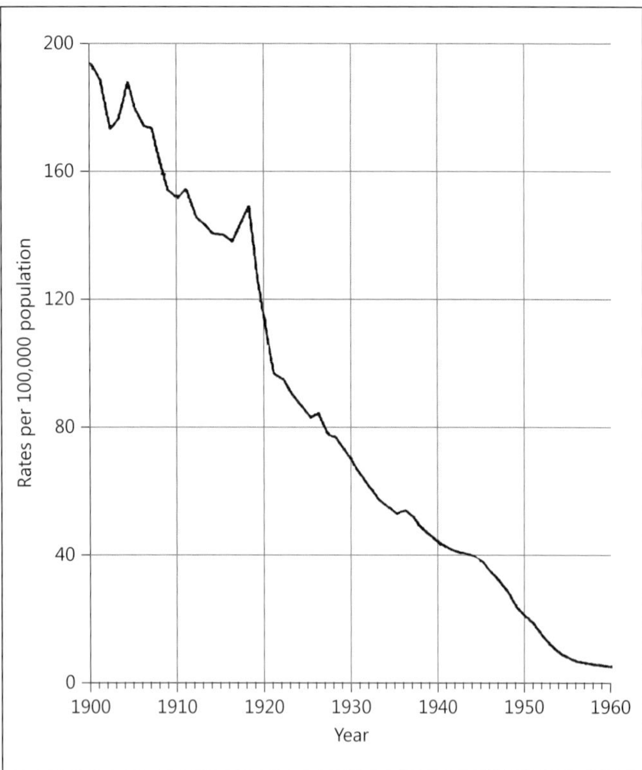

Fig. 1. Death rates for tuberculosis, United States, all forms: Death registration states, 1900–1930; all states 1933–1960 (rates per 100,000 population) [6].

Tuberculosis Trends Prior to the War

It has been widely noted that mortality rates for tuberculosis began decreasing well before the recognition of the infectious and contagious nature of tuberculosis or the discovery of its etiologic agent [4, 5]. However, this steady downward trajectory was interrupted by the First World War, most dramatically in the Western Europe and less strikingly, but still appreciably, in the United States (Fig. 1) [1, 2, 6]. Surprisingly and, largely, inexplicably the tuberculosis mortality rate, following the spike associated with World War I, resumed its downward slope at an even greater rate of decline. (Although the influenza pandemic may have confounded assessment of tuberculosis mortality – both the increase and subsequent sharp decrease in death rates.). By 1920, the mortality rate in the United States was approximately 95/100,000, whereas, a decade earlier it had been about 155/100,000. By 1930, the rate was 71/100,000 and in 1940, the year prior to the entry of the United States into WW II, it was 46/100,000. Thus, insofar as mortality rates reflect disease prevalence, there

was less than half as much tuberculosis in the United States as there had been at the conclusion of the previous war [6].

Validity of the Data

It is important to note that caution should be exercised in interpreting tuberculosis statistics, such as those cited above for the United States. Truly accurate tuberculosis mortality rates for the country have only been available since 1940 and accurate incidence rates since 1953. For the most part, the descriptive epidemiology of tuberculosis was, before the mid-1920s, limited to mortality rates which are dependent on accurate assessments of the cause of death, identification of all deaths caused by tuberculosis throughout the country (generally, only pulmonary tuberculosis deaths were counted), and an accurate count of the total population. All of these data are subject to major limitations in completeness and accuracy. For example, death data for the United States began to be collected in only 10 states and an unknown number of cities in 1900. By 1933, all 48 states were included in vital statistics reports, but it was not until 1940 that the vital statistics were backed by accurate population counts [7]. "Incidence" data began to be collected in the mid 1920s by the National Tuberculosis Association (NTA), but the population base was not clear and both active and inactive cases were counted. In 1953, reporting criteria were changed and only new active cases were included. In spite of these limitations, it is reassuring to note that, prior to the advent of anti-tuberculosis chemotherapy in the late 1940s, the slopes of all the rates – mortality, old incidence calculations, and new incidence calculations – were qualitatively similar so the trends they reflect are probably accurate [8].

Tuberculosis in the Military

Tuberculosis was first recognized as a military problem in WW I. As described by Long [9], screening for tuberculosis among US army inductees was initiated after it was noted that there was a high prevalence of tuberculosis among French troops who had entered the war 3 years earlier. Parenthetically, it should be noted that tuberculosis among French soldiers led to an apparent substantial increase in cases among French civilians [10]. Because radiography was still in its infancy and its role in screening for tuberculosis not yet established, most of the screening of US Army inductees in WW I was done by physical examination. The results of the military screening program for inductees, as well as surveillance for the disease among personnel on active duty, and screening again at the time of discharge provide an interesting window on tuberculosis prevalence and incidence during both world wars. At least for this limited segment of the population, mainly males between 18 and 34 years of age, the data are likely to be accurate, although the rates are subject to inaccuracies of the screening method and are based on the total number of (mainly) men in the military in a given year, not on the population as a whole [9].

Needless to say, the use of physical examination as a screening test was an insensitive means of making a presumptive diagnosis and resulted in the induction of many men with tuberculosis (although some 50,000 men were excluded from service because of presumed tuberculosis, a rejection rate of 2.3% of those screened) and many were mustered out of service because of having tuberculosis [1, 11–13]. During 1917—1918, the annual incidence of tuberculosis in US service men was approximately 12 cases/1,000/military personnel. In total, there were 22,812 separations from service due to tuberculosis in 1917 and 1918 [13]. In addition, a large number of cases were discovered during the demobilization examinations. The military assumed responsibility for the care of these former soldiers, and, at that time, care meant a long stay in a hospital or sanatorium. This left the Army with a large number of patients for whom they were responsible, a number that far out-stripped the capacity of military hospitals.

Although there were a few intermediate steps, it was this large tuberculosis patient load, together with an even larger number of men with "shell-shock" that led to the founding of the veterans administration (VA) system of hospitals in which there was, for many years, an ongoing focus on tuberculosis. In 1917, when the US entered World War I, there were no hospitals specifically for veterans. By 1925, there were 51 in the VA system. The number of patients with tuberculosis in the VA system peaked in 1922 at 44,591. This number had decreased to around 5,000 by 1940, but between 1921 and 1940, a total of 293,761 patients had been admitted to VA hospitals because of tuberculosis [11, 13]. The veterans hospitals together with military hospitals played an important role in tuberculosis research and patient care into and beyond World War II, as will be discussed in more detail subsequently.

During mobilization for WW II, it was decided that chest radiography would be used to screen inductees for tuberculosis. Although the approach proved difficult to implement, in part because of the number of induction stations, ultimately approximately 10 million men received radiographic examinations and about 1% were rejected because of a radiographic diagnosis of tuberculosis [13]. The incidence of tuberculosis during the course of the war was about 1.2/1,000 troops/year or about one tenth of the rate encountered in WW I.

Approaches to Tuberculosis Control up to and Including the War Years

Prior to the late 1800s, although mortality rates were decreasing, there were essentially no effective measures for reducing the transmission of *Mycobacterium tuberculosis* and, thus, no specific tuberculosis control measures. Sanatorium treatment, that began in Europe in the latter half of the 19th century and was subsequently taken up in a limited number of locations in the United States, probably did reduce transmission and decreased mortality rates, but was only very gradually scaled-up to a point where there appeared to be an attributable impact on death rates. Even then the impact of sanatorium treatment remained controversial [14]. Founded in 1904, the National Association for the Study and Prevention of Tuberculosis (NASPT), later the NTA and now the American Lung Association, had, as one of its early programs, advocacy for increasing inpatient beds for tuberculosis. The advocacy effort was successful: Between 1904 and 1919, shortly after the end of World War I, the number of specialized beds for patients with tuberculosis increased from 9,000 to 56,000.

NASPT/NTA had 3 additional areas of activity; creating local societies and, emanating from them, public education on tuberculosis, and advocacy for public health tuberculosis control agencies at county, state, and national levels of government. By 1940, there were approximately 2,500 local tuberculosis societies [15]. The results of public education campaigns are impossible to quantify, but, given the population coverage of local tuberculosis societies and the ubiquity of the Christmas Seal, through which the NTA, largely, was supported, it seems likely that the public was well aware of tuberculosis as a public health problem (Fig. 2). Advocacy for inclusion of tuberculosis control units in public health departments was also very successful, though somewhat slow to be fully implemented. The success was perhaps best demonstrated by the inclusion of an office focused on tuberculosis within the US Public Health Service (USPHS) in 1942. Two years later, Congress established a Tuberculosis Control Division within the Public Health service and in

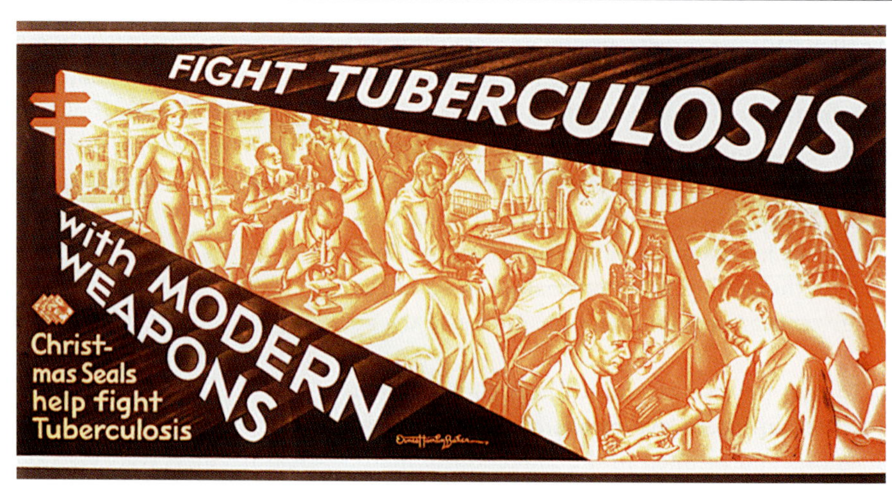

Fig. 2. National Library of Medicine. Visual Culture and Public Health posters: Tuberculosis. https://www.nlm.nih.gov/exhibition/visualculture/tuberculosis.html. From the website description: "This poster by famous portrait artist Ernest Hamlin Baker reflects a distinctive 1930s style of illustration. Rays of light, emanating from the double-barred cross emblem of the NTA, illuminate scenes of health personnel working in laboratories and caring for patients. The figures, design, and composition of this poster reflect a modernist style appropriate for the promotion of newly developed scientific solutions to an age-old problem. A series of illustrations described as "modern weapons" in the fight against tuberculosis include a man looking into a microscope, a nurse and doctor monitoring a woman receiving intravenous treatment, a young boy receiving an injection, and an X-ray displayed prominently in the background. As part of the campaign to solicit contributions, the message in the bottom corner of the poster suggests, "Christmas Seals help fight Tuberculosis."

1960 the Division was incorporated into the National Communicable Disease Center (now, the Center for Disease Control) in Atlanta, GA, USA.

Also, the NASPT/NTA in 1905 gave rise to the American Sanatorium Association, now the American Thoracic Society, as its medical section [16]. Together the 2 organizations conducted local, national, and international scientific meetings and, beginning in 1917, published a scientific journal, both of which enhanced the scientific milieu for tuberculosis research and provided vehicles for dissemination of knowledge about the disease.

Increased understanding of tuberculosis epidemiology and the greater availability of inpatient beds for patients with tuberculosis led to the concept of early case detection and isolation as the underlying principle of tuberculosis control, probably beginning in the 1920s, but increasing in the 1930s and 40s. This concept, plus the increasing availability and utilization of diagnostic radiography provided the rationale for mass radiography campaigns aimed at the general population or targeted to specific risk groups [17]. Both the NTA and, later, the USPHS as well as local organizations conducted campaigns [18]. The development of photofluorography by a Brazilian, Manuel Abreu, in which

the images were recorded on 70 mm film in a continuous roll, enabling rapid scrolling of the films, greatly facilitated the mass campaigns. Mass radiography had 3 objectives: (1) to detect patients earlier in disease progression in an effort to reduce mortality; (2) to reduce transmission by isolating those found to have active tuberculosis; and (3) to identify high-risk tuberculosis suspects. More to the point, the rationale for the campaigns was illustrated by this quote from R. J. Anderson, author of the report for describing the campaigns conducted by the USPHS, "Epidemiologically, it is the hidden case of tuberculosis that represents the chief focus for the continued existence and spread of the disease –" (Fig. 3) [18]. The most comprehensive description of the results is contained in a report on the campaigns conducted by the USPHS in which about 6 million people in 21 mainly urban communities underwent X-ray screening between 1945 and 1948. To summarize the experience, on average, of every 100,000 persons examined 2,202 of the images would be classified as suspected tuberculosis. On further evaluation of the suspect images, 99 would be found to represent active tuberculosis, 90% of which was undiagnosed, and 617 would be considered as inactive [18]. Thus, the prevalence of active tuberculosis in these general population screening campaigns conducted just after the war ended was about 100/100,000 population, very similar to the 120/100,000 incidence observed in the military, and also to the 93/100,000 in the US as a whole. (This last comparison may not be valid, however, because both active and inactive cases were included in the case rate during those years.) Whether the early detection and isolation approach to tuberculosis control had any impact on the incidence of tuberculosis during or just after the war is not known.

The Great Depression, the New Deal, and Public Policy

Although the first decade following the end of WW I in 1919 was one of great prosperity, the crash of 1929, the ensuing Great Depression, and the social and economic upheavals that followed dominated the next 10 years, essentially until the beginning of WW II. It would seem that the conditions brought about by the depression – under nutrition, stress, depression, and a broad inability to afford health care would favor a recrudescence of tuberculosis. This did not happen, at least not during the decade of the depression. Both case and death rates continued on their pre-existing downward course [19]. However, during the decade of the depression, the seeds may have been sown for the increase in case rates that occurred during the war years. Beginning in 1941, there was an increase in case rates from a low of 76/100,000 in 1940 to a high of 94/100,000 in 1944, a 24% increase (Fig. 4).

At its peak in 1933, the unemployment rate was 25% and many individuals and families moved from "comfortable" or "moderate" to "poor" in their economic classification. Levels of stress and depression led to a high rate of suicide. Medical care, at least usual fee for service care, was limited by income but there were many sources of free care. However, care was not sought for many illnesses [20]. The affordability and, thus, accessibility of diagnostic tests such as chest radiographs and sputum microscopy and culture is not known. It could be speculated that for people, especially those in the "poor" category, with reduced incomes seeking care for symptoms of tuberculosis was delayed and, once care was obtained, diagnoses may have been delayed.

In response to the depression, President Franklin Roosevelt, elected in 1932, succeeded in having passed, in 1933, legislation grouped under the "New Deal." The New Deal agenda, among other things, called for increased federal support for public health bureaus and activities, and many

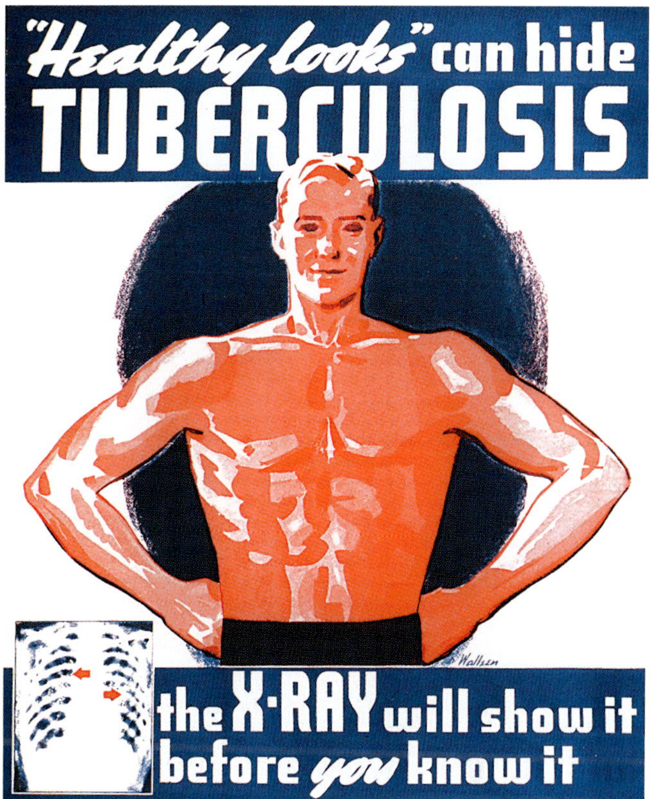

Christmas Seals Fight Tuberculosis

Fig. 3. National Library of Medicine. Visual Culture and Public Health Posters: Tuberculosis. https://www.nlm.nih.gov/exhibition/visual-culture/tuberculosis.html. From the website description: "The National Tuberculosis Association used proceeds from Christmas Seal campaigns to develop educational posters that emphasized both prevention and control. This 1930s poster uses a common technique in public health posters involving the juxtaposition of text and image to create a message that works against viewer expectations. In this poster, the viewer may come to the image with the expectation that it is an advertisement for an exercise program or vitamin supplement, only to learn, by reading the text in the image, that it is a warning that you can look healthy but still have tuberculosis. The image of the healthy man is accompanied by an illustration of how an X-ray machine can be used to identify TB long before symptoms appear. By fostering faith in the value of science and preventive technologies, this technique also confirms the value of the Christmas Seals campaign in supporting additional research."

state governments followed suit. This increased role of government was accompanied (or preceded) by a rising tide of popular support for government programs, including those related to public health. Public health programs, in turn, were intended to foster, mobilize, and consolidate popular support, as well as fight the disease. Thus, during a time of

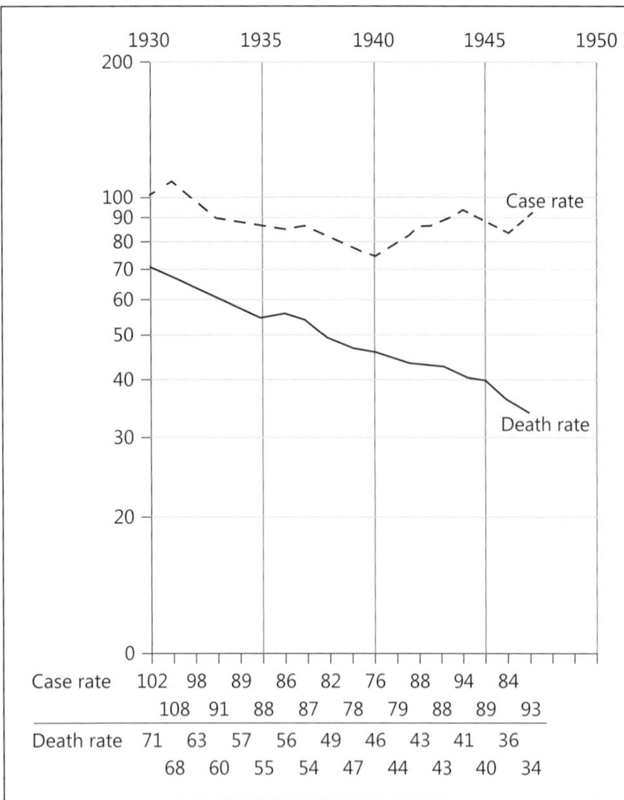

Fig. 4. Tuberculosis case and death rates, United States 1930–1947 (rates per 100,000 population) [19], with permission of the American Thoracic Society.

grave economic crisis, but with popular support, the public health system of the country was strengthened.

The view of tuberculosis as not simply a matter of individual health but of the health of the public, probably dates to at least the first few years of the 20th century with the formation of the NASPT/NTA and its advocacy program for public health tuberculosis control programs and beds for patients with tuberculosis. This concept of tuberculosis as a public health problem may have minimized the potential deleterious consequences of the depression on tuberculosis control, although as noted above, the decade of the 30s may have led to the increased case rates in the 40s.

Chemotherapy

Clearly, the most important event in the evolution of scientific knowledge related to tuberculosis was the discovery of the etiological agent of the disease, *Mycobacterium tuberculosis* [21]. However, although the discovery of the organism

provided a target upon which therapeutic approaches could be focused, little progress was made in identifying chemotherapeutic agents until the 1940s. The failure of tuberculin, advocated by Koch as a therapeutic agent, seemed to discourage further investigations for a time. However, development of penicillin and sulfa drugs, and their spectacular successes during the war reinvigorated efforts to find chemotherapeutic compounds for tuberculosis. Although these efforts were not successful until the development of streptomycin, approaches for testing compounds were greatly facilitated by the methodology used in the clinical trial of sanocrysin (sodium-gold thiosulfate) that was the first, prospective single-blind placebo-controlled trial (Patients were not aware of the study arm to which they were allocated by a coin-flip.) of an anti-infective drug [22]. Although the methods used would not be acceptable by today's rigorous standards for such testing, the study demonstrated the value of a controlled clinical trial and provided the basic framework for testing of subsequent candidate compounds and drug regimens. Needless to say, the trial had negative results and demonstrated that sanocrysin was highly toxic. Thus, going into the era of the war, while there were still no anti-tuberculosis drugs, there was considerable activity, a progressively refined understanding of microbiology, and more sophisticated methodology for animal and human testing of new agents.

It is impossible to know if the war spurred or impeded drug development; however, it was during the war that a group of soil microbiologists, led by Selman Waksman, working at Rutgers University in New Jersey, developed streptomycin that was shown to be effective against *M. tuberculosis,* initially in culture and animal models and, subsequently, in humans [23–25]. During roughly the same time period, Jörgen Lehmann, working in Sweden, synthesized para-amino salicylic acid (PAS), the first orally effective anti-tuberculosis agent. In 1945, Lehmann and his physician partner gave PAS to a patient with TB 3 weeks before Hinshaw et al. first gave streptomycin to a patient. However, for unclear reasons, Lehmann's discovery was not published until 1946, 2 years after the first publication of the effectiveness of streptomycin [26]. Streptomycin and PAS, although effective when used alone, had suboptimal results with frequent relapses and generation of drug resistance. It was not until 1950 with the publication of the results of a British Medical Research Council trial of combination therapy with streptomycin and PAS, that the clear benefits of combining the 2 drugs was demonstrated [27].

As noted earlier in this chapter, the formation of the VA health care system in the early 1920s, based, in part, on the need to care for WW I veterans with tuberculosis provided an important resource for testing innovations in care, including drug trials. Research on tuberculosis was greatly facilitated by the formation of a research subdivision within the VA health care system in the mid-1920s. WW II resulted in a substantial increase in the number of veterans hospitalized in VA hospitals for tuberculosis. The number increased from just over 4,000 in 1940 to 8,000 in 1946 and peaked at nearly 16,000 in 1952 [11]. These patients were, largely, although not entirely, WW II veterans. Recognizing the need for specialized attention to the needs of patients with tuberculosis, the Veterans' Administration hired Dr. John Barnwell, a professor at the University of Michigan and a well-established tuberculosis investigator, to lead clinical and research efforts to improve the care of patients with the disease. Barnwell's hiring came at a crucial time – 1946 – just as streptomycin was becoming available, albeit in very limited quantities. Recognizing the need for clinical studies on streptomycin, Barnwell hired Dr. Arthur Walker who had been part of the group coordinating the study on penicillin and the 2 of them designed the first VA-Armed Forces study of streptomycin that began in 1946. The study utilized a standardized protocol but was observational with the patient's pretreatment course, serving as his/her own "control" rather than being a true controlled clinical trial. The lack of a control group was hotly debated but did not change, surprising in view of the design of the sanocrysin trial some 15 years earlier that did involve a control group. Informed consent was not a part of the protocol [11, 28]. This was the first of an ongoing series of (usually) multicenter cooperative studies on the chemotherapy of tuberculosis. The involvement of the VA in the study of streptomycin led to an annual conference (called simply the "streptomycin conference") that evolved into the VA-Armed Forces Conference on the Chemotherapy of Tuberculosis and subsequently, in 1961, the VA-Armed Forces Pulmonary Disease Research Conference, an annual event until 1972. Even though more generically titled, the conference continued to devote considerable time to tuberculosis.

All of the foregoing is by way of saying that, while anti-tuberculosis drug development was an active and highly productive area of research during the war, effective utilization of the drugs did not occur until after the war and had little impact on either the incidence or mortality during the war. However, it is quite clear that beginning in 1945, the year of the war's end, there is a point of downward inflection in the curves depicting tuberculosis death rates, not only in the United States but also in a number of other countries, including several directly impacted by the war, with rates decreasing substantially more steeply than in prior years (Fig. 5) [29]. Although truly effective chemotherapy was not available until the introduction of isoniazid in 1952, the sustained acceleration of the decline in death rates is highly likely to be the result of effective chemotherapy, as well as improved supportive care in general.

A dramatic demonstration of the impact of chemotherapy, even prior to the wide availability of isoniazid, can be seen in data from the VA hospital system. Over the 12-year period, from 1942 to1953, a period in which admission characteristics of the patients and the supportive care provided had likely changed very little, the percentage of admitted patients who died dropped from 23.2 to 7.5% [29].

In the United States, the decline in tuberculosis death rates continued through the war years. Between 1940 and 1945, the death rate fell from 45.8/100,000 to 40/100,000, a decline of approximately 15%, only slightly less that the 16% decline in the 1935–1940 period (Fig. 2). By 1950, the rate was down to 20/100,000 [29]. Judging by this indicator, the war had very little, if any, impact on tuberculosis in the United States. However, the picture was not so rosy as it might seem. By-and-large since the mid- to late 1800s, the descriptive epidemiology of tuberculosis had focused on death rates. As noted previously, determination of incidence rates did not begin until the mid-1920s and were of questionable accuracy, but over time they became more complete and accurate. Accepting the reported incidence as accurate, between 1940 and 1945 the case rate increased from 76/100,000 to 89/100,000, a 17% increase. In comparison, the case rate decreased from 88/100,000 in 1935 to 76/100,000 in 1940, a 14% decrease. This pattern, decreasing death rates accompanied by increasing case rates, was noted in all parts of the country except the New England and mid-Atlantic states where case rates, as well as death rates, decreased.

The desirability of shifting focus from death rates to incidence is nicely captured in a quote from Edwards and Drolet [29], "Is it not time that we raise our sights from the cemeteries and the premature graves to the living tuberculous who really need our attention and for whom we can still do something?" They go on to say, "It must be obvious that so long as the number of new cases remains constant or, worse, increases, this scourge of mankind is not only under control, but is in fact getting out of control." In 1950, the case rate of 80/100,000 was still 5% higher than it had been in 1940. This raises the question of whether the rapid resumption of the pre-WWI decline in death rates following the war accurately reflected the true situation with regard to tuberculosis control.

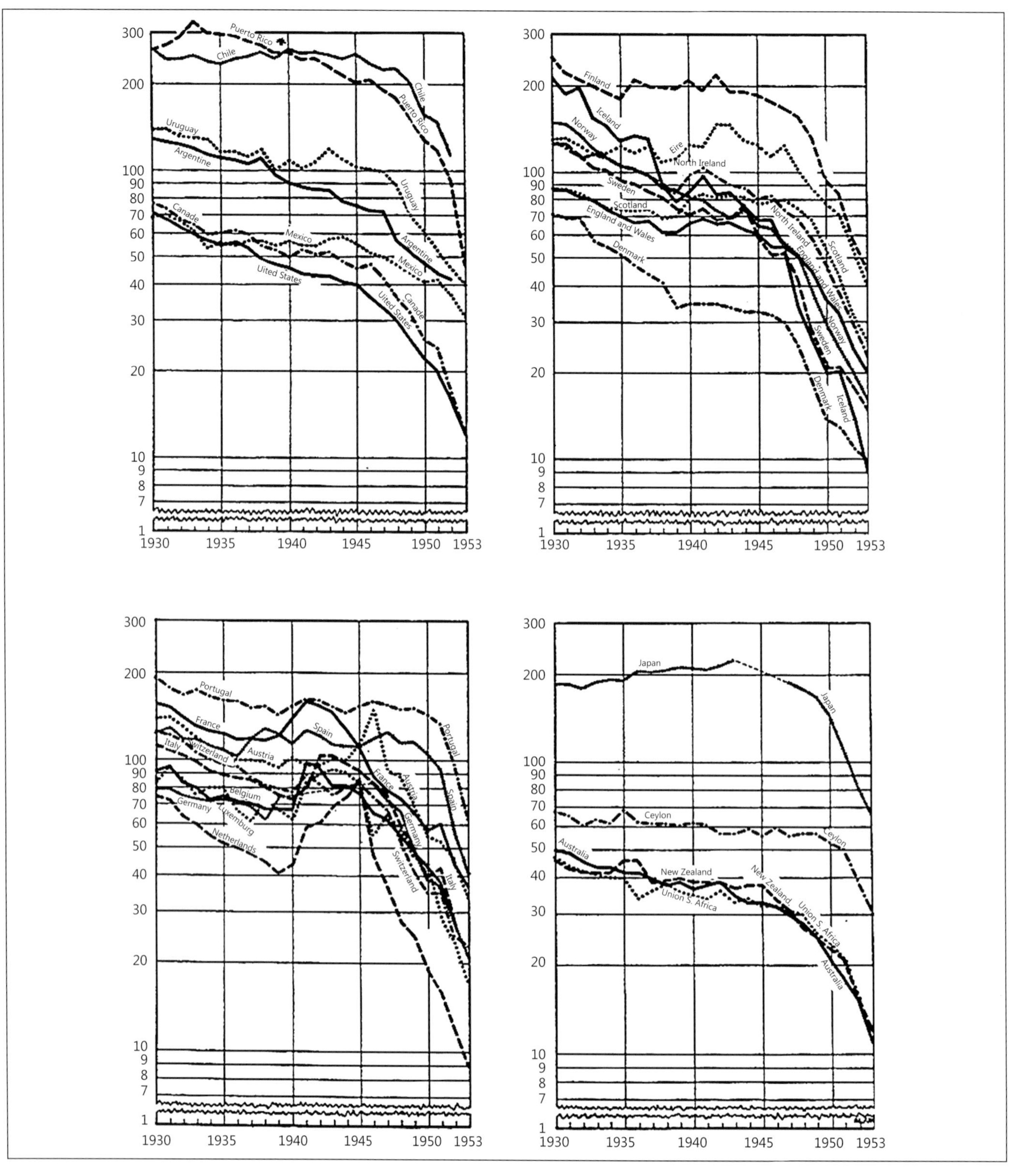

Fig. 5. Tuberculosis death rates, United States and other countries, 1930–1953. United States and other countries of the Americas in left upper panel, England, Wales, Scotland and Scandinavian countries upper right, continental western Europe lower left and Japan, Ceylon (Sri Lanka), Union of South Africa (South Africa), and new Zealand lower right (rates per 100,000 population), with permission of the American Thoracic Society. Copyright © 2017 American Thoracic Society.

References

1 Murray JF: Tuberculosis and World War I. Am J Resp Crit Care Med 2015;192:411–414.
2 Lee WW: The influence of the world war on tuberculosis mortality in civilian populations. Am Rev Tuberc 1931;24:326–339.
3 Quoted in Byerly CR: Good Tuberculosis Men. Office of the Surgeon General, Borden Institute, US Army Medical Department and School, Fort Sam Huston, Texas.
4 Dubos R, Dubos J: The White Plague: Tuberculosis, Man, and Society. New Brunswick, Rutgers University Press, 1996, pp 229–232.
5 Murray JF: The Industrial Revolution and the decline in death rates from tuberculosis. Int J Tuberc Lung Dis 2015;19:502–503.
6 Grove RD, Hetzel AM: Vital Statistics Rates in the United States 1940–1960. US Department of Health Education and Welfare. Washington, Public Health Service, 1968.
7 Linder FE, Grove RD: Vital Statistics Rates in the United States 1900–1940. Washington, Federal Security Agency, United States Public Health Service, National Office of Vital Statistics, 1947 (https://www.cdc.gov/nchs/data/vsus/vsrates1900–40.pdf.
8 Comstock GW: Epidemiology of tuberculosis. Am Rev Respir Dis 1982;125(part 2):8–15.
9 Long ER: Chapter 14, Tuberculosis; Tuberculosis in World War I. US Army Medical Department, Office of Medical History http://amedd.army.mil/bookdocs/wwiiPM4/1444.Tuberculosis.htm.
10 100 years: The Rockefeller Foundation: Tuberculosis in France Peace and Conflict. mht. https://www.rockefellerfoundation.org/about-us/our-history

11 Hays MT: A Historical Look at the establishment of the Department of Veterans Affairs Research and Development program. US, Veterans Administration www.research.va.gov.
12 Marietta SU: Tuberculosis in World War II: the army viewpoint. Chest 1945;11:267–268).
13 Long ER: Chapter 11, Tuberculosis: Part 1, Tuberculosis in the Army. US Army Medical Department, Office of Medical History http://amedd.army.mil/bookdocs/wwiiPM4/1444.Tuberculosis.htm.
14 Daniel TM: The history of tuberculosis. Respir Med 2006;100:1862–1870.
15 Shryock RH: National Tuberculosis Association, 1904–1954. New York, National Tuberculosis Association, 1957.
16 Murray JF, Du Melle F, Hopewell PC: Evolution and revolution: the formation of today's American Thoracic Society, part 1. Am J Respir Crit Care Med 2012;186:948–952.
17 Golub JE, Mohan CI, Comstock GW, Chaisson RE: Active case finding of tuberculosis: historical perspective and future prospects and future prospects. Int J Tuberc Lung Dis 2005;9:1183–1203.
18 Anderson RJ: Community-wide chest X ray survey. Public Health Service Publication No. 222. Washington, United States Government Printing Office, 1952.
19 Edwards HR, Drolet GJ: The implications of changing morbidity and mortality from tuberculosis. Am Rev Tuberc 1950;61:39–50.

20 Perrott GS, Sydenstricker E, Collins SD: Medical care during the depression: a preliminary report upon a survey of wage-earning families in seven large cities. Milbank Q 2005;83:2005–2020. (Reprinted from Milbank Fund Quarterly 1934;12:99–114.)
21 Koch R: Die Aetiologie der Tuberculose, a translation by Berta Pinner and Max Pinner with an introduction by Allen K. Krause. Am Rev Tuberc 1932;25:285–323.
22 Amberson JB, McMahon BT, Pinner M: A clinical trial of sanocrysin in pulmonary tuberculosis. Am Rev Tuberc 1931;24:4401–4435.
23 Schatz AB, Bugie E, Waksman SA: Streptomycin, a substance exhibiting antibiotic activity against gram-positive and gram-negative bacteria. Proc Soc Exp Biol Med 1944;55:66–69.
24 Feldman WH, Hinshaw HC, Mann FC: Streptomycin in experimental tuberculosis. Am Rev Tuberc 1945;52:269–298.
25 Hinshaw HC, Feldman WH, Pfuetze KH: Treatment of tuberculosis with streptomycin; a summary of observations on one hundred cases. J Am Med Assoc 1946;132:778–782.
26 Lehmann J: para-Aminosalicylic acid in the treatment of tuberculosis. Lancet 1946;1:15–16.
27 Treatment of pulmonary tuberculosis with streptomycin and para-aminosalicylic acid; a Medical Research Council investigation. Br Med J 1950;2:1073–1085.
28 Barnwell JB, Bunn PA, Walker AM: The effect of streptomycin upon pulmonary tuberculosis. Am Rev Tuberc 1947;566:4485–4507.
29 Drolet GJ, Lowell AM: Whereto tuberculosis; the first seven years of the antimicrobial era, 1947–1953. Am Rev Tuberc Pulm Dis 1955;72:419–452.

Philip C. Hopewell, MD
Room 5K1
San Francisco General Hospital
San Francisco, CA 94110 (USA)
E-Mail phil.hopewell@ucsf.edu

Murray JF, Loddenkemper R (eds): Tuberculosis and War. Lessons Learned from World War II.
Prog Respir Res. Basel, Karger, 2018, vol 43, pp 188–196 (DOI: 10.1159/000481487)

Tuberculosis in Japan before, during, and after World War II

Toru Mori · Nobukatsu Ishikawa

Research Institute of Tuberculosis/Japan Anti-Tuberculosis Association, Tokyo, Japan

Abstract

Background: During the latter half of the 19th century, Japan experienced a historical epidemic of TB along with the progress of the industrial revolution that accompanied modernization and urbanization. Adolescent women recruited for textile factories were the main victims. After 1910, the epidemic seemed to subside and mortality took a downward, although very slow, course. However, this new trend was soon interrupted as Japan entered the Sino-Japanese War in 1931 followed by World War II in 1941. ***Summary:*** During the war period from 1931 through 1945, the massive mobilization of young males to battle was accompanied by new trends of economy centering on the heavy industry that also mobilized young males to urban factories. TB mortality again began to rise after 1931 until it reached 241 per 100,000 (estimated) in 1944, causing a serious excess of TB deaths over the baseline trends since 1910. This rate is the second highest in Japan's TB history. The main victims were young male soldiers and factory workers. The total number of excess TB deaths during this 15-year period is estimated to be 490,000, i.e., 22% more than the expected number of TB deaths during this period. This excess mortality diminished soon after the end of the war, and the mortality rate returned to the level expected by extrapolation over the basic trend line that had started around 1910. ***Key Notes:*** Governmental and non-governmental organizations made tremendous efforts in public health and clinical services during the war period. These efforts bore fruit only after the end of the war, bringing about the very fast decline of TB mortality exceeding 10% per year. Of course, this improvement was greatly supported by the advent of modern chemotherapy and other preventive measures such as BCG vaccination and X-ray screening that became widely available after the war.

© 2018 S. Karger AG, Basel

Tuberculosis (TB) has existed in Japan since as early as the third century, as signs of TB lesions are evident in bones from that period. Moreover, from feudalistic times until the late 19th century, TB was apparently common or endemic [1]. However, after Japan opened its gate to the world in 1868, the country experienced modernization accompanied by urbanization and industrialization, after which TB gradually became more prevalent, as it did in European countries in the 18th century. From that time through the first half of the 20th century, TB remained the major killer in Japan, and it became known as "the nation-destroying illness."

The patterns and trends of TB in terms of mortality are assumed to remain constant for a certain period due to a balance or equilibrium of various related factors, which are then replaced by different patterns and trends. This change, known as "transition," was initiated in pioneering population studies under the term "demographic transition" [2]. Since the start of industrialization in the late 1800s up to 1980, Japan experienced 3 TB transitions. This chapter discusses the TB transitions in modern Japan that were either modified or not modified by World War II (WWII), and that were affected by the quality and quantity of its effects on TB mortality compared with the baseline demographic trend.

Prelude

The assassination on June 28, 1914 of Archduke Franz Ferdinand and his wife Sophie readied the stage for World War I (WWI), which erupted exactly 1 month later. Among the early belligerents, Germany began its invasion of France via neutral Belgium, and the United Kingdom (UK) declared war on Germany on August 4, 1914. Here is another small but important piece of WWI history that many people have forgotten and most did not know about in the first place: the

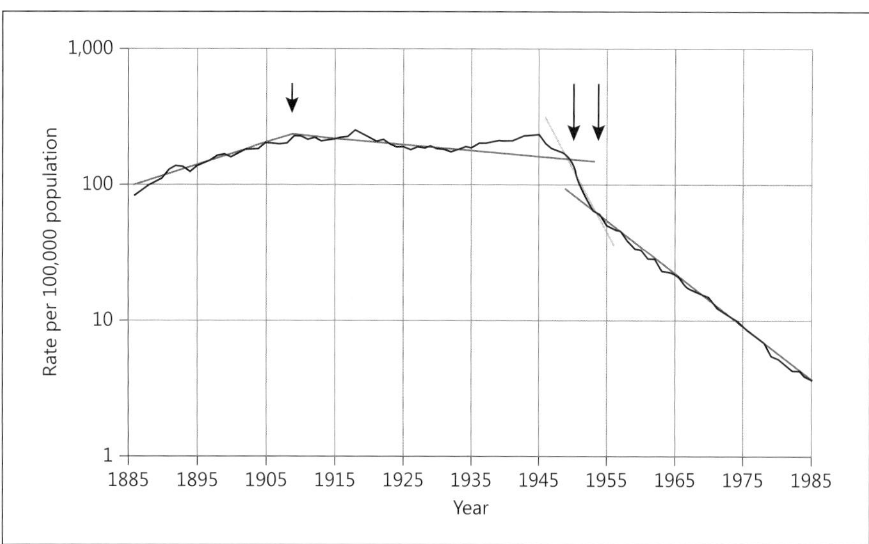

Fig. 1. Secular trends of TB mortality (per 100,000 population), Japan, 1886–1985 (logarithmic presentation). Arrows indicate "Transitions."

Empire of Japan at the time was a valuable member of the Allied powers and made useful contributions to the combined military forces in both Asia and Europe, beginning in mid-August until the end of the war in November 1918.

Three days after it declared war, the UK requested that Japan honor its 1902 Anglo-Japan Alliance, that the 2 governments support each other if either one were involved in a war against more than one power [3]. In agreement, Japan sent an ultimatum to Germany on August 15 demanding that it turn over Tsingtao, its main colony in China, and to withdraw its navy. In the absence of a reply, Japan declared war on Germany on August 23, 1914.

Soon afterward, the Imperial Japanese Navy, with minimum support from the UK army, began to block Tsingtao; next they bombarded it; finally the Imperial Japanese Army laid siege to the city, which surrendered on November 7. In addition, Japan's navy seized coaling depots used by the German navy and captured several German colonies in the Mariana, Caroline, and Marshall Islands. Soldiers from the Japanese army did not see action on the Western front, but the British Admiralty requested and received considerable assistance from Japanese warships in escorting troop ships in the Mediterranean Sea.

American troops joined the WWI allied forces on April 6, 1917: thus linking both United States (US) and Japanese militaries on the same side of the hostilities. Tensions inevitably began to rise, especially over the Japanese army's presence in China and over authority in the Pacific.

In 1918, before the end of WWI, both Japan and the US transferred military units to Siberia to assist White Russian army forces that were fighting against the Bolshevik Red Army. Initially, the Imperial Japanese Army planned to include over 70,000 troops, but after US opposition, the number was greatly reduced. After the Armistice, as a reward for its Japanese military partnership, the UK formalized Japan's territorial holdings in Tsingtao (now called Shantung), China, and the Pacific islands formerly under Germany's control. Japan was also rewarded with a permanent seat on the Council of the League of Nations. But Japan suffered a serious loss and accompanying insult when the "whites-only" Western powers included at the Treaty of Versailles rejected Japan's request for a racial-equality clause in the Treaty [4]. The pale-faced politicians simply refused to acknowledge the belief that non-white persons were intellectually equal to whites. Another reason that Tokyo's plea was denied was because Hong Kong and Singapore were major contributing members of the British Empire.

Epidemiology: before, during, and after WWII

First Transition

In pre-WWII Japan, the TB situation was so serious that it ranked number one among causes of death from 1935 to the end of the war (1945), accounting for more than 10% of all deaths. According to available vital statistics at the time, TB mortality was on the rise until the early 1900s (Fig. 1), when the Japanese industrial revolution was in progress – which started roughly 100 years after Great Britain's – chiefly in the textile industry. The TB epidemic spread first among city factory workers, mainly young women, who were recruited from the countryside, and then spread to the villages when

TB-stricken workers returned home after becoming sick, and eventually spread across the entire country. For example, in Fukui Prefecture, which had many textile factories, the TB mortality rate among females aged 15–19 years was 763/100,000 in 1922. Figure 2 indicates the age-related risk of TB deaths among young females and males in Japan in 1916.

The mortality rate of TB during that time increased 3% annually. The epidemic peaked in 1910, with a mortality rate of 230/100,000, and gradually declined thereafter. Although the annual rate of decline was only 1%, this was the first time in modern Japan that TB was recorded as declining: apparently, during the first TB transition.

This trend was soon interrupted by the worldwide pandemic of influenza in 1918 and 1919, which led to an abrupt and tremendous rise in TB mortality to 257/100,000 in 1918, which was the highest mortality rate ever recorded in Japan (Fig. 1). Note that during WWI, most European countries experienced a striking rise in TB mortality but Japan was not affected. The Japanese economy benefitted during that conflict through market expansion and remained almost untouched by warfare [4]. It is possible that some of this increase in TB deaths may have been due to the over-diagnosis of TB instead of influenza, but it is impossible to differentiate between TB and influenza mortality in the throes of an influenza pandemic.

After 1920, the previous slowly declining trend resumed, as illustrated once again in Figure 1. The decline lasted 11 years but then began to increase again when Japan invaded Manchuria and launched the Sino-Japanese War (1931–1945), which is described more fully in chapter 19, *Tuberculosis during the Sino-Japanese War and World War II in China*.

Second and Third TB Transitions
The second transition began when TB mortality declined soon after the end of the war in 1945 and decreased in 1948 to the level that was expected by extending the base line since 1911 (Fig. 1). After 1948, however, a sharp decline occurred and continued that lasted until 1955: the third TB transition.

The rate of yearly decline from 1948 through 1955 was 19%. This steep decline may have been due to the newly instituted life-saving effect of chemotherapy, which began with small then increasing amounts of streptomycin and para-aminosalicylic acid (PAS) in 1946. Then in 1952 came the long sought-after breakthrough: isoniazid (INH). Soon, combined treatment with all 3 anti-TB drugs – triple therapy – began to cure the majority of patients with TB [5] and proved especially effective for the younger generations

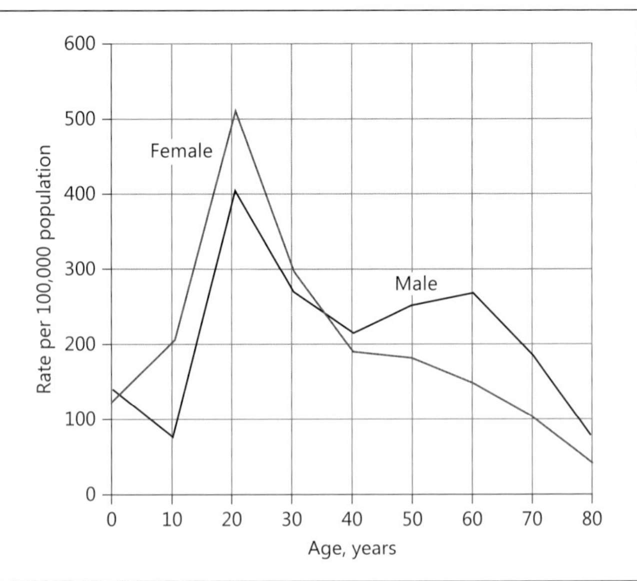

Fig. 2. Age-specific TB mortality (per 100,000 population), Japan, 1916, Male vs Female.

stricken with active disease, at least in terms of reduction of TB deaths (Fig. 3).

The trend in TB after 1955 that followed the third transition was apparently brought about and sustained by improved living standards and intensive implementation of modern TB control measures. The annual rate of decline of TB mortality was 11%. It is interesting to note that this speed of decline is of a scale similar to that of the speed of change in survey-defined prevalence rates of TB, survey-estimated annual risks of infection, and notification-based case rates (incidence rates) (Fig. 4).

Impact of War on TB in Japan

Thirteen years after Japan's involvement in WWI, it launched a new war entirely on its own in 1931, when it invaded Manchuria, in northeast China, and inaugurated the Sino-Japanese War. (More about the Sino-Japanese War between Japan and China [1931–1945], including the roles played by Nationalist China versus Communist China is discussed further in chapter 19 and detailed in Rana Mitter's book, *Forgotten Ally: China's WWII, 1937–1945* [6].) On September 27, 1940, Germany, Italy, and Japan signed the Tripartite Pact, which formally constituted the "Axis Powers," which were subsequently joined by several other countries. The attack on Pearl Harbor and several other Asian military installations on December 7, 1941 greatly widened

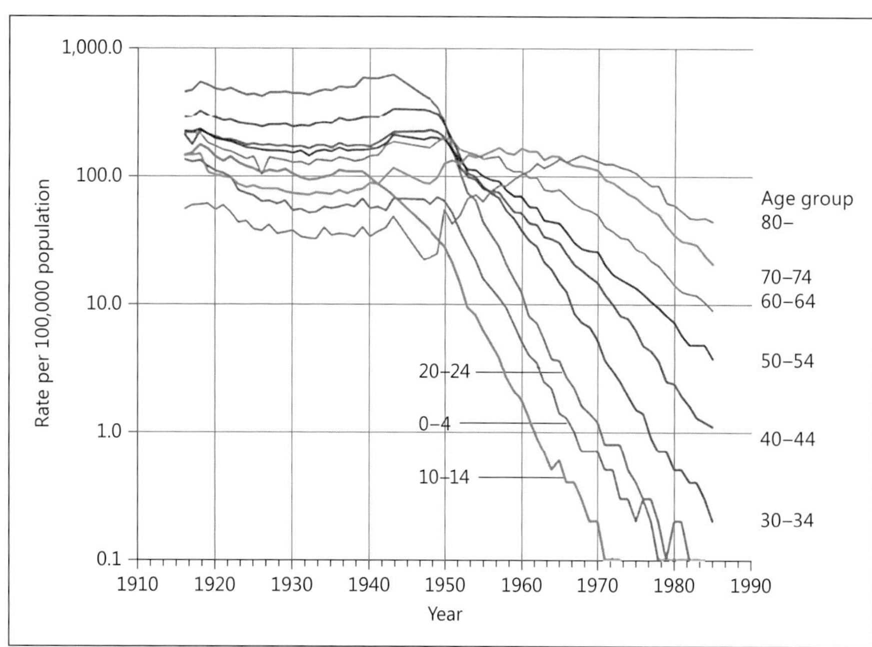

Fig. 3. Age-specific TB mortality (per 100,000 population), Japan, 1915–1985 (logarithmic presentation).

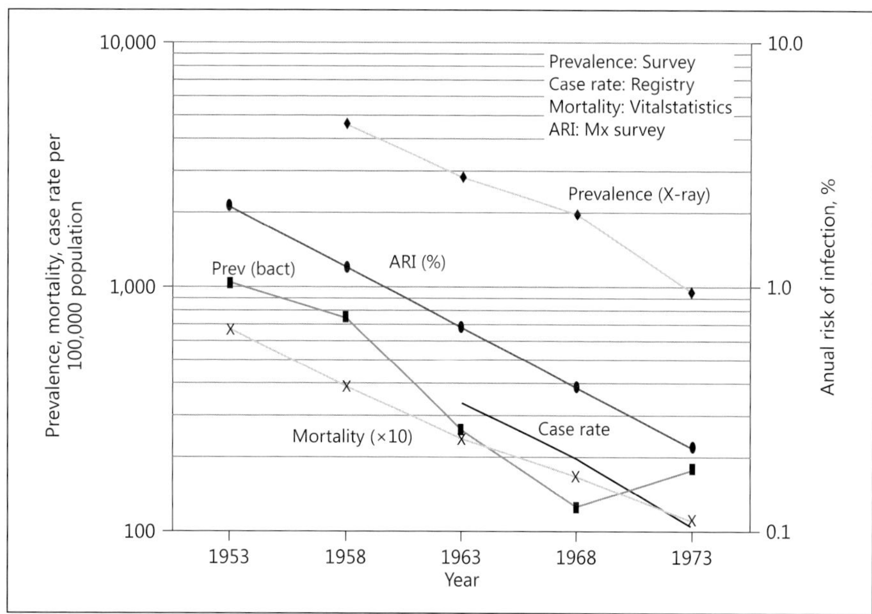

Fig. 4. Trends of various epidemiological parameters for TB, Japan, 1953–1973. Left vertical axis is for survey-defined prevalence (per 100,000 population), registry-defined case rate (per 100,000 population), and mortality (per 1,000,000 population). Right vertical axis is for annual risk of infection (ARI, in %).

Japan's military engagements in WWII. Four years later, Japan's surrender was announced on August 15 and formerly signed on September 2, 1945.

War(s) and Socioeconomic Changes

During and for many years after the beginning of the Sino-Japanese War, the massive mobilization of male adolescents to the battlefields was accompanied by the emergence of new economic trends directly or indirectly related to the war. The workforce was mobilized to the urban environment, resulting in what could be viewed as the late industrial revolution of the country. In contrast with the light industry of the previous industrialization, the heavy chemical industry closely related to the ammunitions industry was the main reason for the mobilization of the young male population to urban factories [1]. Mobilization to the war as well

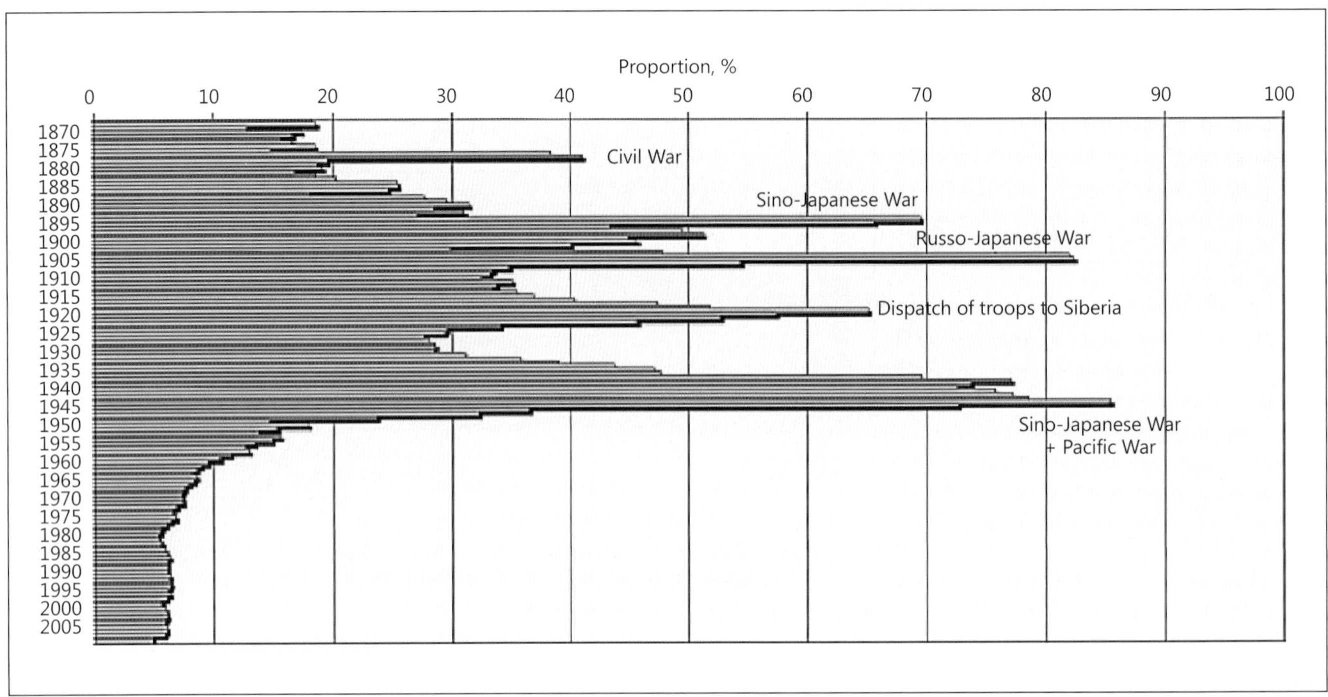

Fig. 5. Trends of proportion of military budget in total government expenditure, Japan, 1868–2009, from Shimao [7], with permission.

as to the industry resulted in TB epidemics among young males during this period.

The economic burden of the war was also tremendous. Figure 5 shows how expensive the wars were, in terms of the impact of military budget on the total national budget in the modern Japan's history. This necessarily led to the poor allocation of budget for public health and welfare [7]. ("Sino-Japanese War" during 1894–1895 refers to the war with Qing Dynasty China.)

But then in August 1942, Japan lost the decisive Battle of Midway near Midway Island, initiating a chain of Pacific Ocean defeats that continued until the end of the war in 1945. In 1944, US forces began to attack mainland Japan's large cities with military and/or political and socioeconomic functions, such as Tokyo and Osaka. Japanese citizens' daily lives were seriously affected. Attacks were mainly air bombardments and occasionally bombardments from the sea, culminating in the atomic bombing of Hiroshima and Nagasaki in 1945. Land warfare was fought on the island of Guadalcanal and other "stepping stone islands," and the prefecture of Okinawa in the South Sea Islands, the keystone in Japan's defense strategy, and the local population was seriously and adversely impacted. These attacks affected not only the military operation of the country, but also the socioeconomic functions that were directly related to the everyday lives of citizens, including their health.

At the end of the war in 1945, Japan had 7,200,000 soldiers, and one of every four Japanese males had been recruited to the war at least once. In other words, every 2 households offered at least one man to the battlefield, comparable to Germany.

Losses due to WWII

According to official statistics, there were between 2,100,000 and 2,300,000 military deaths and 550,000–800,000 civilian deaths [9], and the total population of the country was 71,998,100 in 1945. More than 290,000 civilians lost their lives due to the atomic bombings in Hiroshima and in Nagasaki, and 210,000,000 houses were destroyed. In the Great Tokyo Air Raid, 100,000 citizens were killed and another 1,000,000 lost their homes. In Osaka City, 10,000 died and 1,140,000 lost their homes in August, 1945. (Bureau of War Damage T-LAA, Reconstitution). A total of 123,000 children lost their parents due to WWII (Ministry of Health and Welfare).

In Okinawa, 94,000 Japanese military were killed, and officially 94,000 civilians died. The total population was 492,000. A different estimation indicates that 150,000 civilians died.

General and Infant Mortality during WWII

Figure 6 indicates trends of general mortality and infant mortality from 1900 through 1980, including the war period. No clear deviation from the basic trend occurred during the war period for the either trend line, such as that observed in the TB mortality trend line. Strictly speaking, an increased rate in general mortality may have occurred between 1940 and 1944, but the extent was modest. The influence of war or war-related societal factors seems to be specific to TB, rather than universal to health in general.

TB Mortality during the War Period

After 1931, the mortality curve departed from the downward trending baseline of the 1920s and took an upward course. When Japan entered the Asia-Pacific War in 1941, the mortality rate rose acutely; and in 1944 it was 241/100,000, the second-highest level in history. (Because there are no official vital statistics for 1944, 1945, and 1946 due to administrative disruption, this is an author's estimate based on interpolation of age-specific rates from both sides at that time. The estimated rate is 237 for 1945 and 208 for 1946). Based on observed deviations from the basic trend line from 1931 through 1948, it is calculated that during the 15-year war, approximately 490,000 excess TB deaths occurred, that is, 22% more than the expected number of TB deaths.

Figure 7 indicates the mortality trends for selected age groups from 1916 through 1960. The younger group exhibited the greatest deviation from the basic trend since 1910, and this deviation was less obvious in other age groups. However, the deviation from the baseline was not remarkable among female adolescents, and was not clear for all ages combined. TB mortality was higher for females than for males until the early 1930 for all age groups. This trend reversed beginning in 1935, and male mortality predominated from then until after the war.

In contrast to the early phase of the Industrial Revolution in Japan, mainly in the area of light industry where mobilization of young women as laborers led to higher TB mortality among them, young males were mobilized to the battlefield and to the urban factories, exposing them to the infection and development of TB.

Interestingly, the apparent upsurge of epidemic TB during the war in terms of death seems to have left no obvious long-term impact on mortality rates beyond 3 years after the end of the war (after 1948) [10]. This is similar to the situation in the Netherlands, where during WWII the risk of infection constantly decreased, despite the temporary steep increase of TB mortality and morbidity during this period.

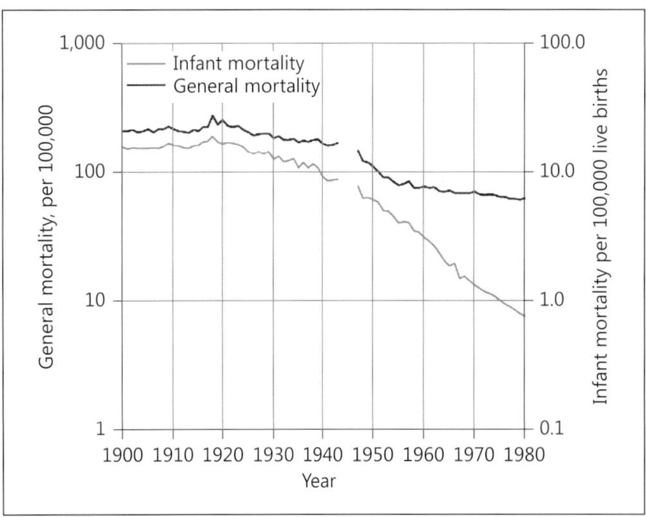

Fig. 6. Trends of general mortality (per 100,000) and infant mortality (per 1,000 live births), Japan, 1900–1980 (Logarithmic presentation).

Styblo et al. [11] explained that the excess incidence of new infection was approximately balanced by the excess incidence of death due to TB, but further infections may not have been produced. In other words, the excessive TB cases or fatal cases were of shorter duration, and so of low infectivity, and thus had less impact on the future trend of epidemics. A similar mechanism may have worked also to the TB upsurge during the influenza pandemic period.

TB Control Efforts during the War

Public efforts to control TB during this period were based on the TB Control Law that was enacted in 1919. This law focused on the isolation of infectious cases and general education, but its implementation in the early years was limited. The founding of the Japanese Society for TB (an academic society) in 1923 symbolized the start of scientific approaches to the TB problem and its control in Japan [12]. Enthusiastic efforts in basic, clinical, and epidemiological research were supported by the government's moves to overcome the national crisis resulting from TB while pursuing warfare and industrial productivity [1].

In 1933, with serious concern over the resurgence of TB mortality, the government reviewed the problem and expressed a clearer commitment to it. The government called for a nationwide anti-TB movement to encourage people to be more alert and more knowledgeable about the problem. At the same time, the government built public sana-

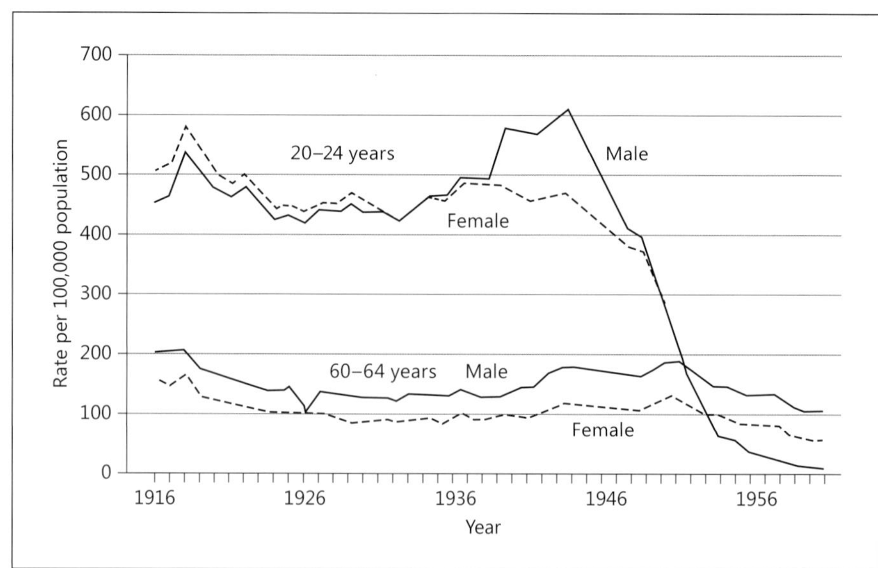

Fig. 7. Sex comparison of TB mortality for selected age-groups (rate per 100,000 population), Japan, 1916–1960.

toria and health centers, with TB control as their main mission to cover the entire country. The total number of TB beds was only 13,900 in 1935 (11 beds per 100 TB deaths). Under the new TB control program, plans were made to construct TB hospitals with a total of 40,000 beds within 10 years. The TB hospitals included those for soldiers disabled with TB. This plan was implemented fairly well, and by 1942 the number of TB beds had reached almost 35,000. The health center network also grew steadily, and by 1944 there were 770 health centers throughout the country. Notification of patients with infectious TB was mandatory; however, actual notifications were limited, possibly due to the stigma of TB and the reluctance of private practitioners to contribute.

In 1938, the departments of government service in charge of health and welfare became independent from the Ministry of the Interior, and were organized as the Ministry of Health and Welfare. This change was in response to the urgent need for healthier workers and stronger soldiers, with TB as the main challenge. Indeed, TB among soldiers was so serious that when the army sent 2 divisions (20,000 soldiers) to China for battle, one battalion of soldiers (500) was sent back with TB.

In 1939, the Japan anti-TB Association was founded as a nationwide non-governmental organization, seeking the voluntary support of government services in advocacy, training and research on TB control. The Research Institute of TB of this association acted as a national TB research center, contributing to policy-making, clinical and basic research, and training TB experts at various levels.

TB control in villages was another important mission for the newly established ministry, because the disease became prevalent in villages as young people returned from military service or urban factories to which they had been recruited. Many of them had TB when they returned home. The program included health screening of the returnees, care for patients and their families, and assistance to help pay medical costs.

In 1940, the Ministry of Health and Welfare launched the National Physical Fitness Improvement Program, which required boys aged 15 through 18 years (later, 15 through 25 years) to undergo fitness screening that included tuberculin skin testing and mass miniature radiophotography, which was developed by Prof. Koga in Japan in 1936. Basically the same technique, Abreugraphy, was invented and named by Prof. Manuel Dias de Abreu of Brazil in the same period [13]. TB mass screening with chest radiophotography was extensively performed to cover more than 10,000,000 subjects a year.

In 1943, national health insurance became mandatory for people who did not have other health insurance coverage. By the end of the war, 70% of all inhabitants were covered by this system, which was the start of universal health coverage in Japan.

Beginning in 1937, extensive studies on the effectiveness of BCG vaccination were conducted in various groups throughout the country until 1943, and the vaccination became obligatory for all graduates of primary school. Later, this requirement was expanded to all young workers and students less than 19 years of age. Records indicate that

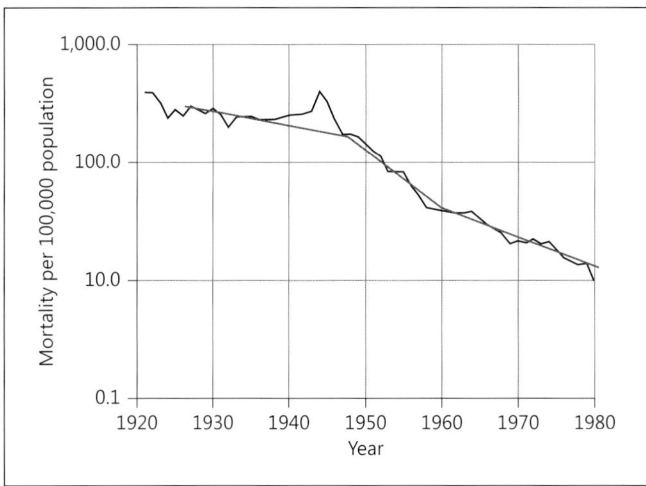

Fig. 8. Trends of TB mortality (per 100,000 population), Singapore, 1921–1980 (logarithmic presentation). Straight lines indicate the estimated baseline trends.

10,000,000 boys and girls were vaccinated in 1 year. Efforts to manufacture a high-quality vaccine during wartime led to the development of the freeze-dried BCG vaccine soon after the war [14].

Appendix

TB in Singapore before, during, and after WWII

As a newly developed Asian country, Singapore is a rare case that has good vital statistics data since before WWII. The country's trend of TB mortality was very similar to that of Japan, with an excess of mortality due to the conflict [15] (Fig. 8).

Singapore's TB mortality had been slowly declining since the 1920s, at a yearly rate of 1%. This rate was similar to that of Japan's baseline trend during 1911–1931. The downward trend in Singapore continued until about 1940, when it was interrupted by the invasion of Japanese military forces. As regards the direct victims of warfare, Rummel estimates that 283,000 citizens (including Malayans) and 1,000 captive Indian soldiers under UK forces were victims [16]. This suggests the severity of impact on people's daily lives and society. By 1947, TB mortality returned to the level expected based on the trend since 1930s. Assuming that the prewar slow decline of TB mortality would have continued if there had been no war, the observed total mortality between1941 and 1946 is calculated as 55% in excess over the expected.

Following the end of the war, the decline of TB mortality occurred, first rapidly at a rate of 12% per year during 1947–1960, owing to the early use of effective chemotherapy, and then more slowly at 5% thereafter. This favorable trend was presumably sustained by the introduction of modern TB control practices, including technologies. The technologies that have been applied with the economic development of the country may have enhanced host anti-TB resistance through better nutrition and housing. The per capita gross national product (GNP) of Singapore was USD 1,300 in 1960 and increased to USD 18,800 by 1988. At the same time, a high level of education and political stability may have contributed to the advanced health infrastructure that enabled the effective working of the newly applied technologies. [17]

Conclusion

WWII plus the preceding Sino-Japan war caused considerable excess TB deaths among the Japanese people recruited to warfare, as well as among workers mobilized to factories in the changing industrial structure accompanying the war. To address this serious national health crisis, both governmental and non-governmental organizations made maximum efforts in public health, clinical services, and research, but were overwhelmed by the accompanying death and destruction of the relentless war. Even though these productive efforts may not have been sufficient to control the ongoing problem, they bore fruit after the end of the war. Accordingly, the modern TB control measures that were developed and implemented enabled the remarkable decline of the current TB mortality.

References

1 Johnston W: The Modern Epidemic: A History of Tuberculosis in Japan. Cambridge, Harvard University Press, 1995.

2 Johansson JR, Mosk C: Exposure, resistance and life expectancy: disease and death during the economic development of Japan, 1900–1960. Population Studies 1987;41:207–235.

3 Dickinson FR: War and National Reinvention: Japan in the Great War, 1913–1919. Harvard University, Asia Center, 1999.

4 Japan during World War I. https://en.wikipedia.org/Japan during World War I (cited March 29, 2017).

5 Iseman MP: Tuberculosis therapy: past, present and future. Eur Respir J 2002;20:87S–94S.

6 Mitter R: Forgotten Ally: China's World War II, 1937–1945. New York, NY, Mariner Books, Houghton Mifflin Harcourt, 2013.

7 Shimao T: Epidemiological Trends of Tuberculosis and History of Tuberculosis Control in Modern Japan. Lecture in Training Course on NTP, Research Institute of Tuberculosis, 2016.

8 Webster D: The Burma Road: The Epic Story of the China-Burma-India Theater in World War II. New York, NY, Farrar, Strauss, Giroux, 2003.

9 Casualties of World War II in Japan. https://en.wikipedia.org/wiki/World War casualties (cited July 12, 2017).

10 Daniels M: Tuberculosis in Europe during and after the Second World War. Brit Med J 1949;2: 1065–1140.

11 Styblo K, Meijer J, Sutherland I: Tuberculosis Surveillance Research Unit Report No. 1: the transmission of tubercle bacilli; its trend in a human population. Bull Int Union Tuberc 1969;42:1–104.

12 Mori T: [Ninety years of the Japanese Society for Tuberculosis – Back to the future for Research and Control of Tuberculosis]. Kekkaku 2015;90: 541–552.

13 Abreugraphy (a Type of Mass Miniature Radiography). https://en.wikipedia.org/wiki/Chest_Photofluorography (cited 8/9/17).

14 Mori T: Role of tuberculosis control technologies in health transition of the productive population; in Furukawa T (ed): High Technology, Population Wealth and Health. Perspectives of Advanced Technology Science 1995;2:73–92, Maruzen Planet.

15 Mori T: Tuberculosis control programme in Singapore. Assignment report. Western Pacific Regional Office, World Health Organization, 1993.

16 Rummel RJ: Statistics of Democide: Genocide and Mass Murder Since 1900. Chapter 3. Statistics of Japanese Democide. Estimates, Calculations, and Sources. 1900 (cited April 4, 2017).

17 Teo SK, Chew CH: Tuberculosis chemotherapy – development in Singapore from 1952–1982. Ann Acad Med 1982;11:1–104.

Toru Mori
Research Institute of Tuberculosis
3-1-24, Matsuyama
Kiyose, Tokyo 204-8533 (Japan)
E-Mail tmori-rit@jata.or.jp

Murray JF, Loddenkemper R (eds): Tuberculosis and War. Lessons Learned from World War II.
Prog Respir Res. Basel, Karger, 2018, vol 43, pp 197–203 (DOI: 10.1159/000481488)

Tuberculosis in Korea during the Japanese Occupation in World War II

Eun Kyung Choi

Institute of Medical History and Culture, Seoul National University Hospital, Seoul, South Korea

Abstract

The Japanese occupied Korea from 1910 to the end of World War II in 1945. For the first 9 years of colonial occupation, Japanese military rule was oppressive and any Korean disapproval was ruthlessly crushed. But after 1919, the Japanese authorities loosened up somewhat. During the period of relative tranquility, beginning in 1936, the Japanese Colonial Government of Korea began tuberculosis (TB) prevention measures. The number of deaths among the Japanese population in Korea increased from 173/100,000 in 1921 to 441/100,000 in 1936. Meanwhile, among the Japanese in Japan and Taiwan, it remained 120–140/100,000 during the 1920s and 1930s. The high mortality rate from TB among the Japanese in Korea had already attracted the attention to the issue, and there was a parallel need to make Korean society and population a "safe, and healthy rear area." The Government organized "The Association to Prevent TB in Korea," a highly-pursued enlightenment campaign. But the renewed fighting during the Second Sino-Japanese War (1937–1945) created exceptional heartlessness against conscripted Korean men and women. The Japanese Government General of Korea kept trying to install sanatoria and anti-TB measures, however, they always failed due to budgetary limitations.   © 2018 S. Karger AG, Basel

Tuberculosis Policy of the Japanese Government of Korea

Epidemic of Tuberculosis in Korea during the Sino-Japanese and Pacific Wars: 1937–1945.
During the Japanese occupation (1910–1945), the Japanese Colonial Government of Korea introduced an efficient sanitary policy based on Western medical practices to deal effectively with contagious diseases in Korean society. Western medicine, which was more "rational" and "scientific," was shown to be highly effective in treating diseases, and a rapid disease response system was established to address acute infection, which introduced mandatory isolation, sterilization, quarantine, and so on. However, sanitary policies were not particularly effective in cases of non-acute infectious diseases, such as tuberculosis (TB), leprosy, and sexually transmitted diseases, which have long bacterial incubation periods and require lengthy treatment. In the case of TB, Western medicine did not have a specific treatment program during the Japanese occupation. Unlike other acute infectious diseases that were believed to be containable with isolation, sterilization, and quarantine, TB was a disease that was difficult for the colonial sanitary policy to address.

TB is believed to have appeared in the Korean Peninsula in the 1st century BC. Korean medicine classic books such as *Donguibogam* (東醫寶鑑), *Jejungshinpyun* (濟衆新編), and *Euijongsonick* (醫宗損益) used the term "*Rochae* 노채 (癆瘵)" or "*Junshi* 전시(傳尸)" to refer to TB. After the introduction of western medicine in the 1870's, physicians from both the US and Japan documented TB in Korea. Records showed that approximately 10% of pulmonary disease patients were diagnosed as TB in Jejungwon, the first western-style national hospital.

The prevalence rate of TB increased after colonization in 1910, as the result of industrialization and urbanization. Korean mass media estimated that in the 1930's the number of TB patients was 400,000 and the number of deaths was 40,000. It is remarkable that the Japanese in Korea showed such a high prevalence of TB. The number of deaths among the Japanese population in Korea increased from 173/100,000 in 1921 to 441/100,000 in 1936. Meanwhile, among the Japanese in Japan and Taiwan, it remained 120–140/100,000 during the 1920s and 1930s. Despite a high prevalence of TB among Japanese in Korea, the Japanese Government General of Korea had done almost nothing until 1936 and there was a parallel need to make Korean society and population a "safe, and healthy rear area" [1]. In 1918, the "Ordinance of Prevention of TB" was enacted, but it was solely about a simple crackdown and isolation that had no effect at all.

It is in this context that the TB epidemic in Korean society during the Japanese colonial period is interesting. From the late 1930s, the Japanese Colonial Government of Korea began to respond to the TB epidemic, but its efforts to establish sanitaria and prevention facilities were extremely slow. Even though the mortality rate from TB of the Japanese people living in Korea during periods of warfare continued to increase, they were not able to create effective countermeasures. While the extermination of TB was considered a critical factor in the construction of a modern nation, there were many difficulties to overcome in the colonial sanitary system. This chapter focuses on the nature of the response to the TB epidemic and the reactions of the Japanese Colonial Government of Korea during WWII. The purpose of this investigation is to point out the limitations of the sanitary policy of the Colonial Government of Korea during this time.

The Threat of TB during War: A Socio-Medical Study of the TB Epidemic among the Japanese in Korea

How serious was the TB epidemic in Korea before and after the war? Taniguchi Yoshinori (谷口芳德) analyzed the geographical distribution of the decrease in life expectancy of the Japanese due to TB based on the mortality tables of Japan; he found that after 1934, Japanese deaths due to TB in Korea were over 2 times the average in Japan [2]. He concluded that the decrease in Japanese life expectancy in Korea due to TB was reaching levels of the 5.54-year life expectancy decrease found in Ishikawa Prefecture (石川縣), which was the highest in Japan. The high mortality rate due to TB

among the Japanese living in Korea showed the "urgency for TB prevention in Korea, which was in the early stages of the industrial revolution" and brought attention to this issue.

The Rural Sanitation of Korea and the *Report on Bul-I(不二) Farm Survey* were both important socio-medical research studies conducted in colonial Korea, which studied the rate of positive reactions to tuberculin in Japanese people and the distribution of tubercle bacilli in rural areas through TB contact. Of the 2, the *Report on Bul-I Farm Survey* was conducted during the Pacific War period and was a study on rural villages composed solely of Japanese inhabitants. The research team tracked the spread and acquisition of TB among Japanese individuals in rural areas by socio-medical personnel from the Japanese Empire. They provided the following background for the study.

The response to tuberculin is 2 times higher in Korean people than in Japanese people. In rural areas, the rate of positive responses in Korean people is almost the same as the rate of positive responses in Japanese cities. On the other hand, for Japanese people living in Korea, despite most of them living in the city, the rate of positive responses to tuberculin is low compared to cities in Japan. The infiltration rate of [tubercle bacilli] in rural Korea is high. … The mortality rate due to TB for Japanese people living in Korea is increasing every year to the point it has reached a rate about 2 times higher than on the Japanese mainland. [3]

Therefore, they found that there was a need for a separate detailed study substantiating the evidence over the high TB mortality rate for Japanese people living in Korea. By studying the acquisition of TB by the Japanese living in rural areas, they aimed to identify the level of "purification of Korea by the Japanese" and use this data for immigration policy.

The results of the study showed that the total rate of positive responses to tuberculin was low at *Fuji* (不二) farm, but in subjects who showed positive responses, many had a high chance of infection within the family. In addition, the prevalence of TB in farms occurred sporadically via infections within families. The results of the analyses of TB families were interpreted as having identified many cases in rural areas from which the younger population contracted TB within heavily populated cities and, upon their return without a period of quarantine, spread TB to their families. The *report on Fuji (不二) Farm Survey* included a demographic analysis of people who had visited cities plus a detailed analysis of the spread of TB after leaving cities, before coming to the definitive conclusion that diagnosis and treatment measures are required for the younger generation who had left rural areas and since returned. The frequent migration of Japanese people could result in TB epidemics, which was an issue of concern for the Japanese Empire.

The *Report on Fuji (不二) Farm Survey* revealed that the high TB mortality rate among the Japanese was the most urgent issue that needed to be addressed to create a stable immigration policy. From the perspective of the Japanese Empire, it was difficult to establish measures regarding immigration and TB without solving this problem. This was because there was a good chance for the younger generation of Japanese people to spread the disease after being exposed to TB in the city during the war and not being quarantined upon their return. It became an important task for Japanese medical science to understand the reality of the high prevalence of TB through detailed studies. However, there were limitations to the actions that the Japanese Colonial Government of Korea could take to prevent TB.

Full-Scale Measures against TB: The Establishment of "The Association to Prevent TB in Korea"

With the establishment of the Association to Prevent TB in Korea on April 7, 1936 under the lead of the Japanese Colonial Government of Korea, TB prevention measures became proactive in comparison with the past. The Japanese Colonial Government of Korea stated that the reason they began full-scale ways to energize TB prevention was the focus on measures against leprosy and drug addiction, which had yielded positive results. Accordingly, it was time to implement full-scale measures to help TB patients [4].

The Association to Prevent TB in Korea had the perception that the extermination of "the enemy of the people," TB, along with the extermination of the "cancer of the peninsula," leprosy, drug addiction, and mental disease, was to revive a "healthy Korea." The main activity of the association was "to construct a TB sanatorium that can accommodate about 40,000 people, and to agree on prevention methods, including expansion of health clinics, protection of weak children, problems in house structure and nutrition, sanitary problems in schools and factories, and so on." Initially, the largest activity was to designate the 3 days from May 26th to 28th to be TB Prevention Week and organize promotion activities.

The fact that the Association to Prevent TB in Korea was established by the Japanese Colonial Government of Korea one year before the Sino-Japanese War had started meant that the TB prevention activities of the Japanese Colonial Government of Korea were becoming viewed as a reaction to the war. As the Sino-Japanese War began in 1937, the Japanese Colonial Government of Korea claimed that TB prevention was of utmost importance for "all people to become one in body and mind" and "to improve the strength of body (體位) of the people." In fact, military terms, such as "prevention formation," "long-term resistance," "mobilization order," and "sanitary formation," were used metaphorically in TB prevention initiatives.

When looking at the state of sanitation so far, I expect you to know that the propagation (保進) of TB prevention facilities is of utmost importance. Especially when seen from the important state that we are in currently, its importance is becoming ever larger. … From long ago, there is the saying that the war is fought with armies and that armies fight on battlefields, however the wars of today are not merely this, but also a war fought between the entire people of both countries. For example, even if crack troops are placed on the battlefield, but the people who are responsible for the rear are not of a single body and mind, it is difficult to achieve final victory. Therefore, all people must come together to not only support soldiers on the battlefield mentally and materially, but they must also improve the efficiency of work in industry, manufacturing, and so on, and faithfully improve national power. …There is no need to reiterate that to achieve the goal of protecting the nation (保國) through one's own livelihood (生業) requires the sound mind and strong body of the people. … The most important reason for the decrease in the strength of body (體位) of the people is the epidemic of TB, and as it is causing considerable damage to national security, industry, education, and so on, there is the need to quickly establish prevention facilities. [5]

As such, there was much concern that TB could become even more widespread due to warfare and its complications. Malnutrition due to war, breakdown of sanitary conditions due to separations of family, the overworking of bodies and minds of soldiers, and the increase of laborers working in military industries could influence the TB epidemic. TB was not merely the problem of soldiers. As TB became increasingly widespread among ordinary people, it could damage the workforce at home. TB was a factor that could lead to unavoidable loss [6].

Compared with the seriousness of the issue, the activities of the Association to Prevent TB were limited, especially after the Korea branch of the Association was established in 1936. At first, it organized associate branches throughout the country in a matter of days and worked on intensive promotion activities for a short period. However, unlike similar chronic infectious disease action organizations, such as the Association to Prevent Leprosy, the Association to Prevent TB failed to have sufficient levels of donation-based membership to promote solicitation of funds. Therefore, the Association to Prevent TB in Korea was limited in resources

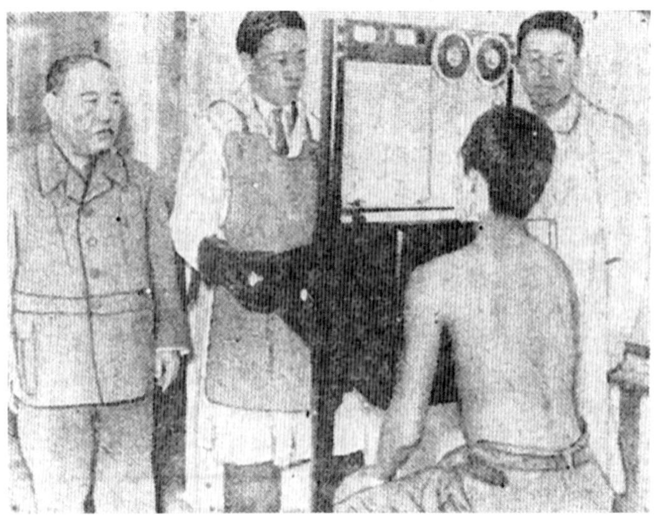

Fig. 1. A medical officer in Gyeongido Sanitary Laboratory takes X-ray examination of a boy in the middle school. This picture shows the scene of group X-ray examination during wartime. *Maeil-Sinbo* 每日申報, May 6, 1942; Korea Press Foundation.

and was unable to select a method of receiving financial support. Thus, the Association to Prevent TB in Korea was unable to conduct any other noteworthy activity other than promotion of TB prevention week.

Large-Scale X-ray Examinations – Expansion of Health Examinations for Government and Public Schools

Among the TB prevention activities that were considered important were medical examinations and sputum examinations, usually conducted on "hospitality personnel (lodging facility personnel)" [7]. Hospitality personnel were summoned to police stations on every TB prevention day to be trained in prevention methods and in the placement of expectoration dishes. At the same time, school personnel became a new target for TB prevention activities. In Japan, it was already known that the prevalence rate of TB among teachers was high. However, it was not until 1936, when a newly conducted survey on TB in schools revealed that 40% of graduates of government and public middle schools and higher education throughout Korea had died of TB, that sanitation in schools became highly emphasized.

Group examinations for TB in schools and workplaces began after 1941 (Fig. 1). With the success of the 3-year trial group examination, which included X-ray studies conducted in 1939 by the Japanese Ministry of Health and Welfare, it was promoted across all of Japan and began being introduced in Korea [8]. Each region, including Pyeongyang, purchased X-ray machines and began group examinations starting with primary and middle school children and teachers, and administered tuberculin skin tests. Starting in August 1942, X-ray group examinations focused on children entering primary school and girls' middle school students. Examinations targeting school-aged women were implemented due to "the importance of sanitary issues related to school-aged women who will become mothers in the future." According to an article that described the atmosphere of the group examinations of the time, it also fulfilled the role of promoting the spirit of TB prevention.

… 120 students from Gyeonggi Middle School 4th Grade Class under the guidance of their homeroom teacher came to the Gyeongido Sanitary Laboratory located in Gwanghwamun all to receive Roentgen examinations. Before this event, in the lawn of this same laboratory they received a round of instruction from the head of Chunan sanitation that "the most important issue in our country right now is securing human resources, and by exterminating the TB bacteria, this issue can somewhat be solved, so you all must be brave and actively exercise, and be close to sunlight to become a soldier that is being raised to drive out TB from schools." Straight after this, all laboratory staff under Dr. Minamioka and medical official Taki were enlisted to conduct indirect Roentgen examinations of all the people over an hour and a half. [9]

Greatest Hurdle for the Japanese Colonial Government of Korea: The Construction of TB Sanatoria

Sanatoria were scarce in Korea during the pre-Sino-Japanese War years. Figure 2 shows a photo of the Haeju Sanatorium, which was built in 1928 and which had "good" facilities and stood virtually alone. Although there were difficulties in procuring resources, the construction of the sanatoria was the most urgent and important issue in TB prevention. From the late 1930s, the installation of sanatoria and plans to introduce a budget for these needs in places such as Pyeongyang and Masan, were discussed in the press [10].

However, despite the will of authorities, there were many examples in which plans to construct sanatoria failed. One of the first sanatoria was planned in Pyeongyang in December 1936; after 3 years of planning, Pyeongyang announced it would establish a TB sanatorium affiliated with the provincial Pyeongyang hospital [11]. This plan initially was expected to spend 21,000 won in 1937 and 44,000 won in 1938, totaling 65,000 won; however, due to skyrocketing construction costs and other reasons, the project was halted and cancelled.

Only a few sanatoria were built during the war. The Yoyangwon Yonsujang (療養院 延壽莊), which was constructed by the Japanese Red Cross, was the first sanatorium to be completed; it was finished after 3 years of planning and construction, and cost around 100,000 won. It had 60–70 beds and was larger in size than the anti-TB sanatoria located in Korea. It placed priority on housing patients who were discharged soldiers, primary school teachers, and police officers, and began receiving patients on November 25, 1940 after having opened on November 20, 1940 [12].

In 1939, the Keijō Imperial University High Altitude Sanatorium and Laboratory was established in Pyeongchang, Gangwon Provence. Pyeongchang was a perfect place for TB study and recuperation, as it was a place where "the landscape is beautiful with plentiful ultraviolet rays and sunlight, and the air is clean." Residents provided about 272,000 m² of land through a supporting association and worked hard to attract the placement of the sanatorium [13]. The major purpose of this facility was the recuperation of TB patients and the study of high-altitude recuperation, but it was also constructed in conjunction with the Korea Postal Life Insurance Sanatorium, which could accommodate 500–600 people [14].

Besides these facilities, other completed sanatoria included the Masan Railway Sanatorium and the Military Masan Sanatorium Veterans. When the results of a health survey of Railway Bureau employees in 1935 found that 85,369 employees suffered from respiratory diseases each year, and of those, 13,888 employees suffered from TB, the Railway Sanatorium was established [15]. The Military Masan Sanatorium for Veterans was established directly under the control of the Japanese Colonial Government with a construction cost of 650,000 won. Construction began in January of 1940, and was completed 2 years later in February of 1942 [16]. At the sanatorium, patients could receive treatment for various work-related diseases, including special infections (peritonitis), as well as TB-related diseases; it was immense with grounds covering 230,000 pyung, and a floor plan measuring 683 pyung.

Other sanatoria were planned, but never constructed. Of note is that none of the national sanatoria for ordinary people proposed by the Japanese Colonial Government in Korea were built. The colonial government had plans to build 3 sanatoria in the north, central, and southern regions; that is Keijo (Seoul), Pyeongyang, and Busan. Twenty thousand won were set aside for the plan to establish national sanatoria in 1939, and after the Japanese royal

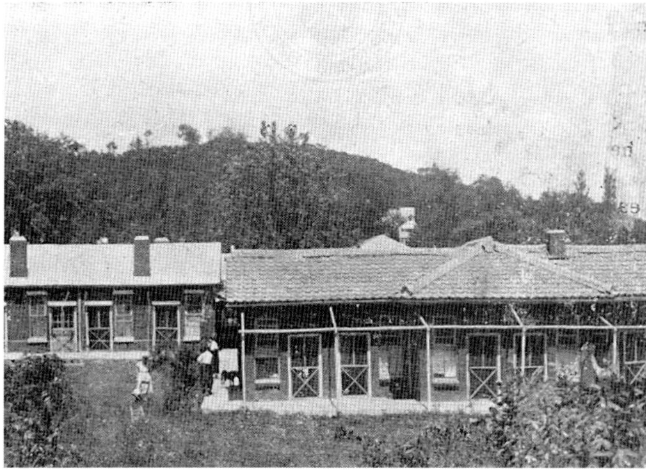

Fig. 2. Haeju Sanatorium in 1940. Haeju Sanatorium was the first modern-style tuberculosis sanatorium in Korea, built by a medical missionary, Sherwood Hall in 1928. During the absence of the Japanese government's efforts in sanatoria construction, Haeju sanatorium was the only sanatorium with good facilities. Korean Mission Field, 1940. No.10 p143.

court bestowed funds, they announced that they would build a sanatorium to house about 500 people [17]. However, these plans were abandoned as the colonial government could not secure the budget to build the sanatoria and had to rely on donations.

When building new sanatoria during times of war was not possible, a temporary stopgap was to acquire existing private sanatoria. In 1943, the Hamheung Jaehae Hospital was acquired and repaired with 191,000 yen in debt as the TB Sanatorium affiliated with the Provincial Hamheung Clinic [18]. In addition, as an emergency wartime measure, a plan was created for Japanese medical teams to utilize all non-operating facilities (inns, restaurants, peacetime industry factories, etc.) to rapidly create 25,000 sanatoria [19]. It is estimated that a sizable amount of private land was used as sanatorium spaces for soldiers who had contracted TB during the war.

From 1936 onward, the Japanese Government General of Korea introduced TB prevention measures to combat the hygienic issue in the war. However, these were almost all temporary measures, including enlightenment and publicity, and TB treatment facilities, such as sanatoria, were barely functional. Sanitary considerations in Korea mostly relied on the police, and they adopted rigorous measures, including isolation and disinfection during the whole colonial period. Nevertheless, such efforts failed to greatly improve the outcome of TB patients, which is not surprising given the hardships and complications of WWII in Korea.

Conclusion

The Japanese Colonial Government enacted full-scale TB prevention measures with the establishment of the Association for TB Prevention in Korea in 1936, 1 year before the start of the Sino-Japanese War. During the Sino-Japanese War and the following Pacific War, measures against TB were related to the idea of protecting the country through protecting livelihoods, within a system where the bodies and the minds of the people were to work as one. That is, education regarding TB was promoted as an attitude and mental weapon that the people must have. The Association for TB Prevention in Korea aimed to employ extensive movements by the people to eradicate TB based on enlightenment and promotion activities with the aim of eradicating the "enemy of the people," TB.

However, despite the urgent situation due to war, and the public demand for accommodating patients with TB, sanatoria for ordinary people established under the Japanese Colonial Government of Korea were not constructed until after the war. The colonial government prepared various law revisions regarding TB prevention, beginning in 1937; however, they did not come into fruition and the same was true for the establishment of sanatoria. In the situation where policies related to TB, such as the modification of laws and systems, and the expansion of facilities were lacking, it was impossible for the colonial government to achieve a "healthy Korea" that would "eradicate the TB bacteria." In context without special legal/institutional/financial support: significant deviation from short-term promotion and enlightenment activities could not be expected.

At the same time, TB prevention activities implemented during WWII that had the longest influence on Korean society were the introduction of group examinations, including X-ray examinations. The early diagnosis, particularly of TB, through group examination was emphasized. Although there were not many Koreans who were able to participate in the group examinations introduced by the Japanese Colonial Government during the Pacific War period, the introduction of group examinations was lauded as a method to quickly identify patients with TB.

References

1 Choi EK: Anti-Tuberculosis Policy of the Government General of Korea during Japanese-Colonial Period (1910–1945): from simple restriction to active enlightenment. Uisahak 2013;22:713–758.

2 Taniguchi, yoshinori 谷口芳德. *honna ni okeru ketkakku shimau ni yoru heikin yomei tanshuku no chiriteki bunpu* 本那二於ケ結核死亡二因ル平均餘命短縮ノ地理的 分布 [geographical distribution of the average reduction in life expectancy due to the tuberculosis in Japan]. *Chosenigakukaijyashi* 朝鮮醫學會雜誌1939;29:41–58.

3 Keijoteikokudaigaku eiseichiyousabu 京城帝國大學衛生調査部 [keijo imperial university hygiene survey team]. "Fuji noujiou chiousa bougoku" 不二農場調査報告 *[Report on Fuji Farm Survey].* (Keijo: Keijo imperial university, 1942)

4 Na-byung, ma-yak twoichi duinieo pyebyung bakmyul-e shinjuryuk" 癩病, 麻藥退治뒤니어 肺病撲滅에 新注力[We will newly concentrate the eradication of pulmonary disease, after the extermination of leprosy and drug addiction], *Maeil-Sinbo* 每日申報, January 23, 1936.

5 Nishigame, Sankei 西龜三圭, "Jikyoku no ketkaku-yobou" 時局と結核豫防[a current situation and the tuberculosis prevention], *Keimuibou* 警務彙報 384, April 1938.

6 Nishigame, Sankei 西龜三圭, "Jyu-go no ketkaku-yobou sisetsu" 銃後の結核豫防施設[The tuberculosis prevention facilities behind the lines] Korea oyo mansyu.

7 The "hospitality personnel" were usually referred as prostitutes, midwives, and nurses in the inns and restaurants. "Kyulhaek yebanggwa jeildan wuisengchuijegesi, jubgaekupja junban-ui gungang jindan" 結核豫防第一彈 衛生取締開始 접객업자 전반의 건강진단 警察部衛生課에서[The first measures in the prevention of tuberculosis will starts. The department of hygien in police station will perform the physical examination among the hospitality personnels] ,*Maeil-Sinbo* 每日申報, May 8, 1936.

8 "Kyulhaek bakmyul-ui daechaek-husengsung jibdangumjin-ui sungsong-ul jungukjuckuro jangryeo" 結核撲滅의 對策-厚生省 集團檢診의 成功을 全國的으로 獎勵[The measures to eradicate tuberculosis-The Ministry of Welfare will promote a group examination on a national-wide scale] , *Maeil-Sinbo* 每日申報, July 30, 1941.

9 "Junghakseng-ui kyulhaek-gumsa-jakil-buteo kyunggido wuisenggwa-eseo silsi" 中學生의 結核檢查 - 昨日부터 京畿道街生課에서 實施 [The department of public hygiene in Kyunggi province performs the tuberculosis test in the middle school students since yesterday], *Maeil-Sinbo* 每日申報, May 6, 1942.

10 "Minjung bokun sang jungdae munjae; gyukjung-haeganun kyulhaek hwanja, jaknyunjung samang guchon-yeo, wuisangdanggukdo yebang-e gosim jung, masan dungji-e yoyangso gyehaek"民衆保健上 重大問題; 激增해가는 結核患者, 昨年中 死亡九千餘, 衛生當局도 豫防에 苦心中, 馬山等地에 療養所計劃 [Important problems in people's health; tuberculosis patients is increasing. Nine thousand patients were died last year and the hygiene authority concerns the prevention. It plans the tuberculosis sanatorium in Masan] *Donga-Ilbo* 東亞日報. Mar 29, 1935.

11 "Pyungyang kyulhaek yoyangso kupsok hyunsil yomang, gongsabi imanichonpalbaek won myunyundo yesan-e gyesang(pyungyang)" 平壤結核療養所 急速實現要望, 공사비 二만二천八백 원 明年度 豫算에 計上(平壤) [Tuberculosis sanatorium in Pyongyang will be realized soon, twenty two thousands and eight hundreds won will be included in next year budget for the costs of construction] *Donga-Ilbo* 東亞日報. February 11, 1936.

12 "Jucksipja kyulhaekyowon isipil-e gaewonsik geohang"赤十字結核療院 二十日에 開院式舉行[Red-Cross tuberculosis sanatorium will be opened in November.20], *Maeil-Sinbo* 每日申報, November 17, 1940.

13 "Gowonjidae pyunggang-e yoyangsosulchi gye-
hwaik miguyensengdel sungdaegowonyoyangso,
juminun kisunghwoi jojik" 高原地帶平康에
療養所設置計劃 未久誕生될 城大高原療
養所 住民은 期成會組織[The authority has
plan to establish sanatorium in the highlands in
Pyungang. Keijo Imperial University sanatorium
will be established soon. The residents in Pyungang organizes the supporting association], *Donga-Ilbo* 東亞日報. September 19, 1938.

14 "Dongyang je il sisul wanbi cheshingukui pyun-
ganggowongyulhaekyoyangso-palwol-e jungong,
sibwolbuteo hwanja suyoung" 東洋第一施設完
備 遞信局의 平康高原結核療養所-八月에
竣工, 十月부터 患者收容[The best facility in
East Asia, The building of Pyungang highland
tuberculosis sanatorium will be completed in August, and it will accommadate the patients in Oc-
tober], *Maeil-Sinbo* 每日申報, January 27, 1943.

15 "Chuldogukwon-gwa gajok-e hohupkibyung
hwanja dasu, jongupwon wuihaya sip-o-manwon
gyungbiro masan-e yoyangso sinsul" 鐵道局
員과 家族에 呼吸器病者多數 종업원 위
하야 十五만원 경비로 馬山에 療養所新
設[Respiratory disease is prevelent among the
employees and family in the railway administration. The administration will establish the sanatorium in Masan with the budget of fifty thousand
won], *Maeil-Sinbo* 每日申報, March 23, 1938.

16 "Sungdae kyulhaek yoyangso pyungangkun-ha-e
gunsul-e chaksu, myungchunsamwol-e-nun jungong" 城大結核療養所 平康郡下에 建設에
着手, 明春三月에는 竣工[Building up Keijo
Imperial University sanatorium in Pyungang kun,
it will be finished in March, next Spring], *Maeil-
Sinbo* 每日申報, April 3, 1941.

17 "Kyulhaek hwanja-e rangbo kuknipyoyangso-rul
sulchi myungnyun jung silhyun giun nonghu isip-
manwon-uro uisun baekmyung suyoung" 結核患
者에 朗報 國立療養所를 設置 明年 中
實現機運 濃厚 廿萬圓으로 爲先 百名 收
容[Good news to the tuberculosis patients: National tuberculosis sanatorium will be established
next year, will it will accomodates hundres people
in twenty thousand won]. *Maeil-Sinbo* 每日申
報, December 25, 1938.

18 "Douritsu hamhung ien husetsu ketkkaku ryouy-
oujiou baisyu ki kisaino ken" 道立咸興醫院附
設結核療養所買收貴 起債ノ件 [Articles
regarding the purchasing plan of the tuberculosis
sanatorium affiliated to the Provincial Hamheung
Clinic] October 6, 1943.

19 "Imanochon-ui-yoyangso kyulhaek twaichi-wui-
hayeo uiryowoneseo jungsul". 二萬五千의療養
所 結核退治爲하여 醫療團에서 增設
[medical institution will establish twenty five
thousands beds in sanatorium to eradicate tuber-
culosis], *Maeil-Sinbo* 每日申報, July 12, 1943.

Eun Kyung Choi
Institute of Medical History and Culture, Seoul National University Hospital
101 Daehak-ro, Jongno-gu
Seoul 03080 (South Korea)
E-Mail qchoiek@gmail.com

Murray JF, Loddenkemper R (eds): Tuberculosis and War. Lessons Learned from World War II.
Prog Respir Res. Basel, Karger, 2018, vol 43, pp 204–212 (DOI: 10.1159/000481489)

Tuberculosis in China before, during, and after the Sino-Japanese War

John F. Murray

University of California San Francisco, San Francisco, CA, USA

Abstract

The second Sino-Japanese War has 2 different start dates, first 1937, and September 18, 1931, the date the Imperial Japanese Army invaded Manchuria. Furthermore, meet 2 Chinese men who played important roles in the civil war that consumed China from the 1920s to its end in 1949: Chiang Kai-shek, leader of the Nationalist Army, and Mao Zedong, active member, then chairman of the Chinese Communist Party. An early key event was the Shanghai War of 1931–1932, which lasted only 33 days and the Chinese lost decisively. Another Shanghai War erupted in 1937, which again led to a major Japanese victory. Meanwhile, because the Japanese were constantly pushing Chiang's army back and the Communists were constantly fighting the Nationalists, the diagnosis and treatment of TB was largely ignored. Currently, TB remains a gigantic burden in the People's Republic of China and has the second largest worldwide problem after India. TB was revolutionized in 1990–1991 with considerable improvement, but a 10-year follow-up revealed poor detection of new smear-positive cases, far lower than the 70% case detection target. Taiwan has had a decreasing incidence of TB, 74.6/100,000 in 2002 and 54/100,000 in 2012, but problems with drug resistance remain.

World War II (WWII) started on September 1, 1939 when the German Army invaded Poland and headed relentlessly and rapidly towards Warsaw; there was no real way of slowing the Nazi forces down. Two days later on September 3, 1939, the United Kingdom (UK) and the Republic of France officially declared war against Nazi Germany, and hours later on the same day, several member countries of the United Kingdom also declared war. Those dates and the

horrific, worldwide disasters that followed the next almost 6 years have long been memorialized in history. Much earlier, however, well before WWII started, a barely known military conflict between China and Japan had been festering for almost a decade. And, moreover, while that nation-to-nation war was taking place, a different epoch-making battle for the domination of China itself was playing out. Sides were drawn in 1921 when the Chinese Communist Party (CCP) launched its first congress. Among the enthusiastic participants was a young man who within the next few years began to attract considerable attention: Mao Zedong. At roughly the same time – and at the opposite end of the revolutionary political universe – a protégé of Sun Yet-sen's Chinese Nationalist Party was also gaining attention: Chiang Kai-shek.

Most historians agree that the Second Sino-Japanese War started on July 7, 1937 between the Republic of China and the Empire of Japan [1]. However, fierce fighting between the 2 nations actually began on September 18, 1931, which was intense in its early years, with huge casualties, especially among the Chinese. Other expert historians believe that the Second Sino-Japanese War started on that fateful September day in 1931 [2]. Moreover, the Chinese Communist Government has tried to extend the "official definition of the Second Sino-Japanese War" back to the exact date of what actually happened that launched the conflict in 1931: the Invasion of Manchuria by Japan on September 18, 1931. That is where our story begins.

Second Sino-Japanese War: Invasion of Manchuria, 1931–1937

The Mukden Incident

The most likely interpretation among the various versions of the Mukden (or Manchurian) incident is that a small group of aggressive young Japanese officers who were supposedly defending the Japanese-owned South Manchurian Railway, decided – among themselves – on September 18, 1931 to sabotage a short section of the track and blame the damage on Chinese troops who were stationed nearby [3]. At roughly 10:20 p.m., a small cache of explosives was detonated close to one side of the paired tracks causing trivial damage. Notably, within a few minutes after the explosion an ordinary passenger train passed over the affected track without noticeable impairment.

At first, the commanding Japanese general of the Kwantung Army protecting the southern Manchurian territory, General Shigeru Honjō, was angry to learn that junior officers carried out the attack without his knowledge or permission, but he realized its strategic benefits and quickly granted approval to dispatch local troops [4]. Furthermore, Honjō sent for immediate reinforcements from Manchuria and Korea and he moved his headquarters to Mukden the next day: all without authorization by the Emperor in Tokyo. Within a few days, all 1,175 km (730 miles) of the South Manchurian Railway and its adjoining cities had been seized.

Five years earlier, on June 5, 1926, Chiang Kai-shek became the head of the National Revolutionary Army (NRA) and later established the National Government in Nanjing. Chiang began a modernization program that improved the Chinese economy and business activities, which focused chiefly on the rich. But there were also many flaws, especially flagrant corruption that affected farmers and the already poor, which gave local CCP members, survivors of the various assassination attempts, something to tell the world about. Then in late September 1931, the Japanese invasion of Manchuria presented Chiang with an unsolvable problem: his Chinese army was no match for the Japanese army and new remedies were needed [1].

Important overlapping developments included a directive from the League of Nations that mandated withdrawal of Japanese forces, which was rejected by Japan who insisted instead on direct negotiations with Chiang Kai-shek and the Chinese Kuomintang Government. Failure of negotiating progress was in part complicated by the recently constituted independent government of Hu Hanmin, then leader of the CCP. In October 1932, the Lytton Report of the League of Nations rejected Japan's assertion that its conquest of Manchuria was not an act of self-defense, but was caused by military aggression in China [5]. Five months later (March 1933), Japan quit the League of Nations.

Shanghai War of 1931–1932

In 1931, serious fighting erupted again, this time in Shanghai between Chinese factory workers and Japanese monks. Capitalizing on this unusual opportunity, Rear Admiral Shiozawa Kôichi of the Imperial Japanese Navy, demanded apologies and compensation in efforts to quell anti-Japanese demonstrations. But they were destined to fail, because privately Chiang had emboldened the Chinese army to retaliate. The fighting in February 1932 lasted only 33 days, but the toll included more than 10,000 civilian deaths plus 14,000 Chinese and 3,000 Japanese casualties [6]. A provision of the subsequent truce agreement limited the NRA's ability to function in Shanghai, which angered the Chinese residents there.

Chiang had no alternative but to discreetly strengthen the Chinese army. In 1934, he recruited a former World War I (WWI) German military officer to rigorously train the officers of his amateur military personnel; in 1935, he hired a replacement German officer for additional training. Meanwhile, the Japanese kept demanding further surrender of Chinese territory. A quasi-truce between Japan and China was arrived at that hugely favored the Japanese, but it provided Chiang vital time to reinforce his army and modernize their weapons and equipment.

The Long March

A slowdown of fighting by the Japanese army allowed the NRA to continue to chip away at the Chinese Communists, but by mid-1934, Chiang's increasingly efficient military forces were causing serious damage. In-fighting among factions of the Red Army added to the worsening confusion. In June 1934, thousands of Communist troops began a spectacular organized retreat from Jiangxi in southeast-central China called *The Long March*. For a while, it was not much to brag about, but at its end it had assumed mythic proportions.

According to one report, the evacuation plan of October 1934 initially consisted of 86,000 troops and the line of marchers stretched for 60 miles [7]. Chiang's army knew exactly where the Communists were coming from and had prepared formidable fortifications and a succession of deadly ways of blocking river crossings and obstructing routes; endless daytime bombings and repeated skirmishes kept adding casualties. Mao Zedong was an involved participant but not in charge during the first months of the retreat, but he regained the chairmanship in January 1935. He changed tactics to split his forces into smaller groups using different escape paths, and he avoided direct engagement with Chiang's forces whenever possible.

Arriving after almost exactly 1 year of travel, the 4,000 surviving troops had crossed 24 rivers, ascended 18 snow-covered mountain ranges, and walked 9,656 km (6,000 miles): "the longest continuous march in the history of warfare" [8]. Mao became the exalted leader of the CCP: the position he attained and presided over until his death in 1976. The Long March became far more than a myth of heroism and fortitude, its reality attracted thousands of young Chinese students, workers, and peasants who then enlisted in the Red Army to fight from 1937 until the end of WWII – first in partnership with Chiang Kai-shek and his Nationalist Army – against the hated Japanese. Immediately afterward, they went back to fighting each other.

History of Tuberculosis

There is not much information about the history of TB in China during the 19th century, according to the comprehensive analysis by Lei [9]. Both Benjamin Hobson [10] in 1840s and Dudeon [11] in 1870s spoke about "phthisis" and "consumption," respectively, as a broad constellation of conditions linked to pulmonary symptoms and emaciation; patients with TB may well have been included in their surveys but the results had no scientific foundation and were proposed more than a decade before Robert Koch discovered *Mycobacterium tuberculosis* in 1882. By 1910, however, Jefferys and Maxwell [12] concluded "tuberculosis is without any shadow of a doubt more prevalent and more fatal among the Chinese than it is in Europe and America." Cadbury [13] "expressed little doubt" that TB was both widespread and deadly in China, but he could only support his views by stating that mortality rates among American victims of TB in China were higher than those in Native Americans and African Americans.

The Qing Dynasty, which ruled from 1642 to 1912, finally fell and the Republic of China was declared on 1 January 1912. Not long afterward, the Republican Government "deliberately avoided" efforts to even begin to limit TB. Meanwhile, much of the rest of the world was showing that financial investment in control of TB led to the better management of cases and fewer deaths. In 1933, the National Anti-Tuberculosis Association of China was founded in Shanghai and one of its goals was to popularize the belief that TB was "epidemic" in China; but the statistics that were marshaled in 1927 to support that supposed premise were wholly inaccurate [14]. It would suffice to say that in 1933 "Tuberculosis was the greatest cause of death in China" [15].

After decades of trying to get the facts straight and to convince authorities that TB was the number one health problem in China up to the mid-1930s, it is time to tackle an unexpected and surprising allegation that the prevalence of TB was reversed in China compared with long standing findings in Western countries of Europe and America. These reports indicated that in China more rich people had TB than poor people – exactly the opposite of long established dogma. This interesting concept is based on data and analyses published by Lei [9].

Differences in the prevalence of TB infection – based on tuberculin skin test surveys in the 1920s – showed that poor children had lower rates of positivity than rich ones, and that among various occupational groups, students had higher rates of tuberculin reactivity than others. In addition, the results of studies of 30,000 patients in 3 different hospitals in Canton (Guangzhou) found that TB infection rates were 3 times greater in patients hospitalized in private rooms than in ordinary wards; also, tuberculin positivity values among professionals were over 3 times above those of laborers. Moreover, results began to mount supporting observations that rich Chinese people who spent considerable time indoors had far more TB than those working outdoors. These findings led to the belief – though not uniformly shared – that the disease was caused by traditional family living habits, including spitting, sharing chopsticks from a common bowl, and presence of multiple family members living in small, poorly ventilated sleeping spaces.

There are reasons to question these conclusions, starting with the gospel that TB is most often transmitted by coughing, sneezing, and other means of generating an aerosol containing minute, invisible, infectious tubercle bacilli that, in turn, remain airborne for hours and cause TB infection when particles are inhaled and deposit in small airways (bronchioles) and/or gas exchange regions (alveoli). Eating contaminated food remains a most unlikely way of spreading infection; drinking unpasteurized milk, however, containing *M. tuberculosis* or *M. bovis* was and still is a means of transmission, though not particularly common. Injection or direct contamination by tubercle bacilli is rare.

As authorities remind us: (1) Spitting is a disgusting, uncivilized, and unhygienic act, but hardly ever causes TB. In the early 1900s, the National Association for the Study and Prevention of Tuberculosis, now the American Lung Association, advertised heavily against spitting because they believed it caused TB: as far as TB is concerned, coughing remains the major factor and spitting is rarely involved.

(2) Sharing the same pair of chopsticks from mouth to mouth and from family member to family member, all from a common bowl transmits saliva and bits of food among participants, but rarely if ever causes TB. (3) On the contrary, the gathering of multiple, cloistered family members sharing limited, unventilated sleeping space provides a classic method of transmitting TB, and may have contributed to its pathogenesis during the 1920s and 1930s. But it is hard to believe that a relatively small community of rich Chinese were consistently more often both suffering and dying from TB than the majority of poor people in the country who were affected by the classical social disadvantages that favor the disease, including malnutrition, crowding, and impaired ventilation. We know that there still are millions of patients with TB in China, and that the current and accurate statistical analyses remind us that susceptibility to TB occurs by the traditional means of exposure to *M. tuberculosis,* fairly often followed by infection less often by disease.

Second Sino-Japanese War: 1937–1945

Marco Polo Bridge
Around the year 1300, Venetian merchant traveler Marco Polo saw and marveled at "one of the finest bridges in the world," about 15 km from today's central Beijing that showed off more than 500 beautifully carved granite lions, a landmark that became forever known as the Marco Polo Bridge [1]. More than 600 years later, the Marco Polo Bridge witnessed another vicious chapter of the Sino-Japanese War, this one starting on July 7, 1937. Unexpectedly, Japanese soldiers began firing more often than was customary in one of their "incidental exchanges," and Chinese Warlord Song Zheyuan's troops began firing back in the belief that the Japanese were on their way to occupying additional Chinese territory. At his headquarters in Nanjing, NRA Commander Chiang Kai-shek did not really know if the incoming cables singled another Japanese invasion or not, but he was increasingly prepared to go to war, even though he desperately needed more time to prepare. Soldiers on both sides of the Marco Polo Bridge were considering a cease-fire, but Chinese leaders in southern China, Japanese leaders in Tokyo, and International experts in Washington and elsewhere were sure war was inevitable, and were preparing for its consequences. On July 26 1937, heavily reinforced Japanese army divisions attacked Beijing and Tianjin, 2 major cities that were quickly conquered, and victorious fighting in the north lasted only another week [1].

Chiang's differences with most of the rival NRA Generals he confronted made him agree to wage war against the Japanese, but under their own jurisdictions. Mao Zedong also encouraged Chiang to continue fighting and agreed to use Red Army personnel but not under Chiang's control. Nationalist military and political authorities were convened who agreed to go to war. The question now for all to ponder was where and when?

Shanghai War, 1937
Further escalation of the Chinese-Japanese war was inevitable, so Chiang Kai-shek decided to make it happen during the month of August 1937 and in Shanghai, where his best troops were stationed and eager for battle. Chiang's decision gave threatened Western foreigners and Chinese residents time to throng into the British-affiliated International Settlement and French Concession zones in Shanghai where, between July 26 and August 5 according to conservative estimates, 50,000 refugees took shelter [16].

Chiang gave the order to defend Shanghai on August 13 [1], but well before that date Japanese warships had already congregated in the port and around 8,000 troops had been relocated to the city, with many more on the way. The very next day after Chiang issued his order, pilots from the Chinese air force launched a surprise attack on the prize cruiser Izumo that turned into a colossal error. Instead of targeting the Izumo, according to the master plan, pilots from 2 different NRA aircraft dropped bombs that landed in crowded, busy districts near the Palace and Cathay hotels in the politically neutral International Settlement in Shanghai. When the smoke had cleared, more than 1,000 people were dead. Needless to say, public support for the Chinese Nationalist Party withered.

The war over Shanghai was fiercely fought street-by-street but the Japanese had a huge advantage owing to their greatly superior air power and relentless bombing of military facilities. Chiang's German-trained troops proved to be excellent fighters but were badly outnumbered and not as well equipped. Rival Chinese generals accepted roles as regional commanders and towards the end of the roughly 4-month war, over 200,000 Chinese soldiers from both southern and central China were fighting in Shanghai. By contrast, Red Army forces were not involved.

Chiang desperately hoped for and needed cooperation from international governments, particularly the UK and US but the only one that pitched in, not surprisingly, was the Soviet Union (USSR), whose motive was to keep China committed to fighting Japan as long as possible. In August 1937, the USSR signed a mutual nonaggression pact with

China, which provided roughly 300 airplanes, ammunition, and support of nearly 250 million US dollars [17]. The Soviets were making a major contribution to China's future whereas the rest of the world had not yet learned that Japan was an international menace.

The Rape of Nanjing

After almost 4 months of steadily losing ground and battles, in early December 1937, the battle for Shanghai was over. On December 12, the last Chinese army defender was forced to sneak out through a narrow door to safety and abandon the capital; the Japanese army took over the city the next day. After Chiang's NRA withdrew westward to defend central China, his military command facility moved to Wuhan and the administrative services to Chongqing, 751 km (466 miles) apart. That left Nanjing – Chiang's national capital and military headquarters – virtually defenseless. In rapid succession, the Japanese began to rain bombs on the city and to establish a Central China Area Army (JCCAA), which allowed troops to extend and augment their control over Nanjing and neighboring regions.

Within a few hours after Nanjing surrendered, the JCCAA lost all semblance of authority throughout the city, including officers supposedly in charge. Tens of thousands of soldiers unleashed a continuous spree-orgy of unrestrained mass killing, torture, robbery, and rape – that endured for the next 6 weeks. The small group of remaining Westerners in Nanjing, a few Germans, and Americans, established a Safety Zone within the campus of Ginling College, which was quickly over run with Chinese inhabitants seeking protection: within a week more than 9,000 people were searching for a place to sleep within the college's confines. Random fires, both large and small – mainly set by the Chinese – broke out in numerous buildings in a last-ditch effort to destroy any structure that could be useful to the invaders. Chief targets of the marauding Japanese were ordinary looking Chinese men who might be soldiers but who were not wearing their uniforms. But there was no means of real verification so the slaughter was indiscriminate and massive.

After the sewage system in Nanjing failed in the early days of the massacre, raw sewage percolated out from drains, which added to the growing, offensive smell throughout the city. Sanitation was, to say the least, inadequate; available stool buckets soon overflowed. As human excrement and urine began to accumulate, the stench worsened as did the health hazard. But the unrelenting pandemonium of gunfire, explosions, shrieking, and moaning gave abundant witness to the deaths and assaults that were taking place.

The massiveness of the cold-blooded savagery of the JCCAA has been written about and lamented over many times [18], but the specification and immensity of the events that characterize the story as it is usually told fully justifies the subheading used in this chapter: *The Rape of Nanjing*. Countless reports tell of women, from 12- to 60-years old, being repeatedly sexually assaulted. John Rabe, one of the few Western witnesses to the ongoing horrors, described the events on 17 December 1937: "Last night up to 1,000 women and girls are said to have been raped, about a hundred girls at Ginling College alone. You hear of nothing but rape" [19]. And rape was indeed interminable; thousands of women were injured, other thousands killed. On December 30, 1937, Japanese guards were stationed to protect foreign embassies, but break-ins and rapes continued. Nearly 1 month later, toward the end of January 1938, the scourge of murders and constant rapes began to diminish, and by mid-February they had supposedly ended. The full story behind Nanjing's 6 weeks of murders and rapes as well as the 200,000–300,000 Chinese deaths, will never be indisputably known, but keeps attracting new books, films and videos. All the attention to *The Rape of Nanjing* underscores the belief that such terrorization should never happen again.

Finally a Victory, Then More Defeats

After the barbaric 6 weeks of Nanjing, Japanese troops kept penetrating ever deeper into central China, but resistance by the Chinese army not only endured but strengthened. Fighting was brutal on both sides, but by April 1938 the NRA had taken charge of the remaining Japanese forces and scored a convincing victory at Taierzhuang. And with it, an accompanying tremendous boost of moral for the Chinese people [1].

The triumph, however, was short lived and Japanese troops began once again advancing, but were slowed down by a desperate measure: the breaching of dikes along the Yellow River, which caused massive flooding and around half-a-million Chinese casualties. Chiang was forced to retreat further west and set up a new temporary capital at Chongqing. Foreign observers – and even the Japanese occupiers themselves – believed the NRA was going to surrender and many thought it should have. But Chiang toughed it out and through it all kept fighting. The CCP held on in the far West and did not contribute to the struggle.

Between the roughly 2-plus years from September 1939 and the Pearl Harbor attack, December 1941, both the Nationalist and Japanese armies each made serious offensive ventures but without much military success in either direction. The Japanese air force, though, continued its incessant bombing attacks, which were far more often aimed at the Nationalists than the Communists. A collaborationist Chinese regime engineered by Wang Jingwei and supported by Tokyo was established in Nanjing, but failed to attract significant support [1].

Meanwhile, as their armies continued to gain strength and firepower, and despite their United Front of mutual support, the NRA was doing its best to stifle the CCP. But the growing Communist forces, along with their appended political influences, had spread from their northwestern headquarters in Yan'an to central China in regions long dominated by Chiang. In August 1940, the Red Army initiated the one and only major series of all-out offensive strikes during the pre-WWII period against strategic military locations; the fighting lasted 3 months and triggered ferocious Japanese counter initiatives.

"A Date That Will Live in Infamy"

The sneak attack on December 7, 1941 by squadrons of Japanese aircraft – that destroyed US ships, airplanes, and military installations in and around Pearl Harbor – led President Franklyn D. Roosevelt to declare war on Japan, Germany, and Italy, the Axis powers, the following day. Please remember that Nazi Germany and the Soviet Union had signed a nonaggression pact on August 23, 1939, protecting each country against an attack from the other, but Germany broke the agreement by invading the Soviets on June 22, 1941, about 6 months before the US joined the Allies. Thus, the number and military might of various international belligerents changed dramatically. Japan, of course, had been at war against China since 1931, but it broadened its adversarial targets and quickly conquered Hong Kong, Thailand, Singapore, Burma, and later the Philippines.

The fall of Singapore in early 1942 was disastrous for the UK. About 80,000 British, Australian, and Indian troops, along with its advanced military port facilities, surrendered to the Japanese. These prisoners joined 50,000 others captured during the Malayan Campaign [20]. In May 1942, about 53,000 American and Philippine military personnel and an uncertain number of civilians were taken prisoners [21]. These and other prisoners of the Japanese spent the remainder of WWII under murderous, often inhumane conditions.

But then in August 1942, the US Navy and Air Force won the decisive 4-day Battle of Midway in which all 4 Japanese aircraft carriers and one heavy cruiser were sunk; in comparison, the US lost one carrier and a destroyer: a crucial turning point that led to a series of subsequent successive victories in the Pacific war.

One year later (1943), the Japanese launched an unusually large offensive in China in an effort to force the NRA to surrender; Chiang suffered multiple defeats but held on. But because of the losses, in the voices of the US and its Allies, the balance between the CCP and Chinese Nationalist Party had greatly shifted in favor of the Communists. One of the chief goals of the 1943–1944 and earlier Imperial Army offensives was to cause the Chinese to sign a truce or surrender, which would allow 600,000 Japanese troops to be redeployed to urgently needed combat zones. But the Chinese managed to hang on and not quit.

After the atom bomb explosions on August 6 and 9, 1945, first in Hiroshima and then Nagasaki had paved the way, the Japanese surrendered on August 15, followed by the signing of surrender documents on September 2 that officially ended WWII. Immediately afterward, however, the Communists and Nationalists resumed their civil war. As the war smoldered on, Chiang seems to have lost his military skills and the CCP army commander, Lin Biao, increasingly prevailed. In May 1949, Chiang retreated to Taiwan and never returned to mainland China. Mao had won big, but his Great Leap Forward (1958–1961) led to a disastrous famine that killed around 20 million people, and soon after was followed by the Cultural Revolution of the 1960s, which pitted "bad" families against "good" families, a sort of internecine bourgeois battle, which left innumerable scars.

Tuberculosis Control in China

In the recently published book entitled "A history of Tuberculosis Control in China" (see the front cover in Fig. 1), Dai et al. give an overview on the development of TB control in China during the last century [22].

They depict mainly the following 3 important steps:

1) In 1929, and based on an estimated Chinese population of 400 million inhabitants, Dr. Lu Yongchun, a pioneer of modern TB control in China, estimated that the prevalence of TB was about 11 million people and that the annual mortality of the disease was 1.22 million. In 1930, TB mortality was updated to 307/100,000. Four years later (1934) in Shanghai, the infection rate of children and young adults with TB, based on positive Mantoux tuberculin skin tests, increased with age to 60.0% at age 10–14 years, and was 94.3% at age 25 years and older.

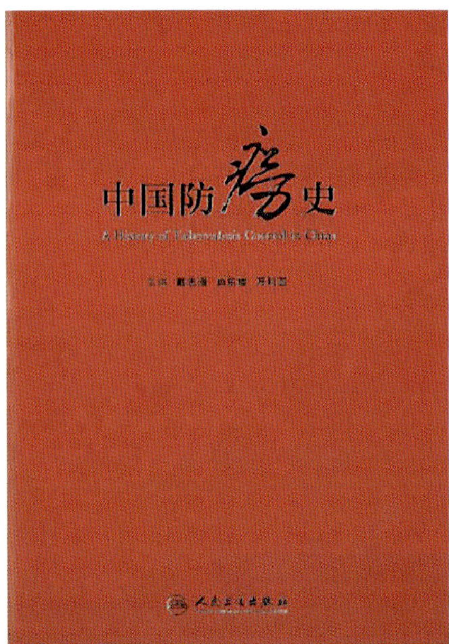

Fig. 1. Front cover in red, showing Chinese characters plus the much less distinct English title of the book "A History of Tuberculosis Control in China", reproduced from [22], with permission.

2) TB sanatoria took off in Europe in the mid-19th century, then spread and reigned throughout most of the world until displaced by anti-TB chemotherapy in the early 1950s. China's sanatoria were established at the beginning of the 20th century, first in Beijing and Shanghai, then spread to other major cities. Some sanatoria were independent institutions; others were affiliated with large, comprehensive hospital facilities.

3) The final table in the chapter includes fascinating details about how the 20 designated Chinese sanatoria system cared for patients stricken with TB. It starts routinely with names and local addresses; but then the so-called "start year" is given in "year of the Republic of China," which was founded in 1912; accordingly, the 20th year of the Republic of China actually indicates 1932. Next, the number of beds, usually 12–30, occasionally 50, is straightforward but criteria of admission are complex: ground rules include "Admit various early-stage TB but no admission of surgical TB patients;" next, "[O]nly admit those accept artificial pneumothorax;" lastly, "[A]dmit both severe and mild cases." Economic costs vary considerably; "Monthly Patient Fee" starts with "More than 10 [cheapest] to 40 yuan," and "100–500 [most expensive] yuan. (In the 1930s, 10 yuan equaled roughly USD 1.50 per month, whereas 500 yuan per month cost USD 75.) Finally, here are the "Traffic Conditions" that define how TB patients locate their chosen sanatorium: "Convenient water and land transportation;" "Take a train to Hanzhou;" "Take a car from Jiujiang to Lianhuadong then take a sedan to go up the mountain;" and lastly, "Car and rickshaw" available.

Tuberculosis and the People's Republic of China
The People's Republic of China (PRC) has the largest number of inhabitants of any country in the world: 1.388 billion, according to the latest census. Life expectancy had lengthened but the One Child policy, 1.55.children per woman, continued to slow the population growth. For at least 2 centuries, China has had an enormous number of patients with TB and mortality from the disease, but inaccurate statistical studies have long clouded demographic data concerning health and disease.

Currently, TB remains a serious problem in the PRC and has the second largest worldwide burden of TB after India, Mao's Great Leap forward and Cultural Revolution were national disasters that not only undermined TB prevention and control efforts, but led to a stagnation of national economic policy measures that hampered progress in the diagnosis and treatment. In 1990–1991, the Government of China, Ministry of Public Health with support from the World Bank and WHO, initiated a review of the TB program performance. This study identified several drawbacks that diminished the benefits of the program. These include, the inability of many patients to pay for their diagnosis and treatment, poor compliance with instructions and unreliable laboratory services. In addition, the reporting and evaluation systems for case finding and for the assessment of treatment outcomes were deficient.

As a basic starting point, the cure rate in TB treatment programs in 1991 and before hovered around 50%. An entirely new program was started that year based on Directly Observed Short-course Chemotherapy (DOTS). Patients with suspected TB were referred to TB dispensaries for physical examination and fluoroscopy. Suspects submitted 3 sputum specimens for AFB smear examinations. Smear-positive patients were treated by village doctors (also known as barefoot doctors) – free of charge – for 2 months with 4-drug standard chemotherapy followed by 2 months of isoniazid and rifampicin. Already treated patients received the same regimen plus ethambutol for the entire 6 months.

Between 1991 and 1994, almost 1.6 million patients with suspected TB had physical examinations and fluoroscopy. There were 104,444 new AFB-positive cases and 95,616 previously treated AFB-positive cases. Short-term cure rates were 89.7% for new cases and 81.1% among those retreated,

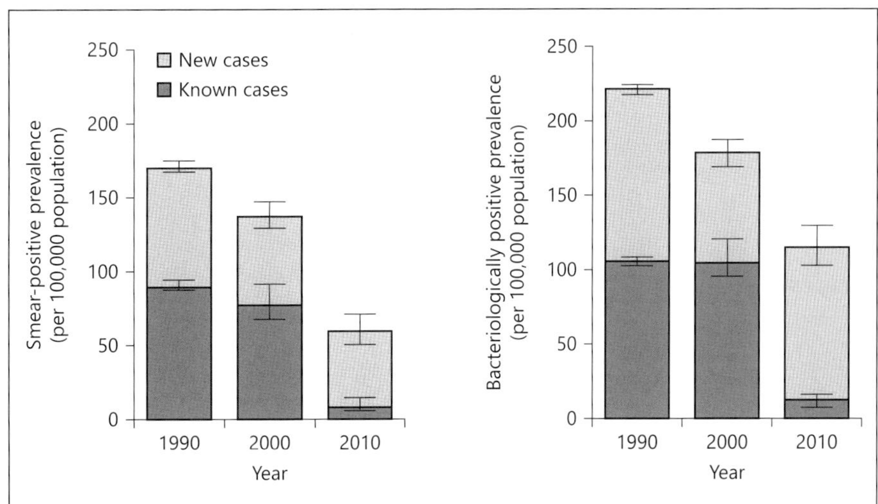

Fig. 2. Prevalence of smear-positive and bacteriologically positive tuberculosis stratified by new and known cases, 1990–2010. Analyzed by use of 1990 diagnostic protocol and unstandardized for age or other variables. Error bars show the 95% CI. Reproduced from The Lancet [25] with permission from Elsevier.

demonstrating that "high rates of compliance and cure" can occur in 6 months in large numbers of TB suspects by DOTS [23].

A subsequent 10-year follow-up of 8 million TB suspects who followed these guidelines was reported in 2002. All had been evaluated at no charge, 1.8 million cases were treated by DOTS, of whom 1.3 million were treated at no cost (i.e., 0.5 million were charged), and over 90% were cured. Downsides of the project were a detection rate of new AFB-smear positive cases of only 54% and 41.2% had lower than the 70% case detection target [24].

The positive effects of the control program were assessed in a study published in Lancet (2014) showing that the prevalence of smear-positive or bacteriologically positive TB in known cases was significantly lower in 2010 than in 1990 (Fig. 2). Thus, the prevalence of TB halved in China in 20 years, a marked improvement in TB treatment – as the authors conclude – due to a major shift in treatment from hospitals to the public health centers after implementation of the DOTS strategy [25].

Tuberculosis in Taiwan

The past history of TB in Taiwan undoubtedly began in 1949 when Chiang Kai-shek and his Nationalist Government left mainland China for the new country. As was the case for my search for information about TB during the formative years of the PRC, I came up empty handed: nothing. So I can only provide some fairly recent information about the status of TB after about 1998 to let readers know where Taiwan stands in the continuum of world TB. Knowledge about health in the country has been greatly assisted by its National Health Insurance program, constituted in 1996, which has provided mandatory medical coverage for 95% of Taiwanese residents.

Data from the Centre for Disease Control, Department of Health, Taiwan and peer-reviewed reports, document that in 2002, the incidence of TB was 74.6/100,000, and was significantly higher in aborigines, 289.8/100,000 and in mountainous regions 256/100,000. The TB mortality rate was 5.68/100,000. A summary of primary drug resistance data from 1990 to 2002 showed a rate of 4.7–12% for INH, 0.7–5.9% for RIF, 1–6% for ethambutol, and 4–11% for SM. Rates of MDRTB among new cases and previously treated cases were 1–3 and 15–46%, respectively [26]. Note that the incidence of TB had fallen in 2012 to 54.5/100,000, but that Taiwan remained an "intermediate incidence setting" for TB [27].

Conclusion

For century after century, TB was by far the most common cause of death in Europe, and for a period of 300 years in England it is believed to have killed over 1 billion men, women, and children. And according to the WHO, TB remains the largest cause of death from an infectious disease in the world. But what about China, the most populated country in the world with its 1.388 billion inhabitants? TB has long had an abundance of TB deaths and disease in China, but reliable data on the exact size of the burden has proved difficult to quantify. A large part of the problem, since at least during the 1920s has been the ongoing vicious warfare among 3 different belligerent forces: the Imperial Japanese Army, Navy and Air Force on one side, and 2 different Chinese armed forces – the Chinese Nationalist Army and the Chinese Communist Army – who took turn fighting the Japanese and also relentlessly kept fighting each other.

The Second Sino-Japanese War and the 4-year long post-WWII civil war between the CCP and NRA created an almost 20 year hiatus of progress in implementing public health measures and applying new techniques for diagnosing and treating TB. Both the PRC and Taiwanese are catching up and making headway, but considerable damage was done and much remains to be accomplished.

References

1 Mitter R: Forgotten Ally: China's World War II, 1937–1945. Boston, Mariner Books, Houghton Mifflin Harcourt, 2013.
2 Coble PM: Facing Japan: Chinese Politics and Japanese Imperialism, 1931–1937. Cambridge, Harvard University Press, 1991.
3 Ferrell RH: The mukden incident: september 18–19, 1931. J Mod Hist 1955;27.1:61–72.
4 General Shigeru Honjo. http://en.wikipedia.org/wiki/ShigeruHonjō (cited June 18, 2016).
5 Lytton Report. http://en.wikipedia.org/wiki/lytton_Report (cited June 18, 2016).
6 Jordan DA: China's Trial by Fire: The Shanghai War of 1932. University Michigan Press, 2001.
7 Watkins T: The Long March of the Communist Party of China, 1934–35. San José State University Department of Economics. www.sjsu.edu/faculty/watkins/longmarch.htm (cited July 21, 2017).
8 This Day in History: October 20, 1935. www.history.com/this-day-in-history/maos-long-march-concludes (cited 18 June 2016).
9 Lei SH: Habituating individuality: the framing of tuberculosis and its material solutions in Republican China. Bull Hist Med 2010;84:248–270.
10 Wang J, Wu L: History of Chinese Medicine: Being a Chronicle of Medical Happenings in China from Ancient Times to the Present Period (ed 2): Southern Materials Center, 1985.
11 Dudeon J: The Diseases of China: Their Causes, Conditions, and Prevalence, Contrasted with Those of Europe. Dunn & Wright, Glasgow, 1877.
12 Jefferys WH, Maxwell JL: The Diseases of China, Including Formosa and Korea. London, Bale and Danielson, 1910.
13 Cadbury WW: "Luilun feiluo summing neishang zheng," (A proposal for an antituberculosis crusade in China), Zhonghua yibao (Chinese medical news) 1921, pp 1–7.
14 Hall GAM: Tuberculosis in China. Br J Tuberc 1935;29:132–144.
15 Oldt F: Tuberculosis in Kwangtung: According to age, sex, occupation, and economic condition. Chinese Med J 1933;47:111–127.
16 North China Herald, August 11, 1937, p 217.
17 Taylor J: The Generalissimo: Chiang Kai-shek and the Struggle for Modern China. Cambridge, Belknap Press of Harvard University Press, 2009.
18 Chang I: The Rape of Nanking: The Forgotten Holocaust of World War II. New York, Penguin Books, 1997.
19 Woods JE: The Good Man of Nanking, the Diaries of John Rabe. New York, Knopf Publishing Corporation, 1998.
20 The British Empire in World War II. https://en.wikipedia.org/wiki/British_Empire_in_World_War_II. Cited July 26, 2017.
21 American Prisoners of war in the Phiippines: Office of the Provost Marshal Report, November 19, 1945. www.mansell.com/pow_resources/camplists/philippines/pows_in_OPMG_report.html (cited August 6, 2017).
22 Dai Z, Xiao D, Wan L, et al: A history of Tuberculosis Control in China. People's Medical Publishing House, March 2013, Beijing, PRC.
23 Results of directly observed short-course chemotherapy in 112,842 Chinese patients with smear-positive tuberculosis. China Tuberculosis Control Collaboration. Lancet 1996;347:358–332.
24 Xianyi C, Fengzeng Z, Hngjin D, et al: The DOTS strategy in China: results and lessons after 10 years. Bull World Health Organ 2002;80:430–436.
25 Wang L, Zhang H, Ruan Y, et al: Tuberculosis prevalence in China, 1990–2010; a longitudinal analysis of national survey data. Lancet 2014;383:2057–2064.
26 Hsueh PR, Liu Yc, So J, et al: Mycobacterium tuberculosis in Taiwan. J Infect 2006;53:77–85.
27 Hung CL, Chien JY, Ou CY: Associated factors for tuberculosis recurrence in Taiwan: a nationwide nested case-control study from 1998 to 2010. PLoS One 2015;10:e0124822.

John F. Murray, MD, Professor Emeritus of Medicine
University of California San Francisco
P.O. Box 0841
San Francisco, CA 94143-0841 (USA)
E-Mail johnfmurr4@aol.com

Conclusion

Murray JF, Loddenkemper R (eds): Tuberculosis and War. Lessons Learned from World War II.
Prog Respir Res. Basel, Karger, 2018, vol 43, pp 214–228 (DOI: 10.1159/000481490)

Tuberculosis and War: Lessons Learned From World War II

Robert Loddenkemper[a] · John F. Murray[b]

[a]German Central Committee against Tuberculosis, Berlin, Germany; [b]University of California San Francisco,
San Francisco, CA, USA

Abstract

Tuberculosis (TB) is one of the most frequent and most dangerous diseases that further complicate the special circumstances of warfare. TB was also the major health disaster of World War II (WWII). Environmental and host-dependent risk factors – usually both combined – contributed to the increase in TB mortality during WWII. The main risk factors included malnutrition, which weakens the host immune defenses; overcrowding, which increases the risk of transmission of tubercle bacilli; and disruption of medical and public health services, which impair control and treatment efforts. Anti-TB drugs were discovered towards the end of WWII, and later refinements dramatically improved the TB epidemic. Years later, 2 big problems emerged: drug resistance and human immunodeficiency virus co-infection. Thanks to the effectiveness of high-tech case-finding and microbiological advances, the possible eradication of TB seems possible sometime in the future, but that goal becomes ever more distant as long as wars continue. This book, *TB and War: Lessons Learned from WWII*, provides an overall assessment of the partnership between TB and war, plus chapter by chapter account of the dramatic events that affected the number of TB cases and the outcomes of the disease in the 26 countries discussed in the book.   © 2018 S. Karger AG, Basel

"War is the Enemy of Health" [1] and tuberculosis (TB) is one of the most frequent and most dangerous diseases ever to accompany the special circumstances of warfare. According to the British TB specialist Marc Daniels, who analyzed the TB outcome in several countries after the war, TB was the major health disaster of World War II (WWII) [2]. There is no doubt that WWII is up to now the deadliest conflict in human history – by far – with an estimated more than 60 million fatalities, including about 20 million military personnel and 40 million civilians. Many of the civilians died because of deliberate genocide, massacres, mass bombings, disease, and starvation [3]. No one knows the total number of casualties in WWII, because countless deaths went unrecorded.

Figure 1 shows which countries were affected by military and civilian deaths due to WWII, and to what extent. Those countries with the highest absolute numbers of deaths include the Soviet Union, Poland, and Germany in Europe, as well as China, Japan, and Indonesia in Asia. Note that many of the same countries also experienced high numbers of war-related excesses in TB mortality, as described in detail in chapters 5–19 (see also Table 1).

Evolution of TB during WWII

In several European countries, the scourge that was called consumption or phthisis affected multitudes of people with real, but not yet discovered TB. However, the numbers also included many others who had a different diagnosis. In addition, many people with real TB were missed and not counted because of their atypical manifestations. At roughly the same time in London, England, mortality rates from supposed TB rose to a peak in the late 1700s–

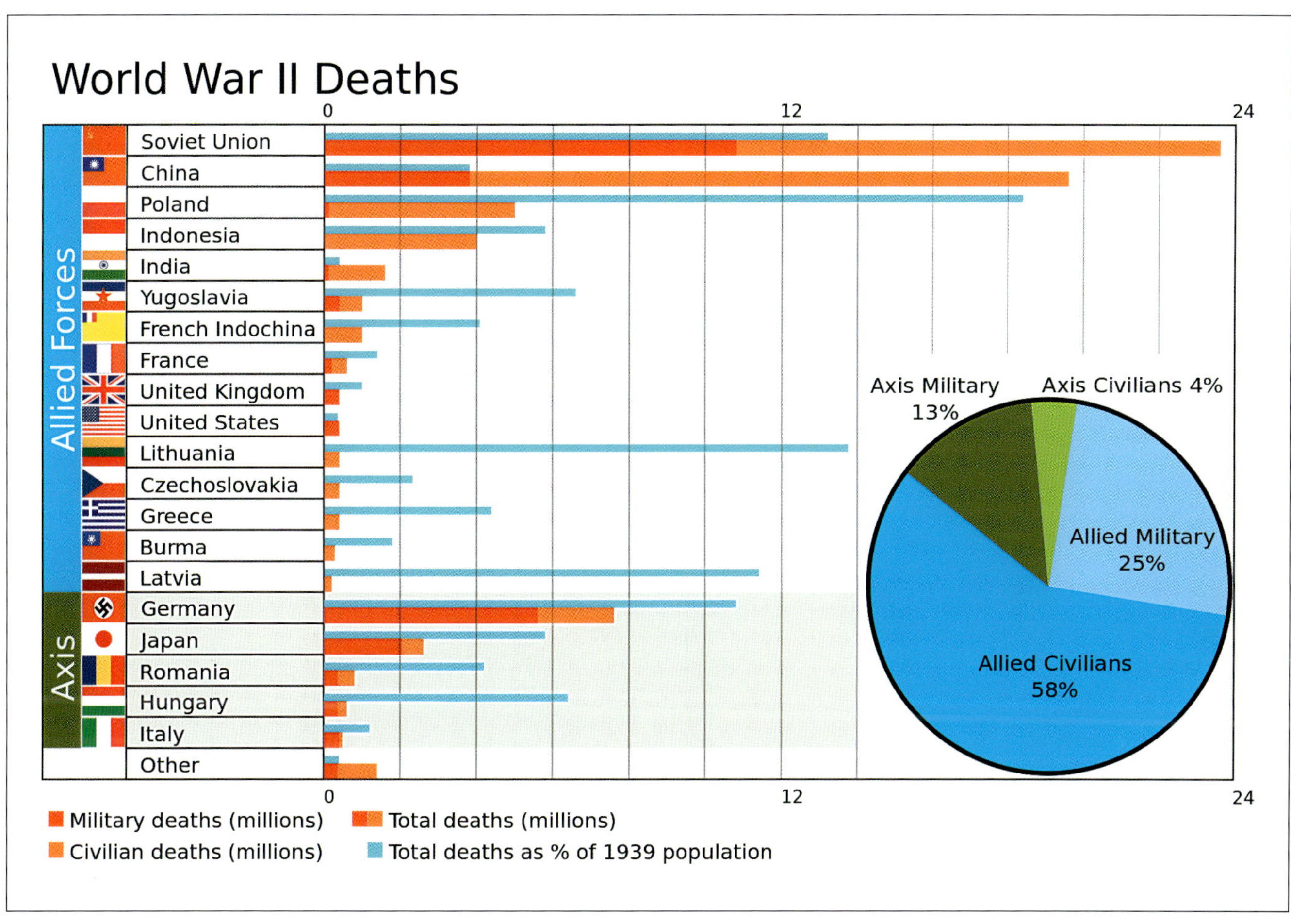

Fig. 1. World War II casualties [3].

early 1800s and then pursued a relatively orderly continuous, slow decline for well over the next 100 years. Other western European countries and major cities reached similar peaks of TB mortality 50 or even 100 years later, but then started their own slow descent. Suddenly though, around the beginning of August 1914, an abrupt and striking upsurge of TB deaths signaled the onset of WWI that lasted through WWI and the overlapping Spanish Influenza pandemic. Note, however, that when the post-WWI downward trend resumed, it picked up as though the war and accompanying flu pandemic had not happened, as illustrated in Figure 2 for UK and Wales and Figures 5 and 6 in chapter 5 [4]. Although the absolute rise in TB mortality that occurred during WWI was not reached in WWII, the increase over the global pre-war rate was proportionately even greater [5]. Although there were exceptions, TB mortality rose during WWII, in some countries soon after the beginning, in others gradually

during or steeply after the war. Even some non-belligerent (neutral) countries observed an increase in TB, whereas a few belligerent countries saw a fall in numbers of TB cases (Bulgaria, Denmark, and England and Wales) [2].

Table 1 summarizes the changes seen in various belligerent and non-belligerent countries comparing the lowest (prewar) mortality rate with the highest estimated rate during or after WWII, bearing in mind all the uncertainties and difficulties in the retrieval of reliable epidemiological data during wartime. As described in Chapter 2, problems include the destruction of the public health infrastructure; the redeployment, transfer or elimination of health resources and personnel; the collapse of communication systems; the lack of diagnostic capabilities; and the presence of censorship, propaganda, and the intentional falsification of information [6]. But at least it is likely that the observed trends delineated in detail in Chapters 5–19 are germane and plausible.

Table 1. Estimated lowest and highest TB mortality rates before and during/after WWII for various belligerent (Allies and Axis) and non-belligerent (occupied and neutral) countries (change in %)

Country	TB-mortality (n/100,000) lowest level	Year	TB-mortality (n/100,000) highest level	Year	Change in %
Occupied countries					
Belgium[w]	68	1939	98	1941	+44
Netherlands[z]	41	1938	86	1945	+109
Luxemburg[x]	63	1940	93	1945	+48
France[z]	143	1938	158	1941	+10
Yugoslavia[y]	190	1937	400	1944	+210
Greece[y]	116	1938	275	1944	+235
Poland[z]	150	1938	240	1945	+60
Czech "Protectorate"[w]	124	1939	156	1942	+26
Norway[w]	86	1939	61	1945	−22
Denmark[w]	34	1939	33	1945	−3
Egypt[w]	51	1939	71	1944	+39
China[x]	400–500	1939	?	1945	?
Allies					
England-Wales[w]	62	1939	73	1941	+18
Scotland[w]	69	1938	83	1941	+21
Northern Ireland[w]	84	1938	104	1941	+24
Malta[w]	57	1939	97	1943	+70
South Africa[z]	250–300	1938	?	1945	+88
Australia[z]	37	1940	33	1944	−11
New Zealand[w]	39	1940	38	1943	−3
UDSSR (SU)	130	1940	?	?	?
in 45 major cities of SU[z]	287	1940	425	1942	+48
USA[z]	46	1940	40	1945	−13
Axis					
Germany[z]	62	1938	100–150	1945	+160–240
Austria[w]	101	1938	151	1945	+49.5
Hungary[z]	136	1939	157	1942	+15
Italy[w]	74	1940	102	1943	+35
Romania[w]	162	1939	191	1942	+18
Slovakia[w]	111	1939	140	1941	+26
Bulgaria[v]	138	1939	143	1940	+4
Finland[w]	196	1939	219	1942	+12
Japan[x, z]	207[x]	1939	241[z]	1944	+16
Neutral					
Ireland[w]	109	1938	147	1942	+34
Sweden[w]	75	1939	59	1945	−21
Switzerland[w]	80	1939	83	1945	+4
Spain[w]	113	1940	126	1941	+11.5
Portugal[w]	143	1939	160	1942	+12

Compiled data from [7][w], [8][x], [9][y], corresponding chapters[z].

Evolution of TB after WWII

Chemotherapy of TB

The European element of WWII ended on May 8, 1945, when Nazi Germany and its Axis collaborators surrendered unconditionally, a date – V. E. Day – that still awakens fervent memories throughout Europe; in many countries, such as France, the glorious victory continues to be celebrated as a national holiday. Five months earlier, however, at a time dominated by the terminal agonies of Nazi Germany, a to-

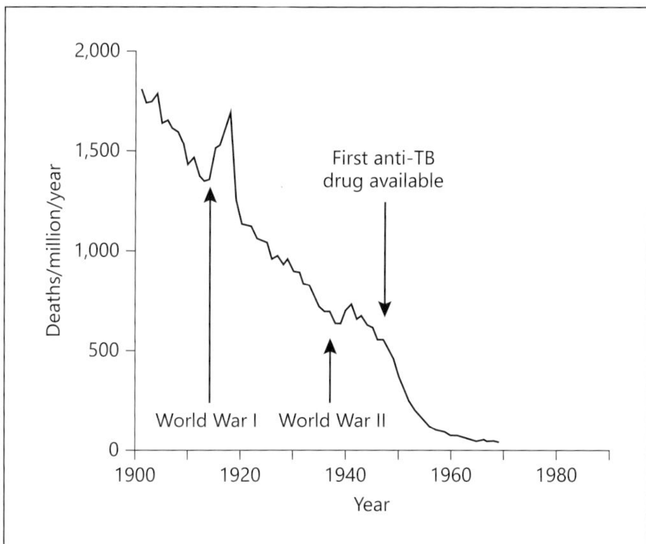

Fig. 2. Decline in TB mortality in England and Wales, and its association in time with the 2 World Wars, and the introduction of chemotherapy against TB [4], with permission.

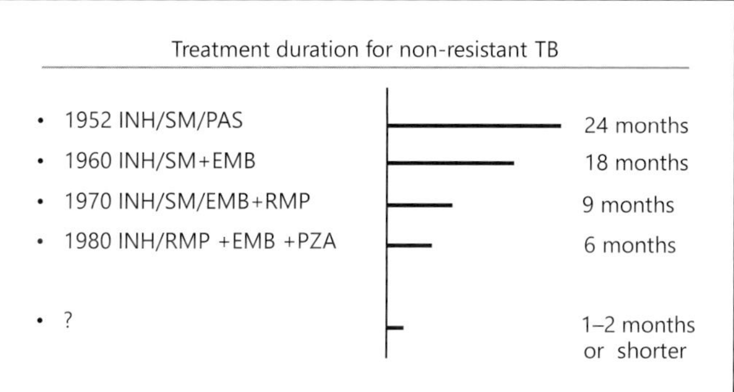

Fig. 3. Stepwise reduction in the duration of standard chemotherapy of drug-susceptible TB, courtesy of Robert Loddenkemper.

tally unrelated pair of world-shaking events passed virtually without notice: on October 30, 1944, Jorgen Lehman and his expert TB partner Gylfe Vallentin administered para-aminosalicylic acid (PAS) to a moribund young Swedish woman. Three weeks later, on November 20, 1944, Corwin Hinshaw and William Feldman partnered with TB specialist Karl Pfuetze and gave streptomycin (SM) to a moribund young American woman. Without fanfare and with considerable angst, this is how the first successful treatments of TB by chemotherapy occurred: both women came back from the brink of death [10].

SM and PAS each had moderate anti-TB activity, but each antibiotic caused significant toxicity, and in addition each alone induced significant drug resistance [11]. Another major advance in the history of TB chemotherapy was highlighted in one of the first statistically controlled clinical trials ever conducted by the British Medical Research Council: that study proved that combined treatment with both SM and PAS was superior to either agent alone. This observation led to the therapeutic maxim: never treat active TB with a single medication [12].

So far so good, but the chemotherapy of TB needed more effective and safer treatment than SM and PAS. Several pharmaceutical organizations were searching for a missing miracle substance, and 3 of them discovered the same chemical agent at practically the same time; this gift to humanity was called isoniazid (INH), and it turned out to be highly effective, safe, and cheap; 2 chemistry students had discovered it years before so it could not be patented. It took a year or 2 to learn how best to use the 3 available medications, which turned out to be "triple therapy" with oral INH and PAS for 18–24 months, supplemented by intramuscular SM for 6 months. This accomplishment was more than an ordinary breakthrough. After over 400 years during which TB had killed more humans than any other disease, triple therapy cured all forms of it. And it saved countless lives for almost 15 years, until newer agents – ethambutol (EMB), rifampicin (RMP), and pyrazinamide (PZA) – were combined with INH, successively shortening the duration of TB therapy to today's 6 months ("short-course chemotherapy"), provided that the patient's TB is fully drug-susceptible (Fig. 3).

Anti-TB Drug Resistance

Among the estimated 10.4 million new (incident) TB cases worldwide in 2016, there were an estimated 490,000 new cases of multidrug-resistant TB (MDR-TB) and an additional 110,000 people with rifampicin-resistant TB who were also declared newly eligible for MDR-TB treatment [13]. Drug resistance was first recognized as a major problem in 1992, when 12% of the TB patients in New York City were found to have MDR-TB, which has been defined as resistance to (at least) the 2 most powerful anti-TB drugs that are currently available: INH and RIF. The incidence of the so-called extensively resistant TB (XDR-TB), which was first described in 2006, is now estimated at 6.2% of MDR-TB cases [13]. By definition, XDR-TB is MDR-TB that is additionally resistant to at least one of the fluoroquinolones and to one of the 3 injectable second-line anti-TB drugs, amikacin, kanamycin, and capreomycin, and therefore difficult to treat. There have even been single cases of extremely resistant (XXDR-TB) and "totally" resistant (TDR-TB) cases reported.

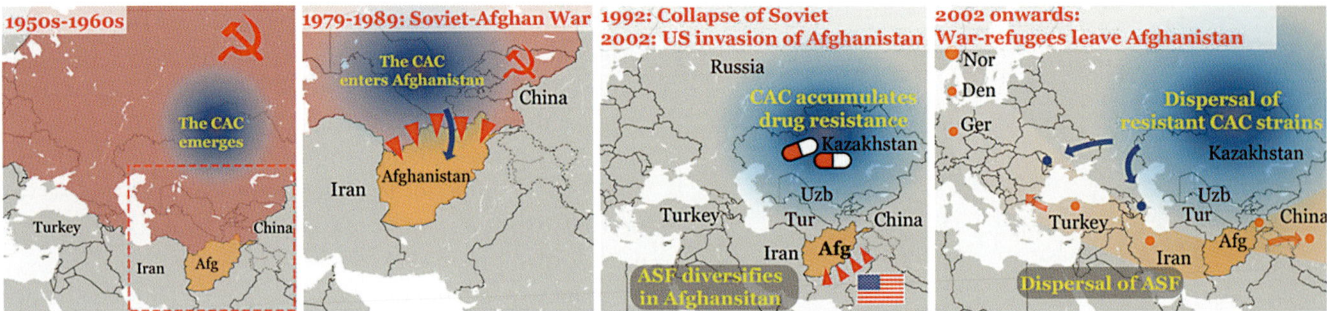

Fig. 4. A scenario for the spread of the CAC and ASF in time and space. Color shading and arrows indicate the emergence and spread of the CAC (blue) and ASF (orange). Dots represent cases or clusters of cases belonging to either the CAC or the ASF based on genome sequences, except the cases in Turkey, China, and Tajikistan, for which only MIRU data were available. Red shading of countries is used to indicate membership in the Soviet Union. Red triangles symbolize armed invasion. Afg, Afghanistan; Den, Denmark; Ger, Germany; Nor, Norway; Tur, Turkmenistan; Uzb, Uzbekistan [15], with permission.

The development of drug resistance is mainly due to the inappropriate treatment, which may have many causes, but is theoretically avoidable. The more widespread TB is in the patient's body, the greater the number of bacteria that are present, and the more likely it is that some of the pathogenic organisms will contain spontaneous mutations conferring drug resistance [14]. One of the main reasons today is the transmission of drug-resistant bacilli to contacts of the patient with infectious TB disease. Major risk factors for MDR-TB are, besides contact with MDR-TB patients, prior (insufficient) anti-TB treatment, immigration from a region with a high prevalence of MDR-TB and imprisonment (prisons require special attention, particularly in the Newly Independent States of the former Soviet Union) [14].

In some regions of the world, the so-called Beijing genotype of *Mycobacterium tuberculosis* is associated with a high resistance rate and, in particular, with a high MDR rate (the "W" strain). These strains may be more virulent, and/or more likely to mutate, and/or able to spread more easily because of poorer TB control in the areas to which they are endemic. In the context of war, a recent publication has shown the spread of the "Beijing" *M. tuberculosis* lineage 2 (L2) to Western Europe [15].

According to the study results, it is estimated that this central Asian clade was introduced into Afghanistan from Soviet Central Asia, coincident with the 1979–1989 Soviet occupation of the country. In the wake of the continued violent conflicts in the country, these strains (central Asian clade) seem to have been brought by Afghan refugees to Western Europe, as shown in Figure 4.

Until 2 or 3 years ago, the standardized treatment of M/XDR-TB led to mixed outcomes and uncertainties. Improved regimens and the addition of 2 new drugs, bedaquiline and delamanid [16], have strengthened the treatment results. In 2016, a new rapid diagnostic test and an improved, shorter and cheaper MDR-TB treatment regimen offered an important new step for those who qualify. Bear in mind, it used to take up to 2 years to assess treatment outcomes that were often poorly tolerated. It thus required a high degree of patient cooperation, and the rate of premature termination of treatment was higher than for non-resistant TB (up to 30%). The possibility of contagion necessitates adequate preventive measures against infection, which is not easy to achieve, particularly in situations of armed conflict [17].

The new rapid diagnostic test is called MTBDRsl, which is a DNA-based test that distinguishes genetic mutations among MDR-TB strains that, in turn, makes them resistant to fluoroquinolones and injectable second-line drugs. This selectivity greatly improves the choice of MDR-TB treatment regimens by avoiding treatment of patients with known resistance to second-line drugs. Test results from, MTBDRsl take only 24–48 hours, another great advantage. The new strategies typically consist of shorter-course (9–12 months), 2-phases (intensive and maintenance), and multiple drugs (up to 7 different agents) [16, 18]. Additional studies are under way as shown in Figure 5 [19].

However, it is estimated that MDR-TB and XDR-TB will still remain a problem for decades (the peak may be reached in 2040), in particular in countries with a high burden of these complex forms of drug resistance [20].

Diagnostic Approach to TB
Radiological Examinations: The importance of radiographic techniques for the diagnosis of active pulmonary TB was acknowledged only a few years after Roentgen

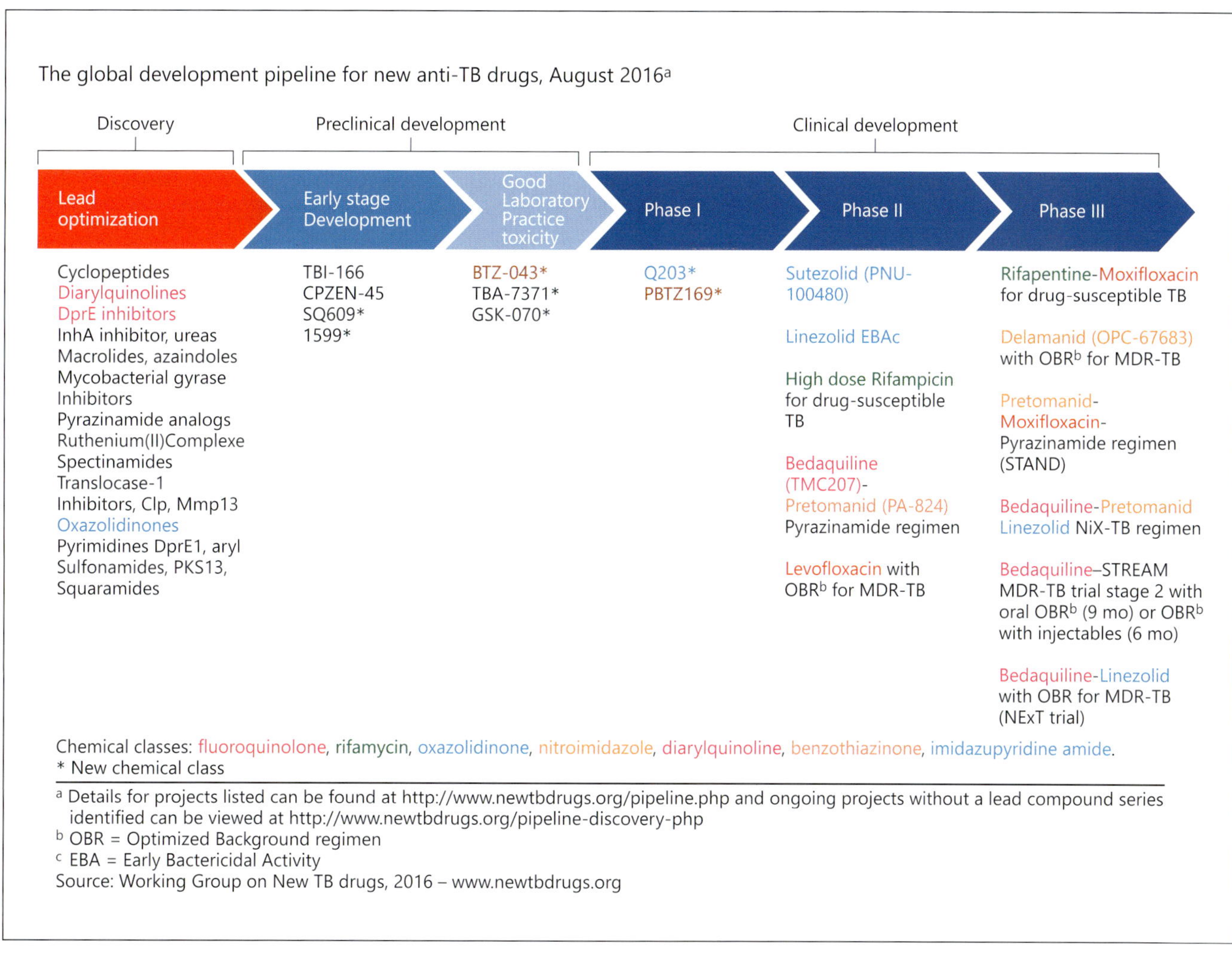

Fig. 5. The global development pipeline for new anti-TB drugs, as of August 2016. WHO Global TB report 2016 [19], with permission.

discovered the value of X-rays, but they were not used on a routine basis until after WWII, either for individuals with suspicion of TB or for screening of large groups of civil or military populations, often for compulsory reasons. Essential prerequisites consisted of combined roentgenologic-fluoroscopic apparatus as well as trained radiologists. Today, computed tomography is sometimes employed in the special evaluation and/or follow-up of TB, but it has not so far been included in national and international guidelines [21]. Literature is lacking and no general consensus exists on the use of ultrasound, computed tomography, and magnetic resonance imaging in TB patients.

Bacteriological Examinations: Before and during WWII, proof of infectivity of a TB case was mainly based on the microscopic examination of sputum. After the war, TB cultures – or even guinea pig inoculations – were gradually introduced into routine practice. Because these methods were more sensitive and specific, more infectious cases were detected. Today, new molecular diagnostic tests are available for earlier and improved diagnosis, especially in patients with smear-negative pulmonary TB, clinically diagnosed TB, and drug-resistant TB; these include rapid molecular methods such as molecular drug susceptibility tests and a variety of rapid and accurate "next generation sequencing" genome sequencing studies, which may well revolutionize the diagnosis and epidemiological study of TB [22]. Figure 6 summarizes the current status of the development of molecular TB diagnostics [19]. These modern techniques show great promise when practiced in sophisticated laboratories, but problems are likely if applied in poor countries and under conditions of warfare [23].

An overview of progress in the development of molecular TB diagnostics, August 2016[a]

Technologies in development for use in reference level laboratories	Technologies in development for use in intermediate level laboratories	Technologies in development for use in peripheral level laboratories
■ m2000 RealTime MTB System, Abbot, USA ■ TruArray® MDR-TB, Akonni, USA ■ INFINITI® System MDR-TB BioFilm Chip® Microarray, AutoGenomics, USA ■ BD ProbeTec® ET Direct TB assay, BD, USA ■ TB drug resistance array, Capital Bio, China ■ AMTD test, Hologic Genprobe, USA ■ Cobas TaqMan MTB test, Roche Switzerland ■ Anyplex™, Seegene, Korea ■ Magicplex™, Seegene, Korea ■ TRC Rapid® MTB, Tosoh Bioscience, Japan ■ MeltPro®, Zeesan Biotech, China	■ FluoroType MTB/FluoroType MTB RNA, Hain Lifesciences, Germany ■ iCubate System, iCubate, USA ■ AdvanSure, LG Life sciences, Korea ■ vereMTB, Veredus Laboratories, Singapore ■ SPEED-OLIGO®, Vircell, Spain ■ MolecuTech REBA, YD Diagnostics, Korea ■ LATE-PCR, Brandeis University, USA ■ GeneXpert XDR cartridge, Cepheid, USA ■ Xpert Ultra, Cepheid, USA ■ Enigma ML, Enigma Diagnostics, UK	■ Genedrive MTB/RIF ID, Epistem, UK ■ HYDRA, Insilixa Inc, USA ■ Truelab/Truenat MTB, Molbio/bigtec Diagnostics, India ■ EasyNAT TB Diagnostic kit, Ustar Biotechnologies, China GenePOC test, GenePOC, Canada ■ Xpert Ommi, Cepheid, USA

a This is not an exhaustive list of technologies in development. Those listed are the ones documented in publications by UNITAID and TAG.
UNITAID. 2014. Tuberculosis Diagnostic Technology and Market Landscape, 3rd edition. Geneva: World Health Organization.
http://www.unitaid.eu/images/marketdynamics/publications/UNITAID_TB_Diagnostics_landscape_3rd-edition.pdf
Frick M., Lessem E., McKenna L., "2016 pipeline report. Tuberculosis (TB) Edition. Diagnostics, treatment, prevention and vaccines in development",
HIV 1-Base/Treatment Action Group. London/New York 2016.
http://www.pipellnereort.org/sites/g/files/g575521/f/201507/2015%20Pipeilne%20Report%20Full.pdl

Fig. 6. Overview of progress in the development of molecular TB diagnostics [19], with permission.

Prevention of TB

Preventive Chemotherapy of Latent TB Infection
Tuberculin testing for the detection of latent TB infection (LTBI) was being used decades before WWII, both for individual diagnostic purposes and for mass screening (e.g., in military recruits). After WWII, tuberculin skin testing was increasingly used for universal screening of the general population and for periodic screening of high-risk populations [24]. The test became very important after it was proven that anti-TB treatment is effective for the eradication of LTBI [25, 26]. Because of their higher sensitivity and specificity, Interferon-Gamma Release Assays (IGRAs) are currently – when available – preferred for the diagnosis of LTBI [27, 28]. Preventive chemotherapy in designated high-risk groups may contribute considerably to the reduction of TB morbidity and to the elimination of TB [29].

Vaccination
BCG vaccination (*BCG: Bacille Calmette-Guérin*) with the attenuated *M. bovis* strain developed by the French researchers Calmette and Guérin, was first used for TB prevention in 1921 [30]. Acceptance was initially slow, and then virtually stopped entirely after the Lübeck disaster in 1930, in which several babies died following the oral application of real *M. tuberculosis* [31]. After WWII, in many countries the routine administration of BCG was implemented somewhat reluctantly, and only because vaccination was vigorously promoted and organized, particularly by the Danish and Swedish Red Cross and expedited by The United Nations International Children's Emergency Fund (UNICEF), it finally became the most frequently applied vaccination worldwide. BCG has its greatest effect in preventing miliary TB and TB meningitis in infants and young children, and is unfortunately much less effective in older persons and against other forms of TB. Both the US and The Netherlands disclaim BCG vaccination, relying instead on the detection and treatment of latent TB through preventive chemotherapy, which was introduced in 1957 [25]. More effective vaccines could contribute decisively to the global elimination of TB, and considerable research is presently being performed in several institutions aimed at developing better anti-TB vaccines [32]. Figure 7 gives an overview of the status of ongoing research projects [19].

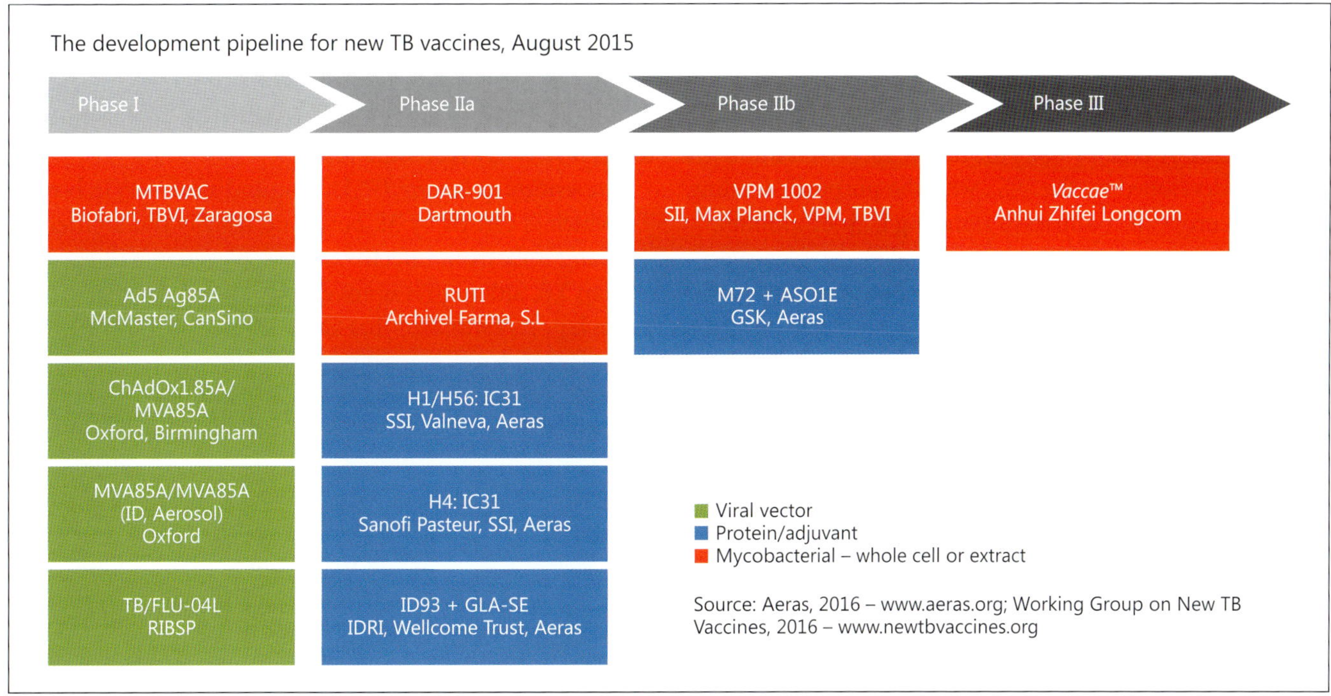

Fig. 7. The development pipeline for new TB vaccines [19], with permission.

Reducing the Risk and Burden of TB after WWII
Both environmental and host-dependent risk factors – usually both combined – were responsible for the increase in TB mortality during WWII. The main risk factors included malnutrition, which weakens the immune defenses of the host; overcrowding, which increases the risk of transmission of tubercle bacilli; and disruption of medical and public health services, which weaken the efforts to control and treat TB [4] (see also Chapter 3).

Improving the Food Supply: TB and malnutrition are interlinked in a complex relationship. The infection may cause malnutrition through either increased metabolic demands or decreased intake, sometimes both, and nutritional deficiencies may worsen TB or delay its recovery by depressing important immune functions. However, there is insufficient research to know whether the routine provision of supplementary food or energy supplements results in better TB treatment outcomes or improved quality of life [33]. According to a systematic literature review, a strong and consistent log-linear relationship has been found between TB incidence and body mass index (BMI) across a variety of settings with different levels of TB burden [34]. However, the authors conclude that more research is required to test the relationship at very low and very high BMI levels, to establish the biological mechanism linking BMI with the risk of TB and to establish the potential impact on the global TB epidemic of changing nutritional status of populations.

Food shortages, and in particular shortages of protein [35] and vitamin-rich food, were an intrinsic problem in most belligerent countries during WWII. Undernutrition may increase the risk of progression from LTBI to disease or the reactivation of previously healed TB, which under wartime conditions may enhance the recurrence of active disease, sometimes in a very acute and severe form, with short survival times from diagnosis to death. Once the supply of food has improved – usually only in the post-war period – it contributes significantly to the decrease of TB morbidity and mortality.

Solving the huge problem of providing sufficient quantities of food during famines, warfare, and other catastrophes, has historically been extremely difficult, but new organizations and technologies have lessened the burden to some extent. Exemplary international models that helped to eliminate famine after WWII are United Nations (UN) organizations such as the United Nations Relief and Rehabilitation Administration (UNRRA), founded in 1943, essentially to organize help for displaced persons and, later, for refugees; its successor organization is the United Nations High Commission for

Refugees (UNHCR). United Nations International Children's Emergency Fund (UNICEF) was created by the United Nations General Assembly in 1946 to provide emergency food and health care to children in countries that had been devastated by WWII. In 1947, the highly successful Marshall Plan was developed by the U.S., with the purpose of aiding Western European countries in restoring their economies.

In addition, many non-governmental charitable organizations supported countries or certain populations (refugees, Jews, prisoners) suffering from hunger and in great need of food. In some countries, to ensure a fair supply of food to the general population, food ration cards were introduced. Obviously, the black market for food, medications, and other essentials flourished in many affected regions, and hoarding of food from agricultural sources was widespread.

Improving the Housing Situation: Overcrowding in small dwellings, such as tents, barracks, bunkers, and destroyed houses, and some large facilities, particularly crammed hospitals and bomb shelters, which are typical of wartime, increases the risk of air-borne transmission through the inhalation of droplet nuclei containing *M. tuberculosis*. In addition, environmental transmission is magnified during warfare, because the higher prevalence of active TB disease leads to greater opportunities for person-to-person spread of *M. tuberculosis*. New infections resulting from enhanced community transmission may sometimes mature to active disease in a few months or sometimes decades later. After 1982, an unusual version of rapid-onset, virulent TB developed in patients with coexisting human immunodeficiency virus (HIV) infection (see "New Problems").

It is always desirable to avoid overcrowding in poorly ventilated settings, especially during wartime. Today the best means of limiting TB transmission is through source control, in other words, by identifying unsuspected infectious cases and promptly beginning effective chemotherapy [36]. Obviously, however, this now current and regularly applied practice had not yet been created during WWII due to the absence of effective anti-TB treatment. Thus, environmental control with improvement of natural or assisted ventilation could be applied as an effective method of air disinfection at low cost, but was not always available. Furthermore, people had to be educated not to cough directly into the faces of their neighbors. During WWII, infectious TB patients were often asked to wear a flimsy surgical mask, which was theoretically believed to prevent the transmission of air-borne infection, but no one knew for sure. The effectiveness of modern surgical masks has recently been demonstrated in MDR-TB patients in whom transmission could be significantly reduced (by 56%) [37]. People with suspicion of TB, and in particular diagnosed infectious patients, should always be separated and, when indicated, isolated. Today, in addition, directly observed swallowing of anti-TB drugs is strongly recommended.

Prevention of Bovine TB: During and after WWII, bovine TB which is caused by *M. bovis* and usually transmitted by drinking milk from infectious cows, played a major role in human TB, although it is not exactly known to what extent. Some reports estimated that about 20% of all TB cases were caused by *M. bovis*, in particular extrapulmonary forms, and especially cervical lymphadenitis in children. There are 2 possible ways of preventing *M. bovis* disease: one is the culling of cattle that are infected by *M. bovis* or *M. tuberculosis*, as proven by a positive tuberculin skin reaction. In some countries this extremely important public health procedure was used as early as before WWI, but in many others it was not until culling became compulsory that it was fully utilized – and generally only after WWII [38].

The second method used to prevent bovine TB is the pasteurization of milk, where by rapidly heating and then cooling the milk all tubercle bacilli are destroyed. During WWII, many milk pasteurization plants were destroyed or damaged in several countries, thus entirely losing or greatly reducing the benefits of pasteurization. Fuel shortages were a further cause of limited pasteurization. Corrective solutions had to be gradually implemented, but today pasteurization is obligatory in most countries. Thus, bovine TB has become rare in countries where cattle herds are routinely tested and pasteurization of dairy products is mandatory [39].

Reorganization of Health Services

Marc Daniels, as a member of the UNRRA, described in detail the problems originating from the disruption of the health services during and after WWII in Europe [40]. All over Europe, public health services were partly and in some countries completely disorganized. Trained TB doctors and nurses had been killed, wounded, imprisoned or otherwise lost during the war, creating an enormous reduction of qualified personnel. Thus, after the war, training programs for TB had to be instituted for specialists and general practitioners as well as post-graduate courses for medical students. The lack of trained nurses was partially resolved by using domestic staff who became responsible for hospital duties that did not require special knowledge. There were also shortages of specialized instruments and equipment, including microscopes, fluoroscopes, and other X-ray apparatus, and analyzers for chemical and microbiologic measurements.

Hospitals: Many TB hospitals and sanatoria had been either destroyed or converted into military hospitals for wounded soldiers [40]. Thousands of infectious TB patients had to be discharged home during the war despite the risks for their families and other close contacts of being infected. During air raids it was often difficult or even impossible to segregate infectious patients from healthy people in shelters or bunkers, even though the latter were afraid of becoming infected. After the war, it took time to restore the destroyed/damaged facilities and, if needed, to build new ones, often with the help from international organizations (see above).

Dispensaries: These facilities run by local or national governmental public health services or by non-governmental private organizations, had become available in many countries long before WWII started and contributed significantly to TB control. They played an important role in providing diagnostic examinations, ambulatory care for patients, and support to their families. During the war, many dispensaries suffered from losses of experienced staff (e.g., doctors, nurses, social workers) and had to be reorganized after the war, usually under governmental responsibility [40].

Intensified International Cooperation

The World Health Organization (WHO) was officially established by the UN in 1948, when malaria, TB, and venereal diseases were declared as the "3 main scourges demanding prior and special attention" (this is still valid today), and an Expert Committee on TB was formed [41]. Among the recommendations of the Expert Committee to the WHO, prepared by an Interim Commission that took almost 2 years to complete [42], were the collection of data on TB morbidity and mortality rates, which were published in 1948 in the WHO *Epidemiological and Vital Statistics Report* [7]. The Expert Committee emphasized the use of mass radiography, tuberculin testing, and BCG vaccination, plus other aspects of epidemiological research. The Expert Committee also indicated that it planned to "develop and recommend uniform procedures on such matters as the classification of TB, X-ray interpretation and mass radiography, bacteriological diagnosis, and evaluation of new chemotherapeutic agents such as SM" [42].

Special Situations

Military Service

TB in the military poses special problems: when predominantly young men and fewer young women, both groups vulnerable to developing TB, are recruited into military service, they often live in cramped, crowded accommodation, including barracks or tents, which facilitates the spread of tubercle bacilli. A principal goal of the recruitment process is therefore to exclude from military service all individuals with active TB after screening by medical examination [43]. Screening during WWI was carried out solely by history and physical examination, including percussion and auscultation of the chest, which was highly inefficient.

Photofluorography was much better suited to screening, and was first used extensively in the military services of the army and navy not long before WWII, in countries such as Germany, U.S., and Switzerland, in part also in the Soviet Union. Recruits who had findings suspicious of active pulmonary TB, if confirmed, were not accepted for military service. In 1942, the rejection rate in the US Army was 1.49%, as in the early months of the war period all men with calcified lesions were routinely excluded through over-rigid interpretation, and this rate had dropped to 0.78% by 1945 [44]. The efficacy of the examination depended on the experience of the radiologists, and it emerged later that in some TB cases X-ray findings suggestive of TB had been overlooked. During WWII, the rate of disease and death from TB in the army was one tenth that discovered in WWI. This dramatic fall can probably be attributed not only to the declining incidence of TB in the general US population, but also to the much improved screening methods for identifying TB cases and excluding them from entry into service [43].

In Germany during WWII, the exact number of TB cases that occurred in the military service were not published; one reason may have been to avoid causing undue anxiety in the army. The TB morbidity and mortality figures were available only of the civilian population; the military services kept their own statistics.

By the time of the Viet Nam war (1955–1975), the US strategy for TB screening of its military forces had shifted from radiography to the TST for the identification and treatment of LTBI in both civilian and military populations; years later, targeted testing shifted again to either TST or IGRAs – and only of recruits considered at increased risk for LTBI or progression to TB disease [43, 45].

The optimum method of TB screening among recruits differs according to need, and should be mainly determined by the actual incidence of TB in each country. In countries with low TB incidence, targeted screening by TST or IGRA is sufficient. By contrast, in countries with high incidence, X-ray screening is indicated in all candidates for military service.

Prisoners of War
Millions of prisoners of war were held in custody during and after WWII on the side of the Axis powers and Allies. Germany alone held more than 11 million prisoners in custody. More than 5 million Soviet soldiers were incarcerated in German camps, 3.3 million of whom died from starvation and infectious diseases, weakened by heavy forced labor. It is not known exactly how many prisoners died from TB, but it can be assumed that the number was remarkably high and depended on the conditions in different camps, and particularly on whether their captors respected the rules of the Geneva convention, an approach that varied to a considerable degree (for more details, see Chapter 5, subchapter "TB in prisoners of war").

Other Populations Afflicted by TB

Inmates of German Concentration Camps: As described in Chapters 4 and 5, about 6 million Jews and 500,000 Sinti and Roma were imprisoned in German concentration camps, and most were murdered during the Holocaust. TB was one of the most common prevailing diseases in concentration camps due to the crowded, filthy living conditions, and the accompanying severe malnutrition. Pulmonary TB was reported to be clinically and/or radiographically present in 5–20% of concentration camp inmates when they were liberated (see Chapter 5 under "TB in concentration camps").

Displaced Persons: Between 11 and 20 million people were displaced from their homes during and after WWII, mainly in Germany (for details, see chapter 5). The majority were inmates of Nazi concentration camps, labor camps, and prisoner-of-war camps that were freed by the Allied armies at the end of WWII [46]. How many suffered from TB is not known, but it can be assumed that huge numbers were affected. However, Daniels mentions that it was not surprising that the prevalence of TB among displaced persons was much lower (about 2%) than the expected 70%, as most had already died from TB in the camps [9].

Slave Workers: During WWII, the Nazis organized a vast slave and forced labor program to supply the much needed labor to the German war and industrial efforts. It is estimated that about 7.8 million foreign workers and prisoners of war were assigned to labor deployment. They, too, were at high risk of becoming infected by tubercle bacilli and progressing to TB disease due to crowded living conditions, malnutrition, and exhaustion (see Chapter 5).

Refugees:

Mass evacuation, forced displacement, expulsion, and deportation of millions of people took place across most countries involved in WWII. A number of these phenomena were categorized as violations of fundamental human values and norms by the Nuremberg Tribunal after the war ended. The mass movement of people – most of them refugees – was either caused by the hostilities, or enforced by the former Axis and the Allied powers according to ideologies of race and ethnicity, culminating in the postwar border changes enacted by the international settlements. The refugee crisis created across formerly occupied territories in WWII provided the context for much of the new international refugee and global human rights architecture existing today. The belligerents on both sides engaged in ethnic cleansing of people perceived as being associated with the enemy. The major location for the wartime displacements was the East-Central zone (*Editor's note: one of the editors [RL] was among the refugees from Silesia*) and the Eastern European zone. In addition, displaced Japanese people were expelled during and after the war by Allied powers from locations in Asia, including India. The Holocaust also involved deportations and expulsions of Jews aside from the subsequent genocide perpetrated by Nazi Germany. [47]

It is not exactly known to what degree the exodus of the many millions of refugees contributed to the rise in TB mortality, but it must have been immense (for details, see chapters 4 and 5). From recent wars in the Balkan States in the 1990s, the ongoing war in Afghanistan, and the many other, more recent conflicts, it is known that refugees from these areas have been transporting TB to neighboring and distant countries, always bringing with them the inherent burden of the TB prevalence in their parent country, which escalates as the combined hazards of dangerous living plus new physical depredations quickly increase the risk of developing TB.

The progression of TB in refugees has consistently been higher than among people with stable living conditions. Moreover, a related risk accompanies the emigration of foreign nationals – especially from those with a high background incidence of TB – to a rich country in Western Europe or North America. Credentials, qualifications, and abundant supporting documents were required, including a medical examination to ensure the absence of active TB. In the US and Germany, both low-incidence countries, it has been shown for a decade or more that among the small total number of annual TB cases, a steadily increasing proportion comprises immigrants from high-incidence countries. In addition, a recent study from the Netherlands has shown that the incidence rates of pulmonary TB from high-incidence countries remain high for at least a decade after immigration into the Netherlands. Possible explanations are reactivation of old infections and new infection transmitted after immigration [48]. Similarly, evidence from Berlin shows that there are higher rates of TB even among second-generation immigrants compared to native residents [49]. Thus, the impact of TB in the first-generation migrants may even be greater than formerly anticipated. These important new studies need to be taken into account when undertaking TB screening, surveillance, and control in immigrants and refugees from high-incidence countries [50].

New Problems

In the 1970s, TB was thought to have been nearly vanquished, and yet it remains the most common acute bacterial infectious disease worldwide. One of the main reasons for this astonishing rise is the relentless increase in drug resistance [19], which has been discussed earlier in this chapter; the other is TB and HIV coinfection, a condition that is most common in sub-Saharan Africa but is also intensifying in other regions of the world [19]. Because of the remarkable growth of the coexistence of TB and HIV in the middle of the 1990s, the WHO declared TB a global emergency. And as a postscript to the ongoing confederation between TB and war, we summarize the current status (1995–2014) of post-WWII conflicts (see below).

Human Immunodeficiency Virus Coinfection
The human immunodeficiency virus causes HIV infection, and over time, without treatment, leads to the acquired immune-deficiency syndrome (AIDS). AIDS, which was first observed in 1981 in the USA, is a condition in humans in which progressive failure of the CD4-dependent immune system allows opportunistic infections to thrive, particularly TB, and certain malignancies. In addition to the estimated 1.3 million TB deaths in 2016, there were 400,000 deaths resulting from active TB among people living with HIV [13]. In some sub-Saharan African countries, the TB-HIV coinfection rate has risen dramatically, to 50–80%. The rates of HIV infection are also rising in Eastern Europe, particularly in the Russian Federation and the Ukraine. In these countries, again, prisons are high-risk areas for dual infection because of increasing rates of drug addiction. HIV-positive persons harboring latent *M. tuberculosis* infection (LTBI) are at markedly higher risk of developing TB.

"These 2 infections undoubtedly present the most serious challenge to public health across the world, and are likely to be controlled only by a global mobilization of resources not seen since the end of the last European war" [51].

When crises occur in areas with a high burden of HIV, the epidemiological model becomes more complicated [17]. As reported by the UNHCR, WHO, and UNAIDS: "Screening methods for TB, including symptomatic screening, sputum analysis, tuberculin skin testing, and chest radiography become less sensitive and specific as HIV disease progresses.

Missed cases of TB contribute significantly to HIV mortality and HIV infection increases the case fatality rate of TB." The authors conclude: "TB control is not judged to be a top priority in the emergency phase of relief, and, until the recommendations for TB control in emergencies from WHO and UN High Commissioner for Refugees (UNHCR) it had not been addressed systematically in policy" [52]. Lawn et al. provided an up-to-date review of the current medical management of adult patients with HIV-associated TB and observed great challenges of managing HIV-associated drug-resistant TB in resource-limited settings [53].

TB Control Measures in Recent Post-WWII Conflicts
Figure 8 shows the many armed conflicts by type, which have occurred starting from the end of WWII to 2015 [compiled by the University of Uppsala/Sweden].

Only a few studies have analyzed the impact of control measures in some of these conflicts with particular focus on TB. Heldal et al. (1997) described the successful management of a TB program in Nicaragua under conditions of war by the introduction of short-course chemotherapy, with the support of The Union and Norway [55]. Martins et al. reported on a successful non-governmental TB control program in conflict-affected East Timor [56], coming to the conclusion that coordination, cooperation, and collaboration were major contributors to the success of the TB program. The existing local structure and experience of the local non-governmental organization, the commitment among local personnel and international advisors to establishing an effective program, and the willingness of international advisors and local counterparts to be flexible in their approach, were also important factors [57].

After reviewing several armed conflicts, Drobniewski and Verlander concluded in 2000 that in the modern era war may not significantly damage efforts to control TB in the long term [58]. They suggest that this might be due to the limited scale of most of these conflicts compared to the large-scale civilian disruption associated with "world wars," and that the management of TB should be taken into account in planning post-conflict refugee and reconstruction programs.

After the outbreak of armed conflict in the republics of former Yugoslavia in 1991, the WHO took part in emergency relief operations in the area from July 1992 [59]. The WHO designed a prepacked kit with anti-TB drugs and material for sputum smear examination for use, in combination with policy recommendations and a treatment protocol. It is suggested that support of TB control with essential supplies and strictly focusing on priority measures is the

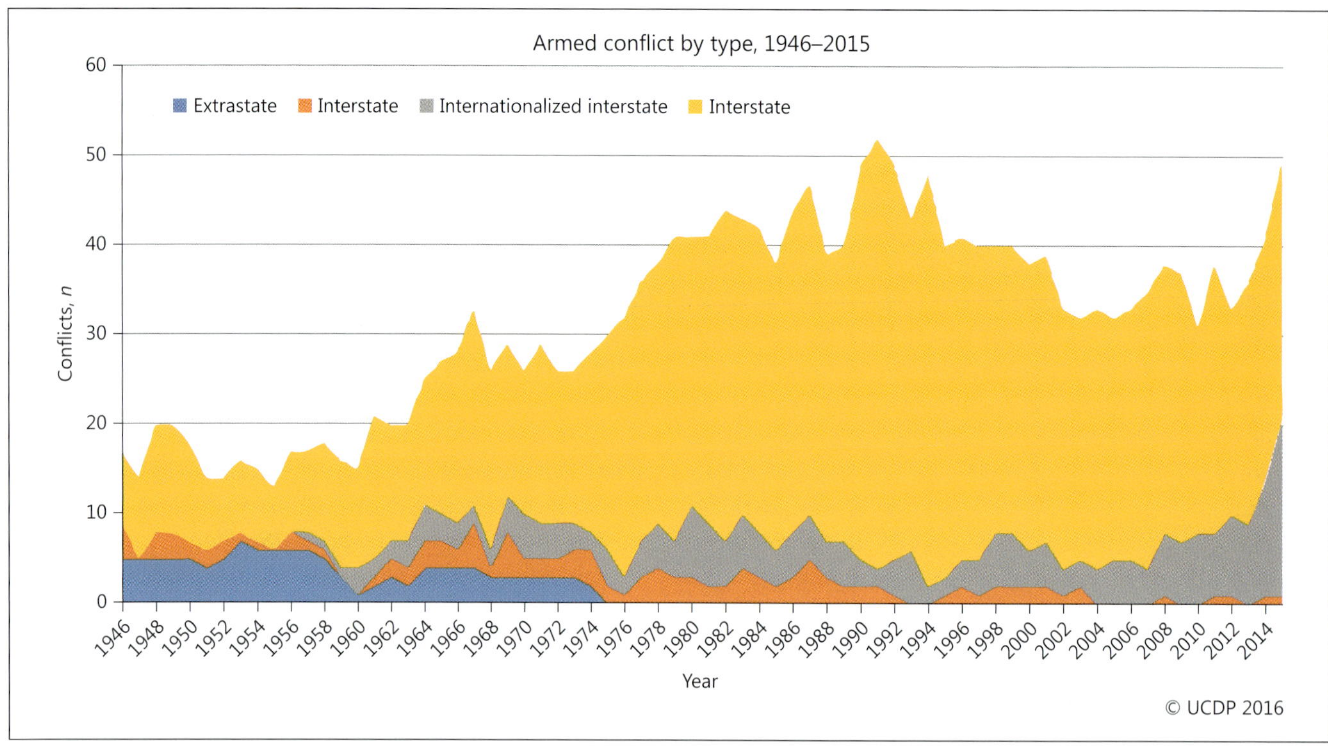

Fig. 8. Armed conflicts by type, from the end of WWII to 2015, compiled by the University of Uppsala/Sweden. Uppsala Conflict Data Program 2016 [54], with permission.

most adequate strategy when dealing with a developed country dependent on humanitarian assistance.

In Afghanistan, which has faced health consequences of war for over 3 decades, including those due to displacement of populations, breakdown of health and social services, and increased risks of disease transmission, it was possible to restructure the National Tuberculosis Control Program (NTP), integrate TB treatment into primary health care, and achieve most of its targets by the year 2011 [60]. The authors conclude that the NTP of Afghanistan is an example of public health programs that can be implemented effectively in fragile states, and that high political commitment and strong local leadership are essential factors for such programs. To ensure the long-term effectiveness of the NTP, they postulate that international support should be withdrawn in a phased manner, coupled with a sequential increase in resources allocated to the NTP by the Government of Afghanistan.

In a study in the Somali Regional State of Ethiopia, Gele and Bjune found that patients from conflict zones experience longer delays in receiving a diagnosis of TB and have higher levels of self-treatment utilization [61]. They suggest that access to TB care should be improved by the expansion of user-friendly DOTS in the conflict zones of the region [2].

Warsame et al. found that fragile, conflict-affected states received on average less funding per capita than non-conflict-affected states (USD 144 vs. 203, respectively), despite worse development indicators, and that such states also received on average only 70% of the TB funds that had already been committed [62].

Conclusions

Future of TB

The worldwide reach of the WHO, founded by the UN, as mentioned, in 1948, has expanded throughout the world and now plays the leading global role in TB prevention and control. "It provides an assessment of the TB epidemic and progress in TB diagnosis, treatment and prevention efforts, as well as an overview of TB-specific financing and research" [19]. Now, in addition, the WHO receives considerable help from literally hundreds of affiliated and independent TB programs, such as the International Union against TB and Lung Disease (The Union), Doctors without Borders, and the Stop TB Partnership, with its nearly 1,500 partners. Much more could be accomplished with additional funding, but the good news is that although the TB epidemic is larger than previously estimated, owing chiefly to new survey data from India, the WHO can confidently boast that "the number of TB deaths and the TB incidence rate continue to fall globally and in India" [19].

From the 17th through the 20th centuries in western Europe and later the eastern US, TB was by far the leading cause of mortality, and was said to have killed over one billion people. And it is still the top cause of adult infectious disease deaths. New scientific techniques of diagnosis and treatment of virtually all patients with TB – if and when modern methods are practiced – should allow ultimate control and eradication of this 70,000-year-old plague.

The Future of War

The future of TB looks much more promising than the future of war. Wars beget wars: there does not seem to be any other valid reason. During the almost 2 million years during which hunter-gatherers managed to survive, and coinciding with the shift from a nomadic life to a settled one of farming and domestication of animals, as well as the major increase in the size of the population, 2 epoch-defining transformations took place at roughly the same time during the Neolithic Revolution. First, the earliest hints appeared of what became known as *civilization*, and second, the beginning of *war*. Inherent but opposite human activities – one creating unbelievable progress and improved well-being, the other of steadily mounting death and destruction, including the possibility of human extinction.

The Future of TB and War

This book, *TB and War: Lessons Learned from WWII,* has provided an overall assessment of the partnership between TB and war, as well as chapter by chapter account of the dramatic events that affected numbers of cases of TB and the outcome of the disease in the 26 countries discussed in the book. But, as is also recounted in the book, the ruinous TB-war alliance keeps recurring and it is all happening on our television screens and reported in other media. Several wars are ongoing as we write this conclusion; the catastrophic war in Syria is causing the most significant worldwide impact today, and we have focused particular attention on this situation in Chapter 1.

Between the end of WWII and the year 2015, a horrifically high number of armed conflicts of different types were observed, as shown in Figure 8 [54].

It repeats the same old story: as death and destruction due to war multiplies, TB strikes and kills more and more people. There is no means of counting the casualties within the country, but Syrian refugees fleeing neighboring Jordan and Lebanon [63] as well as countries of the European Union and elsewhere, have already added to the number of cases.

In conclusion, thanks to the effectiveness of high-tech case-finding and microbiological advances, we forecast the possible eradication of TB at some time late in the future, but that goal becomes ever more distant as long as wars continue.

References

1 Sahloul MZ, Monla-Hassan J, Sankari A, et al: War is the Enemy of Health. Pulmonary, Critical Care, and Sleep Medicine in War-Torn Syria. Ann Am Thorac Soc 2016;13:147–155.

2 Daniels M: Tuberculosis in Europe during and after the Second World War. Br Med J 1949;2: 1065–1072.

3 World War II casualties – Wikipedia. https:// en.wikipedia.org/wiki/World_War_II_casualties.

4 Lönnroth K, Jaramillo E, Williams BG, Dye C, Raviglione M: Drivers of tuberculosis epidemics: the role of risk factors and social determinants. Soc Sci Med 2009;68:2240–2246.

5 Sartwell PE, Moseley CH, Long ER: Tuberculosis in the German population, United States Zone of Germany. Am Rev Tuberc 1949;59:481–493.

6 Smallman-Raynor M, Cliff A: War and disease: some perspectives on the spatial and temporal occurence of tuberculosis in wartime; in Chapter 4 in Gandy M, Zumia A (eds): The Return of the White Plague: Global Poverty and the "New" Tuberculosis New York, Verso, 2003, pp 70–92.

7 World Health Organization: Monthly supplement to the weekly epidemiological record. Epidemiol Vital Statistics Rep 1948;1:223–227.

8 Kröger E, Reuter H: Entwicklung und gegenwärtiger stand der tuberkulose in deutschen und anderen Ländern. Dtsch Med Wochenschr 1949;74: 721–725.

9 Daniels M: Tuberculosis in post-war Europe; an international problem. Tubercle 1947;28:201.

10 Comroe JH Jr: Pay dirt: the story of streptomycin. Part II. Feldman and Hinshaw; Lehmann. Am Rev Respir Dis 1978;117:957–968.

11 Murray JF, Schraufnagel DE, Hopewell PC: Treatment of Tuberculosis. A Historical Perspective. Ann Am Thorac Soc 2015;12:1749–1759.

12 Treatment of pulmonary tuberculosis with streptomycin and para-aminosalicylic acid; a Medical Research Council investigation. Br Med J 1950;2: 1073–1085.

13 World Health Organization: Global Tuberculosis Report 2017. Geneva: World Health Organization, 2017.

14 Loddenkemper R, Hauer B: Drug-resistant tuberculosis: a worldwide epidemic poses a new challenge. Dtsch Arztebl Int 2010;107:10–19.

15 Eldholm V, Pettersson JH, Brynildsrud OB, et al: Armed conflict and population displacement as drivers of the evolution and dispersal of Mycobacterium tuberculosis. Proc Natl Acad Sci U S A 2016;113:13881–13886.

16 Borisov SE, Dheda K, Enwerem M, et al: Effectiveness and safety of bedaquiline-containing regimens in the treatment of MDR- and XDR-TB: a multicentre study. Eur Respir J 2017;49. pii:1700387.

17 Kimbrough W, Saliba V, Dahab M, Haskew C, Checchi F: The burden of tuberculosis in crisis-affected populations: a systematic review. Lancet Infect Dis 2012;12:950–965.

18 Falzon D, Schunemann HJ, Harausz E, et al: World Health Organization treatment guidelines for drug-resistant tuberculosis, 2016 update. Eur Respir J 2017;49:pii:1602308.

19 World Health Organization: Global Tuberculosis Report 2016. World Health Organization Document, 2016;WHO/HTM/TB/2016;13:1–201.

20 Sharma A, Hill A, Kurbatova E, et al: Estimating the future burden of multidrug-resistant and extensively drug-resistant tuberculosis in India, the Philippines, Russia, and South Africa: a mathematical modelling study. Lancet Infect Dis 2017;17:707–175.

21 Bhalla AS, Goyal A, Guleria R, Gupta AK: Chest tuberculosis: radiological review and imaging recommendations. Indian J Radiol Imaging 2015;25:213–225.

22 Jeanes C, O'Grady J: Diagnosing tuberculosis in the 21st century - dawn of a genomics revolution? Int J Mycobacteriol 2016;5:384–391.

23 Engstrom A: Fighting an old disease with modern tools: characteristics and molecular detection methods of drug-resistant Mycobacterium tuberculosis. Infect Dis (Lond) 2016;48:1–17.

24 Holm J: Tuberculosis in Europe after the second World War. Am Rev Tuberc 1948;57:115–128.

25 Ferebee S, Mount FW, Anastasiades A: Prophylactic effects of isoniazid on primary tuberculosis in children. Am Rev Tuberc 1957;76:942–963.

26 Ferebee SH: Controlled chemoprophylaxis trials in tuberculosis. A general review. Bibl Tuberc 1970; 26:28–106.

27 Getahun H, Matteelli A, Chaisson RE, Raviglione M: Latent Mycobacterium tuberculosis infection. N Engl J Med 2015;372:2127–2135.

28 Jamil SM, Oren E, Garrison GW, et al: Diagnosis of Tuberculosis in Adults and Children. Ann Am Thorac Soc 2017;14:275–278.

29 Diel R, Loddenkemper R, Zellweger JP, et al: Old ideas to innovate tuberculosis control: preventive treatment to achieve elimination. Eur Respir J 2013;42:785–801.

30 Calmette A: La vaccination préventive de la tuberculose par le BCG dans les familles de médecins 1924–1932. Ann Inst Pasteur 1932;49(suppl):1–62.

31 The Lubeck Disaster. Science 1930;72:198–199.

32 Andersen P, Kaufmann SH: Novel vaccination strategies against tuberculosis. Cold Spring Harb Perspect Med 2014;4:pii:a018523.

33 Sinclair D, Abba K, Grobler L, Sudarsanam TD: Nutritional supplements for people being treated for active tuberculosis. Cochrane Database Syst Rev 2011; 11:CD006086.

34 Lönnroth K, Williams BG, Cegielski P, Dye C: A consistent log-linear relationship between tuberculosis incidence and body mass index. Int J Epidemiol 2010;39:149–155.

35 Hood ML: A narrative review of recent progress in understanding the relationship between tuberculosis and protein energy malnutrition. Eur J Clin Nutr 2013;67:1122–1128.

36 Jensen PA, Lambert LA, Iademarco MF, Ridzon R; CDC: Guidelines for preventing the transmission of Mycobacterium tuberculosis in health-care settings, 2005. MMWR Recomm Rep 2005;54(RR-17):1–141.

37 Nardell EA: Indoor environmental control of tuberculosis and other airborne infections. Indoor Air 2016;26:79–87.

38 Boland ER: Administration of medicine. Br Med J 1948;2:9–19.

39 LoBue PA, Enarson DA, Thoen CO: Tuberculosis in humans and animals: an overview [Serialised article. Tuberculosis: a re-emerging disease in animals and humans. Number 1 in the series]. Int J Tuberc Lung Dis 2010;14:1075–1078.

40 Daniels M: Tuberculosis in Europe during and after the second World War. Br Med J 1949;2:1135–1140.

41 McDougall JB: Tuberculosis and the World Health Organization. Tubercle 1948;29:208–214.

42 Expert Committee on Tuberculosis Report of the Expert Committee on Tuberculosis. Bull World Health Organ 1948;1:205–212.

43 Mancuso JD: Tuberculosis Screening and Control in the US Military in War and Peace. Am J Public Health 2017;107:60–67.

44 Long ER, Hamilton EL: A review of induction and discharge examinations for tuberculosis in the Army. Am J Public Health Nations Health 1947;37:412–420.

45 American Thoracic Society, Centers for Disease Control and Prevention. Targeted tuberculin testing and treatment of latent tuberculosis infection. Am J Respir Crit Care Med 2000;161(suppl):S221–S247.

46 Wyman M: DPs: Europe's displaced persons, 1945–1951 (reprinted). New York, Cornell University Press, 1998.

47 World War II evacuation and expulsion – Wikipedia. http://en.wikipedia.org/wiki/World_War_ii_evacuation_and_expulsion.

48 Vos AM, Meima A, Verver S, et al: High incidence of pulmonary tuberculosis persists a decade after immigration, The Netherlands. Emerg Infect Dis 2004;10:736–739.

49 Marx FM, Fiebig L, Hauer B, et al: Higher rate of tuberculosis in second generation migrants compared to native residents in a metropolitan setting in Western Europe. PLoS One 2015;10:e0119693.

50 Arshad S, Bavan L, Gajari K, Paget SN, Baussano I: Active screening at entry for tuberculosis among new immigrants: a systematic review and meta-analysis. Eur Respir J 2010;35:1336–1345.

51 Gazzard B: Tuberculosis, HIV and the developing world. Clin Med (Lond) 2001;1:62–68.

52 UNHCR, WHO, UNAIDS. Policy statement on HIV testing and counselling in health facilities for refugees, internally displaced persons and other persons of concern.htpp://www.unhcr.org/hivaids.

53 Lawn SD, Meintjes G, McIlleron H, Harries AD, Wood R: Management of HIV-associated tuberculosis in resource-limited settings: a state-of-the-art review. BMC Med 2013;11:253.

54 Melander E, Pettersson T, Themnér L: Organized violence, 1989–2015. J Peace Res 2016;53:727–742.

55 Heldal E, Cruz JR, Arnadottir T, Tardencilla A, Enarson DA: Successful management of a National Tuberculosis Programme under conditions of war. Int J Tuberc Lung Dis 1997;1:16–24.

56 Martins N, Heldal E, Sarmento J, Araujo RM, Rolandsen EB, Kelly PM: Tuberculosis control in conflict-affected East Timor, 1996-2004. Int J Tuberc Lung Dis 2006;10:975–981.

57 Martins N, Kelly PM, Grace JA, Zwi AB: Reconstructing tuberculosis services after major conflict: experiences and lessons learned in East Timor. PLoS Med 2006;3:e383.

58 Drobniewski FA, Verlander NQ: Tuberculosis and the role of war in the modern era. Int J Tuberc Lung Dis 2000;4:1120–1125.

59 Felten MK, Forte GB: Prepacked kits for diagnosis and treatment of tuberculosis in former Yugoslavia. Tuber Lung Dis 1995;76:360–366.

60 Seddiq K, Enarson DA, Shah K, Haq Z, Khan WM: Implementing a successful tuberculosis programme within primary care services in a conflict area using the stop TB strategy: afghanistan case study. Confl Health 2014;8:3.

61 Gele AA, Bjune GA: Armed conflicts have an impact on the spread of tuberculosis: the case of the Somali Regional State of Ethiopia. Confl Health 2010;4:1.

62 Warsame A, Patel P, Checchi F: Patterns of funding allocation for tuberculosis control in fragile states. Int J Tuberc Lung Dis 2014;18:61–66.

63 Ismail SA, Abbara A, Collin SM, et al: Communicable disease surveillance and control in the context of conflict and mass displacement in Syria. Int J Infect Dis 2016;47:15–22.

Robert Loddenkemper
German Central Committee against Tuberculosis
Hertastrasse 3
DE–14169 Berlin (Germany)
E-Mail robert.loddenkemper@pneumologie.de

Author Index

Subject Index

mortality 119–121
post-World War II 122
pre-World War II 116, 117

Germany, *see also* Nazis
displaced person tuberculosis during World War II
73, 74, 224
mortality rates of tuberculosis
during World War II 60, 61
post-World War II
Berlin 76, 77
British occupation zone 80
French occupation zone 80, 81
Soviet occupation zone 81, 82
United States occupation zone
77–79
tuberculosis control
during World War II 69, 70
pre-World War II 66–68
tuberculosis epidemiology
during World War II 68, 69
post- World War II 75, 76
pre-World War II 64–66
Great Depression 183, 184
Greece, tuberculosis
control and treatment 157, 158
epidemiology 156, 157

Hippocrates, tuberculosis observations 5
HIV, *see* Human immunodeficiency virus
Human evolution
hunter-gathers 3, 4
Neolithic Demographic Revolution 4, 5
prehistory 3
tuberculosis introduction 2
Human immunodeficiency virus (HIV), tuberculosis risk in
wartime 40, 41, 222, 225
Hundred Years' War 14
Hungary, tuberculosis
continuum of disease 168–170
during World War II 166–168
pre-World War II 166

Ireland
industrialization 111, 112
tuberculosis in and around World War II
bovine tuberculosis 113
drug development 113
health policy reforms 112, 113
medical advances 113
ISIS 17
Italy, tuberculosis
control and treatment 154–156
epidemiology 152–154

Japan, tuberculosis
control during World War II 193–195
epidemiology 189, 190
Korea occupation, *see* Korea
overview 188, 189
Pearl Harbor attack 209
Sino-Japanese War, *see* China
war impact
socioeconomic changes 191, 192
World War II deaths 192, 193
Jericho 14

Korea, tuberculosis during Japanese occupation during World
War II
Association to Prevent TB in Korea 199, 200
epidemic 197, 198
sanatoria construction 200, 201
socioeconomic study of Japanese in Korea 198, 199
X-ray screenings 200

Malnutrition, tuberculosis risk in wartime 37, 38, 110, 111, 221,
222
Morbidity, assessment for tuberculosis 23–26
Mortality, tuberculosis
case fatality determination 26, 27
case-to-death ratio 27–30
Nazi Germany 60, 61, 76–82
trends in Western Europe 7, 8, 12
World War II participant countries 216
Mortality, World War II casualties 215
Mycobacterium, isolation by Koch 6

Nazis
case histories of slave laborers
Cohen, Ruth 56, 57
Minza, Simcha 55, 56
overview 224
concentration camps 51–53, 57–59, 71–73, 224
euthanasia and racial hygiene 45–48
ghettos and segregation 49–51
Hitler view of Jews as racial tuberculosis of the nations 44
Nuremberg trials 59, 60
prisoner of war tuberculosis 70, 71
tuberculosis experiments on humans 53–55, 74, 99
tuberculosis mortality 60, 61
Wehrmacht tuberculosis cases 70, 223
Neolithic Demographic Revolution 4, 5
Netherlands, tuberculosis
clinics 140, 141
epidemiology 134–136
post-World War II 141, 142
risk factors 137, 138
treatment and control 138–140
Nuremberg trials 59, 60, 71–73